OBESITY

The Report of the British Nutrition Foundation Task Force

Blackwell Science

© 1999
Blackwell Science Ltd
Editorial Offices:
Osney Mead, Oxford OX2 0EL
25 John Street, London WC1N 2BL
23 Ainslie Place, Edinburgh EH3 6AJ
350 Main Street, Malden
　MA 02148 5018, USA
54 University Street, Carlton
　Victoria 3053, Australia
10, rue Casimir Delavigne
　75006 Paris, France

Other Editorial Offices:

Blackwell Wissenschafts-Verlag GmbH
Kurfürstendamm 57
10707 Berlin, Germany

Blackwell Science KK
MG Kodenmacho Building
7–10 Kodenmacho Nihombashi
Chuo-ku, Tokyo 104, Japan

First published 1999

Set in 9.5/11.5 Times
by DP Photosetting, Aylesbury, Bucks
Printed and bound in Great Britain by
MPG Books Ltd, Bodmin, Cornwall

The Blackwell Science logo is a trade mark of
Blackwell Science Ltd, registered at the United Kingdom
Trade Marks Registry

DISTRIBUTORS

Marston Book Services Ltd
PO Box 269
Abingdon
Oxon OX14 4YN
(*Orders:* Tel: 01235 465500
　　　　　Fax: 01235 465555)

USA
Blackwell Science, Inc.
Commerce Place
350 Main Street
Malden, MA 02148 5018
(*Orders:* Tel: 800 759 6102
　　　　　　　781 388 8250
　　　Fax: 781 388 8255)

Canada
Login Brothers Book Company
324 Saulteaux Crescent
Winnipeg, Manitoba R3J 3T2
(*Orders:* Tel: 204 837-2987
　　　　　Fax: 204 837-3116)

Australia
Blackwell Science Pty Ltd
54 University Street
Carlton, Victoria 3053
(*Orders:* Tel: 03 9347 0300
　　　　　Fax: 03 9347 5001)

A catalogue record for this title
is available from the British Library

ISBN 0-632-05298-8

Library of Congress
Cataloging-in-Publication Data
is available

For further information on Blackwell Science, visit our
website: www.blackwell-science.com

Contents

This report is the collective work of all the members of the Task Force.
Authors of the first draft of each chapter are given below.

Contents

18 Treatment of Obesity I: Introduction   **145**

Professor John Garrow

19 Treatment of Obesity II: Dietary Treatment of Obesity   **151**

Professor John Garrow, Ms Mary O'Kane

20 Treatment of Obesity III: Physical Activity and Exercise   **165**

Professor Kenneth Fox

Terms of Reference

The Task Force was invited by the Council of the British Nutrition Foundation to:

(1) Review the present state of knowledge of the causes, consequences, prevention and treatment of obesity.

(2) Prepare a report and, should it see fit, draw conclusions, make recommendations and identify areas for future research.

British Nutrition Foundation Obesity Task Force Membership

Chairman:

Professor John Garrow, The Dial House, 93 Uxbridge Road, Rickmansworth, Hertfordshire WD3 2DQ

Members:

Dr Ann Fehily
HJ Heinz Company Limited
Kitt Green
Wigan
Lancashire WN5 0JL

Professor Kenneth Fox
  (from August 1999)
Department of Exercise and
  Health Sciences
University of Bristol
Priory House
Woodlands Road
Bristol BS8 2UL

Professor Peter Kopelman
St Bartholomew's and the Royal
  London School of Medicine
  and Dentistry
Turner Street
Whitechapel
London E1 2AD

Dr David Mela
Consumer Science Unit
Unilever Research Vlaardingen
PO Box 114
3130 AC Vlaardingen
The Netherlands

Dr Andrew Prentice
MRC International Nutrition
  Group
Public Health Nutrition Unit
Department of Epidemiology
  and Population Health
London School of Hygiene and
  Tropical Medicine
49–51 Bedford Square
London WC1B 3DP

Professor Mike Stock
Department of Physiology
St George's Medical School
Tooting
London SW17 0RE

Professor Jane Wardle
Health Behaviour Unit
Department of Epidemiology
  and Public Health
University College London
2–16 Torrington Place
London WC1E 6BT

Observers:

Dr Joyce Hughes
Nutrition Unit
Department of Health
Room 638B
Skipton House
80 London Road
London SE1 6LW

Miss Mary O'Kane
Department of Nutrition and
  Dietetics
The General Infirmary at Leeds
Great George Street
Leeds LS1 3EX

Miss Sue Oldreive
Nutrition Unit
MAFF
Room 306B, Ergon House
c/o Nobel House
17 Smith Square
London SW1P 3JR

Corresponding members:

Dr Claude Bouchard
Laboratoire des Sciences
De l'Activité Physique
PEPS, Université Laval
Ste-Foy
Quebec
Canada G1K 7P4

Dr Lauren Lissner
SOS Secretariat
Sahigrenska Hospital
S413 45 Gothenburg
Sweden

Contributors:

The Task Force is most grateful to the following people, who made a significant contribution to writing material for this report.

Dr Tim Cole
Department of Epidemiology
Institute of Child Health
30 Guilford Street
London WC1 N1

Dr Nick Finer
Department of Endocrinology
Luton and Dunstable Hospital
    NHS Trust
Lewsey Road
Luton LU4 OD2

Dr Mary Flynn
Dublin Institute of Technology
Kevin Street
Dublin 8

Ms Gail Goldberg
MRC Dunn Clinical Nutrition
    Centre
Hills Road
Cambridge CB2 2DH

Dr Susan Jebb
MRC Human Nutrition
    Research
Downhams Lane
Milton Road
Cambridge CB4 1XJ

Ms Sharon Kuznesof
Faculty of Agriculture and
    Biological Sciences
University of Newcastle-upon-
    Tyne
Newcastle-upon-Tyne NE1 7RU

Professor Christopher Ritson
Faculty of Agriculture and
    Biological Sciences
University of Newcastle-upon-
    Tyne
Newcastle-upon-Tyne NE1 7RU

Dr James Stubbs
Rowett Research Institute
Greenburn Road
Bucksburn
Aberdeen AB21 9SB

BNF Secretariat:

Ms Amanda Wynne (editor)
Nutrition Scientist
British Nutrition Foundation
Task Force Secretariat
    (from Dec 1997)

Dr Michéle Sadler
Senior Nutrition Scientist and
Task Force Secretariat
    (until Dec 1997)
Institute of Grocery Distribution
Grange Lane
Letchmore Heath
Watford
Hertfordshire WD2 8DG

Dr Judy Buttriss
Science Director
British Nutrition Foundation

Professor Robert Pickard
Director-General
    (from Oct 1997)
British Nutrition Foundation

Professor Brian Wharton
Director-General
    (until Oct 1997)
British Nutrition Foundation

Ms Priscilla Appiah
Science Secretary
British Nutrition Foundation

Ms Maxine Ide
Science Secretary
British Nutrition Foundation

Acknowledgements

The British Nutrition Foundation Task Force is grateful to the following for permission to reproduce copyrighted material on which the following figures and tables are based:

Academic Press for Fig. 10.1; *Acta Medica Scandinavia* for Fig. 20.1; *Acta Physiologica Scandinavia* for Table 15.9; *Age and Ageing* for Table 4.3; the American Society for Clinical Nutrition for Figs 7.3, 7.4, 7.5, 7.6, 13.4 and 20.2; BBSCR for Tables 14.2 and 14.3; Blackwell Science for Figs 8.5, 8.6 and 20.7; and Table 4.7; the BMJ for Figs 13.1, 13.2, 13.3, 13.5, 15.6 and 15.8; BNF for Fig. 14.3; CABI Publishing for Figs 7.8, 7.9, 16.3 and 16.4; the Child Growth Foundation for Figs 2.3 and 2.4; Churchill Livingstone for Figs 2.2, 2.5, 2.6, 16.1, 16.5 and 17.1; the Guilford Press for Figs 23.1 and 23.2; the Health Education Authority for Table 15.2 and Figs 15.4, 15.5 and 20.5; *Journal of the American Medical Association* for Table 2.2; Lippincott, Williams and Wilkins for Fig. 10.2; Massachusetts Medical Society for Table 2.1; MRC Epidemiology Unit, South Wales (Mr Peter Sweetnam) for Table 4.2; The Novalis Foundation for Table 4.6; Oxford University Press for Fig. 2.1; The Royal College of Physicians for Fig. 17.2; Stockton Press for Tables 2.3, 15.3, 15.4, 24.1 and 24.2, and Figs 8.2, 8.3, 8.4, 8.9, 9.1, 10.3 and 23.3; Taylor and Francis for Fig. 7.1; and W.B. Saunders Co. for Fig. 16.2.

Crown Copyright material in Figs 4.1, 4.4 and 19.1 is reproduced with the permission of the Controller of Her Majesty's Stationery Office. Other figures and tables are acknowledged in the text.

1
Introduction

Obesity, defined as a body mass index (BMI) above 30, is recognised in many countries as a major public health problem. BMI can be calculated using Equation (1.1) below:

$$BMI = Weight (kg) : Height (m)^2 \quad (1.1)$$

The prevalence of obesity is rising steadily in many developed countries and also in eastern countries such as China and Japan. The global trend of increasing prevalence demonstrates that current measures to prevent and treat obesity are failing. Despite a vast research effort there are no practical population-based solutions on the immediate horizon.

It is a paradox that, in developed countries, the increasing prevalence of obesity is occurring in an environment of decreasing energy intakes. This reflects increasingly sedentary lifestyles. However, it remains unexplained that not everyone exposed to this environment becomes obese. This highlights our current inability to pinpoint precisely the aetiology of specific eating and lifestyle behaviours, and perhaps why the body's regulatory systems might function better in some individuals than in others. This has undoubtedly contributed to the slow rate of progress in terms of the effective management of obesity.

The need to tackle the obesity problem with some urgency also relates to the undisputed evidence that obesity is a risk factor for a range of medical consequences. Risk of coronary heart disease and diabetes increase with increasing body weight and obesity increases the risk of respiratory disease, osteoarthritis and certain cancers. Yet the perception of obesity as a medical problem is not universal.

In the course of the Task Force's work, health journalists were contacted as representative of those communicating these issues to the public. This exercise (Appendix) highlighted that journalists, and presumably the public, do not perceive obesity in the context of a public health problem. This reflects a different perspective to that of scientists working in the field. Public perception clearly needs to change if progress is to be made.

The health risks of obesity in the UK were first officially recognised in an expert report by the Medical Research Council (MRC) and Department of Health and Social Security (DHSS) in 1976. This report opened with the statement:

'We are unanimous in our belief that obesity is a hazard to health and a detriment to wellbeing. It is common enough to constitute one of the most important public health problems of our time.' (Waterlow, 1976)

At that time there had been no systematic measurement of the prevalence of obesity in a nationally representative sample of adults in the UK. In the last two decades there has been a series of expert reports, which highlight the mounting evidence of the ever-increasing prevalence of obesity, and of the mortality and morbidity that it causes.

In 1983, a Royal College of Physicians working party identified the problem of overweight and obesity in Britain, at this time, as 'substantial' (34%

of men and 24% of women were overweight, and 6% of men and 8% of women were obese). The working party's recommendations included public health measures, based on adjusting nutrient consumption in the population, as well as health education and medical advice for individuals.

The need to remain physically active throughout life was also highlighted, and recommendations were made to encourage the food industry to promote the consumption of foods that were lower in fat and sugar content than those on offer at the time. In 1987 the government's advisory Committee on Medical Aspects of Food Policy (COMA) published a report on *The Use of Very Low Calorie Diets in Obesity*, which reflected increasing concern about the safety and efficacy of 'quick and easy' ways to lose weight.

By the time the report from The Nutrition and Physical Activity Task Forces of the Department of Health, entitled *Obesity – reversing the increasing problem of obesity in England*, was published in 1995, the prevalence of obesity had risen to 13% of men and 16% of women, with over half of the population being either overweight or obese (data from a 1993 survey). This was despite a target to reduce the prevalence of obesity to that of 1980, i.e. 6% of men and 8% of women, set out in the UK government's Health of the Nation White Paper, published in 1992, which provided a comprehensive strategy for promoting public health.

This 1995 report on obesity set out the need for a preventive approach, to make it less likely that people in general will become obese, with targeted measures for those at greatest risk of becoming obese and new therapeutic strategies to help those who are already obese. The need to increase physical activity and to reduce the energy density of the diet, by reducing fat intake, were suggested as the two principal ways to limit excess weight gain.

By 1996 the prevalence of obesity in England had risen further to 16% of men and 18% of women (Prescott-Clarke & Primatesta, 1998). The lack of progress in containing the obesity problem is explained by a number of factors.

- Unchanged environment that combines ready access to energy-dense food with limited need for physical activity.
- Lack of perception of obesity as a public health problem for those above a certain range of

weight-for-height, or above a certain maximum waist circumference.
- Lack of knowledge and public understanding about the aetiology of obesity.
- Need for improved knowledge about the aetiology of obesity.

Considering this background, the British Nutrition Foundation recognised the need for a comprehensive and authoritative report on the problem. A Task Force was convened with experts from many different fields, including biochemistry, clinical medicine, dietetics, endocrinology, epidemiology, food technology, genetics, health education, health service administration, the media, pharmacology, physical education, physiology and psychology. The aim was to draw together in one report the scientific evidence on all relevant aspects of obesity as a basis for assessing what could be done, and for identifying ways forward.

The Task Force identified a number of objectives.

- to consider the issue of obesity in a social context;
- to ensure integration of knowledge across the disciplines;
- to produce an informative report that is easily accessible;
- to help identify and remove barriers to progress;
- to consider future concerns;
- to make realistic recommendations.

The report is aimed at communicators; including the food industry, general practitioners and other medics, the government, health and local authorities, health care professionals, journalists and researchers in relevant disciplines.

To emphasise the importance of the obesity problem and the urgency with which it should be tackled, the report begins by identifying the health risks of obesity, followed by definitions of how obesity is measured. The epidemiology of obesity is considered, followed by a thoroughly comprehensive assessment of our current knowledge about the aetiology of obesity. The significance of individual weight variation is tackled, along with the issue of weight cycling. A section on the prevention of obesity is followed by a full discussion of different approaches to the treatment of obesity. This includes dietary, pharmacotherapy and surgical treatments, in addition to consideration of the role of exercise, behavioural aspects of treatment, and of course the important issue of the goals of treatment. The Task Force's recommendations and suggestions for further research are based on the detailed consideration of all of the above aspects of the obesity problem.

2
Health Risks of Obesity

2.1 Relation of overweight to mortality and morbidity

Life insurance companies need to identify those individuals who are at increased risk of dying young and hence are unprofitable to insure. As early as 1913, the Society of Actuaries published analyses showing that being overweight was an important predictor of decreased longevity. At intervals since then, the Metropolitan Life insurance agency has published tables of 'desirable weight' for men and women of a given height; the most recent of which was the Build Study (Society of Actuaries, 1959). In some publications the range was subdivided according to large, medium and small 'frame' size. There is, however, no agreement about how frame size should be measured. Neither is there any evidence that this refinement improves the accuracy with which mortality, or total body fat, can be predicted for a person of given age, sex and height (Rookus *et al.*, 1985).

There is international consensus that tables showing weight-for-height can conveniently be replaced by a single index. The Belgian astronomer Quetelet observed in 1869 that, among adults of normal body build, weight was proportional to the square of height; in other words weight in kilograms (kg) divided by the square of height in metres $(m)^2$ was constant. Keys *et al.* (1972) made a similar observation, and named the relationship Body Mass Index (BMI). The relation of BMI to body fat, and methods for measuring the amount and distribution of body fat, are considered further in Chapter 3. For the purpose of considering the health risks of obesity in this chapter, three simple anthropometric indices will be used: BMI, waist circumference in centimetres (cm) and waist–hip ratio.

Figure 2.1 shows the general relation of BMI to mortality ratio. The curve is J-shaped, with minimum mortality ratio in the BMI range 20–25. This relationship is similar in both men and women.

2.1.1 The effect of age on desirable weight for longevity

The curve shown in Fig. 2.1 applies to young adults, but the BMI at which mortality is lowest changes with age. Between the ages of 20 and 50 years, it increases linearly from a BMI of 20 to a BMI of 25, which in a person 1.73 m tall, implies an increase in body weight from 60–75 kg. This does not mean, as has been suggested, that there is a health benefit from a gain of 15 kg during adult life (Andres *et al.*, 1985). In fact, there is good evidence that, for an individual, minimum mortality is associated with a constant weight between the ages of 20 and 50 years.

Many confounding factors operate.

- Some people who are very overweight at age 20 years will already have died by age 50 years.

- The degenerative diseases, which are the main cause of excess mortality in obese people, take many years to develop. The life expectancy of a young person is, therefore, more likely to be limited than that of an old person.

- Malignant disease, bowel diseases and chronic infections tend to cause weight loss and thus increase the mortality ratio in the lower weight ranges.

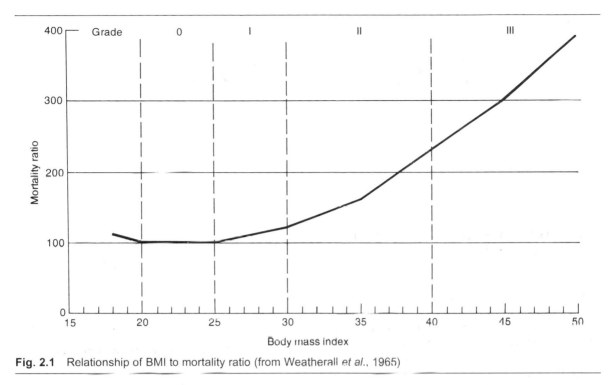

Fig. 2.1 Relationship of BMI to mortality ratio (from Weatherall *et al.*, 1965)

● Body composition changes with age, therefore, even without weight gain, there is an increase in body fat, particularly intra-abdominal fat, with increasing age in men and post-menopausal women.

2.1.2 Confounding effect of disease, smoking and ethnicity

The J-shaped curve in Fig. 2.1 indicates that the mortality risk is lowest within the BMI range of 20 and 25, and increases at BMIs above and below this range. However, detailed analysis of large epidemiological studies shows that the increased relative mortality risk at low weights may disappear if data for people who do not smoke cigarettes, and who maintain a constant weight during adult life, are separately analysed. This is well illustrated in the Nurses Health Study, which recruited 121 700 registered female nurses (almost all white) aged 30–55 years in 1976. Of these, 115 818 were initially free from diagnosed cardiovascular disease or cancer and were followed-up for 14 years. Manson *et al.* (1995) analysed the influence of BMI on relative mortality risk, results of which are sum-

marised in Table 2.1. Taking data from all the women in the study, there is a familiar J-shaped curve with increased relative mortality risk above and below a BMI range of 20–29, which agrees with data from insurance societies and the American Cancer Society study (Lew, 1985). When the analysis is confined to women who never smoked, the J-shape disappears. Minimum mortality risk is present in the lowest BMI groups, and there is a significant increase in risk at and above a BMI of 27. When data concerning women who died in the first 4 years of the study and women who smoked are removed from the analysis, the number of deaths decreases to 1168. The minimum mortality rate occurs in the thinnest women and the multivariate relative risk increased with increasing weight. The increase in relative risk became statistically significant above a BMI of 27. This strongly suggests that the J-shaped curve, with a nadir (lowest point of the curve) of a BMI of about 25, is caused by deaths among smokers or among those with pre-existing disease.

Ethnic effects on the prevalence of obesity are discussed in Section 4.6; however, there are also ethnic differences in body fat distribution, which in

Table 2.1 Influence of BMI, history of cigarette smoking and of adult weight gain, on relative mortality risk in 30–55 year old women, followed for 14 years (adapted with permission from: Manson *et al.* 1995).

BMI	< 19	19.0–21.9	22.0–24.9	22.0–26.9	27.0–28.9	29.0–31.9	> 32.0
All women							
Adj. RR[a]	1.0	0.8	0.8	0.8	1.0	1.2	1.5
95% CI[b]		0.7–0.9	0.7–0.9	0.7–0.9	0.9–1.1	1.0–1.3	1.3–1.7
Women who never smoked							
Adj. RR	1.0	1.0	1.1	1.1	1.4	1.7	1.9
95% CI		0.8–1.3	0.9–1.3	0.8–1.3	1.1–1.8	1.4–2.2	1.5–2.5
Women who never smoked and had stable weight							
Adj. RR[c]	1.0	1.2	1.2	1.3	1.6	2.1	2.2
95% CI		0.8–0.6	0.9–1.7	0.9–1.9	1.1–2.5	1.4–3.2	1.4–3.4

[a] Relative risk of death from all causes adjusted for age, smoking, menopausal status, use of oral contraceptives and post-menopausal hormones, and parental history of myocardial infarction before age 60 years.
[b] 95% confidence interval for relative risk.
[c] Excluding first 4 years of follow-up and women with > 4 kg weight change during those 4 years.

turn cause differences in the consequences of obesity. For a given BMI, mortality and morbidity from coronary heart disease is particularly high among South Asian people (Bangladeshi, Indian and Pakistani). These people tend to have a central fat distribution (McKeigue *et al.*, 1991). Hypertension and diabetes are also very common among Afro-Caribbean people, especially among women (Forrester *et al.*, 1996), but in this case the differences cannot easily be explained by differences in body composition.

2.1.3 Relation of obesity to morbidity

The relation of obesity to mortality, shown in Fig. 2.1, indicates that obesity begins to be of clinical importance at a BMI of about 30. However, examination of morbidity data shows that health penalties start at a much lower level. Rissanen *et al.*, (1990) analysed data from the Finnish Social Security system and found that the risk of drawing a disability pension increased significantly among individuals with a higher BMI, even within the 'desirable' BMI range of 20–25. The cause of the disability was mainly either cardiovascular or musculo-skeletal disease.

The relation of heart disease to obesity is probably one of increasing risk with increasing weight, or with increasing weight gain, in adult life. In the Nurses Health Study there were 991 non-fatal and 389 fatal myocardial infarcts (MI) during 14 years of follow-up (Willett *et al.*, 1995). After controlling for age,

smoking, menopausal status, post-menopausal hormone use and parental history of heart disease, the risk of MI with increasing obesity is shown in Table 2.2. When also adjusted for reported weight at age 18 years, and the other risk factors, there was a clear increase in risk of MI in women who gained >5 kg of weight after age 18 years compared with those who did not. For a weight gain of 5–8 kg, 8–11 kg, 11–19 kg and 20+ kg the relative risks were 1.25 (1.01–1.55), 1.65 (1.33–2.05), 1.92 (1.61–2.29) and 2.65 (2.17–3.22), respectively.

Similar conclusions can be drawn from the British Regional Heart Study, which recruited 7735 men aged 40–59 years and followed them for an average of 14.8 years (Shaper *et al.*, 1997). All-cause mortality was significantly increased among men with a BMI of <20 or >30, but the risk of cardiovascular death, heart attack and diabetes increased progressively from a BMI of <20, even after adjustments were made for age, smoking, social class, alcohol consumption and physical activity. These results are similar to those obtained for men and women in Japan (Tokunaga *et al.*, 1991) and in Framingham in the USA (Kannel *et al.*, 1996).

2.2 Operational definition of obesity in adults

It is evident from Fig. 2.1 that obesity can be arbitrarily divided into three grades. A significant effect on longevity begins somewhere in the BMI

Table 2.2 Influence of BMI on risk of coronary heart disease in 35–40 year old women followed for 14 years (data from: Willett *et al.* 1995, reproduced with permission).

BMI	< 21	21.0–22.9	23.0–24.9	25–28.9	> 29
Adj.RR[a]	1.0	1.19	1.46	2.06	3.56
95% CI[b]		0.97–1.44	1.20–1.77	1.72–2.48	2.96–4.29

[a] Relative risk of coronary heart disease adjusted for age, smoking, menopausal status, use of oral contraceptives and post-menopausal hormones, and parental history of myocardial infarction before age 60 years.
[b] 95% confidence interval for relative risk.

range 25–29.9, which is Grade I. Within this BMI range the health risk is related to the pattern of fat distribution. Intra-abdominal fat is associated with greater metabolic disturbance than an equal amount of fat subcutaneously in the limbs (Section 2.5). The mortality risk is obviously increased above a BMI of 30 (Grade II), and above a BMI of 40 (Grade III) the effect on health is severe. Figure 2.2 shows the bands of weight and height that define these grades. It is a form of presentation that people find easy to understand and on which it is possible to indicate an obese patient's present situation and also a reasonable target weight which he or she might profitably try to achieve (Garrow, 1981).

There are obvious practical disadvantages in using an operational definition of obesity that is changed with each reported epidemiological study. The J-shaped curve relating BMI to mortality or morbidity varies with differences in the age and gender of the subjects studied and with the correction for confounding factors such as cigarette smoking and the duration of follow-up. The American Health Foundation selected the BMI range of 19–25 as a 'reasonable goal' (Meisler & St Jeor, 1996) and the Scottish Intercollegiate Guidelines Networks (SIGN) suggest a BMI range of 18.5-25 (SIGN, 1996). The World Health Organisation (WHO) guidelines classify individuals with a BMI of <18.5 as underweight, 18.5–24.9 as a healthy weight, 25.0–29.9 as overweight, 30.0–39.9 as obese and >40 as morbidly obese (WHO, 1997). In this report we use the round values for BMI of 20, 25 and 30 as the boundaries, i.e. >25 is overweight and >30 is obese. This is not to imply that any especially important changes in health risk occur exactly at these levels, but the classification is convenient and fits the data well (Garrow, 1981).

2.3 Complications of obesity

2.3.1 Non-insulin-dependent diabetes mellitus

It has now been clearly shown in animal studies that the metabolic abnormalities, which are seen in obese animals, arise primarily as a result of decreased sensitivity of peripheral tissues to the action of insulin. This in turn has profound effects on the pattern of substrate utilisation and of 'counter-regulatory' hormone secretion. That this is also true in man was shown by the studies of experimental obesity in human volunteers conducted by Sims *et al.* (1973). Normal young men with no personal or family history of obesity or diabetes were overfed for six months; as a result they increased their body weight by 21%, of which 73% was fat. There was a significant increase in fasting insulin, glucose, triacylglycerol, cholesterol and amino acids, along with a decrease in oral and intravenous glucose tolerance. These are all changes of the type that characterise the non-insulin-dependent diabetic. The subjects did not become frankly diabetic but their BMI at maximum weight was only about 28. The overfeeding was then stopped, they lost weight and the insulin insensitivity reverted towards normal.

Closely similar observations have been made in rhesus monkeys that spontaneously develop obesity-associated non-insulin-dependent diabetes mellitus (NIDDM), which is preceded by the development of obesity and insulin resistance (Hansen & Bodkin, 1986; Ortmeyer *et al.*, 1996). It is unreasonable to ask for a more convincing demonstration that obesity causes (and is not merely associated with) insulin insensitivity.

In epidemiological studies, the prevalence of diabetes increases with increasing severity of obesity, with increasing duration of obesity and

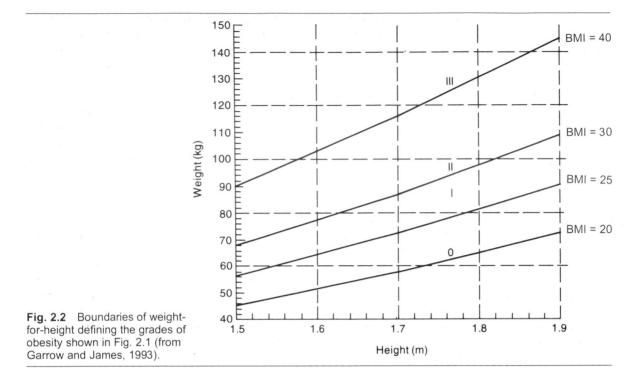

Fig. 2.2 Boundaries of weight-for-height defining the grades of obesity shown in Fig. 2.1 (from Garrow and James, 1993).

with increasing age. Analysis of the National Health and Nutrition Examination Study (NHANES) data shows that, for each kilogram increase in weight of the population, the risk of diabetes increases by 4.5% (Ford *et al.*, 1997). The prevalence is higher among American black than white people (Bonham & Brock, 1985). Even among pre-pubertal children, obesity is associated with peripheral and hepatic insulin resistance (Hoffman & Armstrong, 1996). For a given age, sex and ethnic group, the prevalence among overweight people (BMI >28.5) is about three times greater than among normal weight people (BMI <24.4). However, the association between being overweight and the prevalence of obesity underestimates the contribution of obesity to the incidence of diabetes because there is often substantial weight loss when diabetes develops. Knowler *et al.* (1981) showed that, among the Pima Indians, the age- and sex-adjusted prevalence of diabetes was virtually constant at about 25% over the BMI range of 28–45. However, the incidence (new cases/1,000 person years) increased steeply from a BMI of 28 at age 20 years, to a BMI of 45 at age 75 years.

Although diabetes is not directly the cause of most of the excess mortality among obese people, the metabolic defect underlying NIDDM is clearly the result of obesity (Scheen *et al.*, 1995), which itself predisposes to hypertension and heart disease (Reaven, 1995). These defects are reversible with weight loss, with a corresponding improvement in mortality. In overweight diabetics, the excess mortality risk is reversed by a 15–20% weight loss in the first year after diagnosis (Lean *et al.*, 1990). A deliberate weight loss of 0.5–9.0 kg is associated with a 30–40% reduction in diabetes-related mortality (Williamson *et al.*, 1995).

2.3.2 Coronary heart disease

The main cause of the excess mortality among obese people is coronary heart disease (CHD). Myocardial infarction (MI), hypertension and congestive failure are all significantly more common among obese people than among people of normal weight. In women, obesity (following age and blood pressure) is the third most powerful predictor of cardiovascular disease (Hubert *et al.*, 1983). It is ironic, therefore, that Keys *et al.* (1984)

concluded, from their very influential seven countries study, that obesity was not an independent predictor of CHD. This conclusion arose because, when age, cigarette smoking, blood pressure and serum cholesterol were included in a multiple regression equation, relative weight did not significantly predict heart attacks in men who were recruited at the age of 40–59 years.

This paradoxical situation arises because obesity is itself strongly related to hypertension and stroke, particularly in young people (Chen *et al.*, 1995). Obese people also have an adverse blood lipid profile, and therefore, in Keys' multiple regression equation, part of the effect of obesity has already been 'explained' by the hypertension and cholesterol. However, these risk factors improve when obese people lose weight (Stamler *et al.*, 1980; Dattilo & Kris-Etherton, 1992). After adjustment for age and smoking, the risk of a fatal or non-fatal MI among women with BMI >29 is three times that among lean women (Manson *et al.*, 1990, 1995).

High blood pressure, a high triacylglycerol concentration and a high low-density lipoprotein level favour the formation of atheromatous lesions, but obese people have the added hazard of abnormalities of blood clotting factors, which further increase the risk of thrombosis and MI (Meade *et al.*, 1993). It is not known why these abnormalities improve with therapeutic weight reduction (Ernst & Matrai, 1987).

2.3.3 Cancer

A very large survey by the American Cancer Society found that the mortality ratio for cancer among men who were 40% overweight was 1.33, among women, the corresponding figure was 1.55. The most important increase is for breast cancer in post-menopausal women, but there is also an increased risk of cancers of the endometrium, uterus, cervix, ovary and gall-bladder in women; and of the colon, rectum and prostate cancers in men (Garfinkel, 1985). Intentional weight loss of 0.5–9.0 kg is associated with a decrease of 40–50% in mortality from obesity related cancers (Williamson *et al.*, 1995).

2.3.4 Osteoarthritis

Degenerative disease of weight-bearing joints is a very common complication of obesity, particularly in the knees of middle-aged women (Hartz *et al.*, 1986; Seidell *et al.*, 1986) and causes significant disability (Rissanen *et al.*, 1990). Unlike the risk of heart disease or diabetes, the risk of osteoarthritis is related to the total amount of fat, and not in particular to the amount of intra-abdominal fat (Davis *et al.*, 1990). It seems that the excess weight, rather than any metabolic effect, causes the disease. Weight loss usually brings considerable relief of pain.

2.3.5 Gallstones

Obese people have a higher output of cholesterol in bile, with a lower concentration of bile salts, as such, their bile is constantly in danger of forming gallstones (Whiting *et al.*, 1984). Rapid weight loss increases the release of cholesterol from adipose tissue, and hence increases the load to be excreted in bile (Spirt *et al.*, 1995). Bile stasis contributes to biliary infections and also to the risk of gall-bladder cancer, mentioned above.

2.3.6 Sleep apnoea

Obesity causes inefficiency of respiratory function by several mechanisms. The mechanical load of fat on the chest wall increases the mechanical work of inspiration, especially when the subject is recumbent, and a large mass of intra-abdominal fat tends to push the liver upward, thus decreasing the intrathoracic space. There is also a mismatch of pulmonary ventilation and perfusion. Therefore, much of the blood flowing through the lung capillaries is at the base of the lung, where ventilation is poor. These problems may cause the Pickwickian syndrome of chronic hypoxia and carbon dioxide retention, which may manifest itself as inappropriate somnolence (vividly described by Dickens in the fat boy in *Pickwick Papers*) and obstructive sleep apnoea (OSA). This is a serious condition, which is associated with pulmonary hypertension and right-sided heart failure. Rossner *et al.* (1991) report a prospective study on 34 men with OSA, who had an average age 46 years and average BMI 41.6. In 4 years of follow-up there were 5 deaths, 3 from myocardial infarction and 2 from pulmonary oedema, despite normal blood lipid profiles. Lung compliance was reduced to 50% of normal.

Grunstein *et al.* (1995) reported from the Swedish Obese Subjects (SOS) study that OSA was an important contributor to morbidity in severe obesity and contributed to cardiovascular mortality. Respiratory function improves when obese people lose weight (Harman & Block, 1986).

2.3.7 Reproductive disorders

Significant associations are seen in reproductive endocrinology between excess body fat and ovulatory dysfunction, hyperandrogenism and hormone sensitive carcinomas (Kirschner *et al.*, 1982). The topography of fat distribution is correlated with these changes (Evans *et al.*, 1983). The differences in fat distribution relate to differences in androgenicity and to the variations in insulin action seen between upper body and lower body types of obesity. However, obesity influences the menstrual cycle independently of fat distribution (Kopelman *et al.*, 1980). Menarche frequently occurs at a younger age in obese girls and menstrual abnormalities are common in adulthood (Hartz *et al.*, 1979). Weight loss has a salutary effect on ovulatory function, with the return of menses in previously amenorrhoeic obese women (Kopelman *et al.*, 1981). Obese women may be characterised by distinct alterations in circulating sex hormone levels (Kopelman *et al.*, 1981). Androstenedione and testosterone concentrations are commonly elevated whereas sex hormone binding globulin (SHBG) is reduced. The plasma ratio of oestrone to oestradiol is also increased in obesity. Interestingly, a similar pattern of changes in sex steroid concentrations and binding are found in women with polycystic ovary syndrome (PCOS), with which obesity is frequently an accompaniment (Baird, 1978).

Subnormal plasma testosterone concentrations and reduced SHBG levels occur in massively obese men, with an inverse relationship between plasma testosterone and body weight. In these men, it has been proposed that a rise in plasma oestrogens, which result from increased aromatization of androgen precursers by adipose tissue, results in a negative feedback on the hypothalamo-pituitary axis with subnormal luteinizing hormone (LH) and follicle stimulating hormone (FSH) levels. Partial support for this hypothesis is the reversal of the reduced gonadotrophin levels following cortico-suppressive doses of dexamethasone, but this was not accompanied by a change in testosterone (Zumoff *et al.*, 1988).

2.3.8 Effect of obesity on pregnancy

The effect of obesity on endocrine function, and hence fertility, has been discussed above. However, once a pregnancy is established, an obese woman is at increased risk of complications (Garbaciak *et al.*, 1985). To some extent these complications apply also in the non-pregnant state, but examination of obese pregnant women is particularly difficult whether by abdominal palpation, ultrasound or laparoscopy. The difficulty in monitoring fetal well-being in severely obese mothers partly explains their increased rate of caesarean section. However, even moderate degrees of obesity are associated with an increased incidence of hypertension, toxaemia, gestational diabetes, urinary tract infections and fetal macrosomia (Galtier-Dereure *et al.*, 1995). Table 2.3 shows the incidence of maternal complications in pregnant obese women. Perinatal mortality is also increased in the babies of obese mothers. In an analysis of 56 000 births from the US collaborative Perinatal Study, it was shown that perinatal death was three times more common in obese than in thin women (Naeye, 1990). More recently, there has emerged strong evidence that obese women are at increased risk of having babies with congenital malformations, in particular neural tube defects (Prentice & Goldberg, 1996). Among women over 70 kg in weight, dietary intake of folic acid does not have the same protective effect that it has in leaner women (Shaw *et al.*, 1996; Werler *et al.*, 1996).

2.3.9 Psychological disorders

Any clinician with experience of obese patients realises that there are many psychological and social penalties associated with the condition. However, there is little consensus about the aetiology of these problems; are they innate characteristics of obese people, or are they induced by pressures from others either to be unreasonably thin or to adopt an unreasonably restricted diet?

Orbach (1978) maintains that the typically female anxiety about slimness is a manifestation of low self-esteem, which has been promoted by the media in a male-dominated society. This problem,

Table 2.3 Obesity and incidence of maternal complications during pregnancy (adapted from: Galtier Dereure *et al.*, 1995).

	Normal	Overweight	Obese	Massively obese	*p* value
Number of subjects	54	48	34	30	
Hypertension (%)	9.3	33.3[a]	54.6[a]	79.3[a]	< 0.0001
Toxaemia (%)	3.7	17.8	30.3[a]	42.9[a]	< 0.0001
Gestational diabetes (%)	1.9	12.3	39.4[a]	44.8[a]	< 0.0001
Insulin (% patients)	0	2.1	12.1[a]	20.7[a]	< 0.001
Insulin (% diabetics)	0	16.8	30.7[a]	46.2[a]	< 0.001
Urinary infection (%)	16.7	8.7	29.0	37.5	< 0.02
Preterm labour (%)	14.8	13.0	22.6	28.0	NS
Caesarean section (%)	9.3	16.7	15.1	42.9[a]	< 0.002
1st caesarean section (%)	7.4	10.4	5.9	33.3[a]	< 0.006
Hospitalisation					
Outpatients (%)	7.4	33.3[a]	45.5[a]	61.5[a]	< 0.0001
Inpatients (%)	9.3	33.3[a]	36.4[a]	66.6[a]	< 0.0001
Hospitalisation					
Outpatients (days)	0.2	1.5[a]	2.9[a]	4.7[a]	< 0.0001
Inpatients (days)	0.6	2.9[a]	3.7[a]	8.6[a]	< 0.0001
Overall cost[b]	5.7	9.6[a]	11.0[a]	18.4[a]	< 0.0001

Normal = BMI of 18–24.9; Overweight = BMI of 25–29.9; Obese = BMI of 30 34.9; Massively obese – BMI of > 35.
[a] – significantly different from normal weight group, [b] = cost assessed as equivalent outpatient hospitalisation.

which concerns mainly young women, has caused some psychiatrists to condemn all dieting as misguided and to maintain that it is the cause of eating disorders (Garner & Wooley, 1991). Selection bias is very likely to affect the opinion of professionals in this field, as the patients who are referred to psychiatrists with an interest in eating disorders are likely to have these disorders. Furthermore, psychiatric patients who are on treatment with neuroleptic drugs, such as flupenthixol or fluphenazine, are very likely to be obese (Silverstone & Goodall, 1987). Psychiatrists, therefore, have good reason to believe that obesity and dieting are strongly related to neurosis and psychosis.

The key question is: are obese people more likely than normal to be anxious or depressed, and does dieting make their anxiety better or worse? In a survey of 393 girls in a local school (average age 15.8 years), Wadden *et al.* (1989) found no association between measures of anxiety or depression and weight category. The overweight girls were, however, significantly more dissatisfied with their figures and more of them were trying to lose weight. Rothschild *et al.* (1989) recruited, by advertisement, 63 men aged 25–36 years, who ranged from very

thin to very fat. They found that there was a significant positive association between obesity and depression (measured by the Beck depression inventory) but that the average scores for the obese, overweight and normal weight subjects were all within the normal ranges.

Among the severely obese volunteers for the Swedish SOS study, both men and women showed very poor ratings for mental well-being and more symptoms of anxiety and depression than the reference population. The scores on psychometric scales were as bad as, or worse than, those of patients with chronic pain, generalised malignant melanoma or tetraplegia after neck injury (Sullivan *et al.*, 1993).

Wadden & Stunkard (1985) monitored the psychological state of 17 severely obese women before, during and after a 6-month period of dieting. Weight loss at the end of this period was on average 20.5 ± 9.2 kg. They administered both the Beck depression inventory and the Minnesota Multiphasic Personality Inventory. The scores on all the scales were within normal ranges at all times, but there was a significant improvement in all scales (except anxiety) at six weeks and in all the ratings (including anxiety) at six months.

It is, therefore, not true to say, in general, that obese people, or people on diets, are significantly depressed or anxious, but of course these traits are frequently seen in patients who are referred to hospital. When it has been carefully monitored, the effect of dieting in obese people has been to improve psychological function rather than to induce neurosis.

The relation of obesity to psychiatric disorders is discussed in more detail in Chapter 12, including the extent to which these disorders may be caused by obesity or methods for the treatment of obesity. The extent to which the obesity may be caused by psychiatric disorders or by psychotropic medication is also discussed.

2.3.10 Social penalties

There is compelling evidence that our society discriminates against fat people. This is particularly damaging to the psychological well-being of obese children, who are believed by their peers at school to be lazy, dirty, stupid, ugly, cheats and liars (Wadden & Stunkard, 1985). Parental support may be counter-productive. Bruch (1974) drew attention to the over-cared-for child who was given food as a comfort in any stressful situation. The child was never allowed to experience hunger, and was strongly conditioned to expect food whenever anything went wrong. Bruch hypothesised that this was the mechanism by which such children became fat adults.

Social discrimination continues into adult life. Sonne-Holm & Sorensen (1986) showed that for a given parental social class, intelligence and education, severely obese people achieved less favourable social status than non-obese people did. Overweight in adolescence is associated with less social success in later life. In the USA, Gortmaker *et al.* (1993) studied a nationally representative sample of 10 039 men and women, who were 16–24 years of age in 1981, and obtained follow-up data on 65–79% of the cohort 7 years later. Women who were initially above the 95th centile for BMI had completed fewer years in school, were less likely to be married and had higher rates of household poverty than the women who had not been overweight. These findings were independent of their baseline socio-economic status and aptitude test scores. However, people with chronic conditions

such as asthma and musculo-skeletal abnormalities did not differ from non-overweight people in these ways. There was no evidence of an effect of being overweight on self-esteem. Evidence that social deprivation in children predicts obesity comes from a Danish study by Lissau & Sorensen (1994). They found that indices of parental neglect were strong predictors of the development of obesity ten years later, whereas the level of education or occupation of the parents had no predictive value.

2.4 Obesity in children and adolescents

2.4.1 Measurement of obesity in children and adolescents

The bands of BMI, which define grades of adult obesity (Fig. 2.2) do not apply to children and adolescents. Between the ages of 1 and 5 years there is a decrease in BMI, because children are increasing in height relatively faster than they are increasing in weight. But after the age of 5 years, weight gain is more rapid than height gain, until the adult ranges are reached, by which time height gain has ceased. Indeed the situation is still more complex because fatter children enter the pubertal growth spurt at an earlier age than do thinner children. Consequently fat, fat-free mass and height are all changing quite rapidly, and at different rates, especially around the age of puberty. Indices of weight-for-height are not, therefore, very good indices of adiposity (Lazarus *et al.*, 1996).

The traditional method for assessing the nutritional status of children is to compare the observed weight and height of the child with standard growth curves for gender and age. A child who is on a higher centile for weight than for height is overweight. This is a cumbersome method for assessing obesity, which is more easily done by BMI, but it has the merit of indicating if the abnormality is in weight alone, or if stature is also affected. Conditions that lead to obesity in childhood, such as single-gene defects (e.g. Prader-Willi syndrome) or hypothyroidism, also cause a decrease in height growth. Thus, a normal or above-normal height in an obese child virtually eliminates the possibility of a genetically determined obesity syndrome.

Despite the limitations of weight–height indices as indicators of obesity in children, BMI is often used in epidemiological studies. The centiles of

BMI among British children up to the age of 20 years are shown in Figs 2.3 and 2.4, for boys and girls respectively (Cole *et al.*, 1995). Similar curves have been derived for Italian children (Luciano *et al.*, 1997). Very fat or very thin children lie outside the range of the centile charts, so it is common to express extreme results as standard deviation score (SDS, or Z-scores). However, centiles for BMI are not normally distributed about the 50th centile. Therefore, Cole (1990) introduced the LMS method for deriving exact centiles from skewed data. The assumption made is that there is a power transformation that will make the distribution normal; the name of the method is derived from L (for lambda, the power transformation), M (æ, the median) and S (å, the coefficient of variation).

An alternative method for assessing the fatness of children is to measure skinfold thickness (Section 3.3.1.). At age 7–15 years there is only a moderate correlation ($r = 0.70$–0.85) between adiposity calculated from BMI and from the sum of four skinfolds, and probably the skinfolds give a more reliable estimate of fatness (Lazarus *et al.*, 1996). In practice, the triceps skinfold is probably the most convenient measure of fatness in children and adolescents. Standard curves for triceps skinfolds for boys and girls are shown in Figs 2.5 and 2.6, respectively.

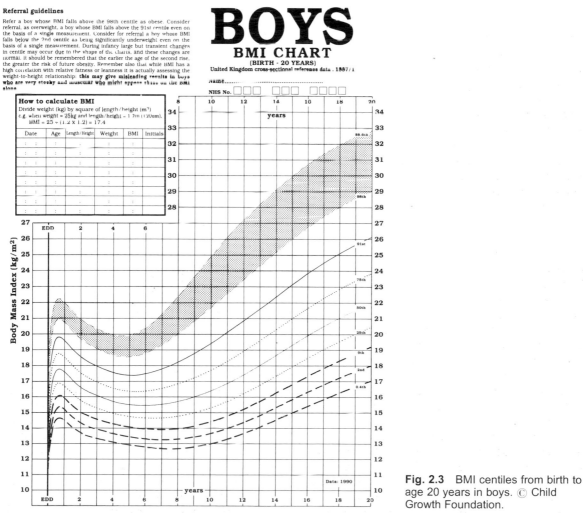

Fig. 2.3 BMI centiles from birth to age 20 years in boys. © Child Growth Foundation.

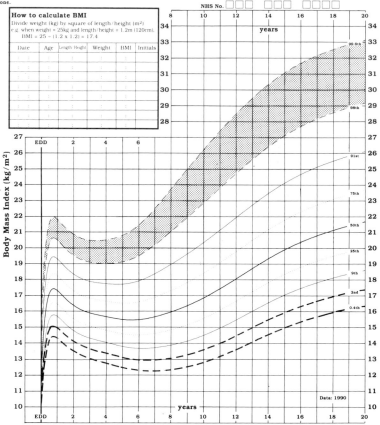

Referral guidelines

Refer a girl whose BMI falls above the 98th centile as obese. Consider referral, as overweight, a girl whose BMI falls above the 91st centile even on the basis of a single measurement. Consider for referral a girl whose BMI falls below the 2nd centile as being significantly underweight even on the basis of a single measurement. During infancy large but transient changes in centile may occur due to the shape of the charts, and these changes are normal. It should be remembered that the earlier the age of the second rise, the greater the risk of future obesity. Remember also that while BMI has a high correlation with relative fatness or leanness it is actually assessing the weight-to-height relationship, **this may give misleading results in girls who are very stocky and muscular who might appear obese on the BMI alone.**

How to calculate BMI
Divide weight (kg) by square of length/height (m²)
e.g. when weight = 25kg and length/height = 1.2m (120cm),
BMI = 25 ÷ (1.2 × 1.2) = 17.4

GIRLS
BMI CHART
(BIRTH - 20 YEARS)
United Kingdom cross-sectional reference data : 1997/1

Fig. 2.4 BMI centiles from birth to age 20 years in girls. © Child Growth Foundation.

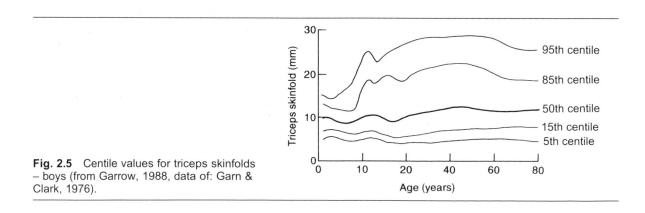

Fig. 2.5 Centile values for triceps skinfolds – boys (from Garrow, 1988, data of: Garn & Clark, 1976).

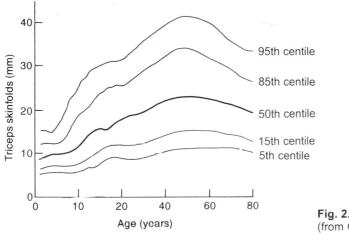

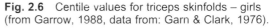

Fig. 2.6 Centile values for triceps skinfolds – girls (from Garrow, 1988, data from: Garn & Clark, 1976).

2.4.2 Health risks of obesity in children and adolescents

In adults, the grades of obesity are calculated on the basis of the severity of the health hazards associated with a given weight-for-height. However, we do not have the data on which to make such a calculation for children. If we knew that obese children always became obese adults we could reasonably argue that, by treating or preventing excessive fatness in children, we were preventing disease and disability in adult life. The extent to which obesity in childhood predicts obesity in adult life is discussed in detail in Section 7.3.2.

Characteristic metabolic defects in obese adults (peripheral and hepatic insulin resistance) can be detected in obese pre-pubertal children (Hoffman & Armstrong, 1996). By the age of 9 years, obese boys and girls have higher blood pressure and plasma cholesterol concentration than non-obese controls (McMurray *et al.*, 1995). Obese adolescents have a greatly increased prevalence of hypertension, of sleep-disordered breathing and of orthopaedic disorders of the hips and knees (Lusky *et al.*, 1996; Marcus *et al.*, 1996).

However, the most prevalent consequences of obesity among children are psychosocial (Dietz, 1992). There are many reports from the USA about social stigmatisation of obese children (Section 2.3.10), but this also is prevalent in the UK. Among 9-year-old children there is widespread dissatisfaction with body shape (Hill *et al.*, 1994). Girls (except for the very thinnest) would prefer to be thinner, whereas boys (except for the very overweight) would prefer to be heavier. Dietz (1996b) has drawn attention to the epidemiology of inactivity, which is often associated with obesity in children. Inactivity has its own health risks, such as insulin resistance, which may confound the association between obesity and health consequences in children.

The long-term effects of obesity in adolescents has been investigated by Must *et al.* (1992), who in 1988 followed up 508 participants from the Harvard Growth Study of adolescents of 1922–1935. They found that the group of men, but not women, who had been obese adolescents, had an increased mortality from all causes (RR 1.8, CI 1.2–2.7) and from CHD (RR 2.3, CI 1.4–4.1). Among those who had been obese as adolescents, the risk of colorectal cancer and gout was increased in men and the risk of arthritis was increased in women. They concluded that overweight in adolescence has adverse health effects, which are independent of adult weight 55 years later.

2.5 Relation of fat distribution to health risk

It has been suspected for many years that excess fat on the trunk, in particular within the peritoneal cavity, is metabolically more damaging than a similar amount of subcutaneous fat on the limbs (Vague, 1953). Interest was reawakened by the report of a study in Gothenburg in which, in both men (Larsson *et al.*, 1984) and women (Lapidus *et al.*, 1984), a high ratio of waist to hip circumference was more important than BMI as a risk factor for cardiovascular disease and death during 12 years of follow-up. Scanning techniques (discussed below) have shown that waist circumference is a good indicator of intra-abdominal fat for groups of subjects, but not for individuals.

There are several plausible mechanisms by which intra-abdominal fat might contribute to disease risk (Björntorp, 1996). Portal adipose tissue is highly sensitive to stimulation of lipid mobilisation, thus causing a high concentration of free fatty acids (FFA) in the portal vein. This stimulates gluconeogenesis in the liver and also increases secretion of very low density lipoprotein (VLDL). It may also decrease insulin clearance by the liver. This direct mechanism of increased portal FFA concentration goes a long way towards explaining the cardiovascular and diabetic risk factors associated with intra-abdominal obesity. However, there are many other mechanisms that can contribute to insulin resistance, which is an important characteristic of intra-abdominal obesity. Insulin sensitivity is affected by changes in the distribution of the microcirculation in muscle, which is in turn affected by physical training and also by hyperinsulinaemia. In visceral obesity, there is also an increase in cortisol and a decrease in both growth hormone and sex steroids. These hormonal changes may be induced by lifestyle factors such as stress, cigarette smoking and a high alcohol intake. Further analysis of the health risks associated with a high waist–hip ratio in the Gothenburg studies showed that these findings were confounded by cigarette smoking and high alcohol intake (Larsson, 1987). It has also been shown that a high waist–hip ratio reflected small hips as well as a large waist (Seidell *et al.*, 1989). It is now emerging, that waist circumference alone may be a better indicator of intra-abdominal fat (Lean *et al.*, 1995, 1998; Section 3.3.2). Fat distribution may itself reflect the quantity and type of dietary fat. Although the association between visceral fat deposition and health risk is very clearly shown in many studies, it is not yet known to what extent the health risk is a direct effect of the visceral fat, or if disease risk and the visceral fat are both indicators of other risk factors (Van Loan, 1996).

2.6 Summary

- Insurance companies have known for nearly a century that people who are very heavy (or very light) for their height are liable to die young, and hence are unprofitable to insure.

- Life insurance data show that the range of weight-for-height associated with least mortality before retirement age is a BMI in the range of 20–25.

- The main cause of excess mortality in people with a BMI above 25 is cardiovascular disease, but recent research shows that the excess mortality below a BMI of 20 is associated with cigarette smoking and cancers. For young non-smokers, the least risk of heart disease is in the BMI range 20–22.

- In this report we use the round BMI values of 20, 25 and 30 as the boundaries, where >25 is overweight and >30 is obese. This classification is convenient and fits the data well.

- The mechanisms by which obesity causes ill health and early death are becoming clear. Excessive body fat (especially intra-abdominal fat) decreases the sensitivity of tissues to the action of insulin. This leads to an increased liability to non-insulin-dependent diabetes, and also to raised blood lipids and blood pressure, which are important risk factors for cardiovascular disease and stroke.

- Obese people are also at increased risk of diseases which do not necessarily decrease life expectancy: reproductive endocrine disorders and some sex-hormone sensitive cancers; osteoarthritis of weight-bearing joints; sleep apnoea syndrome; and gall-stone formation. Apart from these physical disabilities, obese people suffer from adverse social discrimination. This is particularly evident among women and schoolchildren.

3
Clinical Assessment of Obesity

3.1 Reference methods for measuring total body fat

In the previous chapter, BMI was used to obtain an operational definition of obesity in adults. BMI is easy to measure and for many purposes it is quite satisfactory. For example, the life insurance companies use weight-for-height to calculate insurance risks and many epidemiological studies show that weight-for-height correlates well with morbidity and mortality from many diseases. The assumption that BMI indicates fatness is to a large extent true, but there are exceptions. For example, heavily muscled athletes, such as weight lifters or boxers, have a high BMI but are not obese. At the other extreme, elderly people have a low lean body mass; therefore, even if they have a normal BMI, they may have a high percentage body fat. It is evident that excess weight does not necessarily indicate excess fatness and certainly does not tell us anything about the anatomical distribution of body fat. In this chapter we shall consider the reliability and usefulness of methods for measuring total body fat and the distribution of body fat. There are three reference methods by which the fat content of a living subject can be measured, each of which depends on different assumptions.

3.1.1 Body density

The approximate weight, volume and density of main components of the human body in a normal adult male are shown in Table 3.1. Fat has a density of 0.90 kg/l, and the normal 'fat-free mass' is a mixture of water, protein and mineral that has a density of 1.10 kg/l. Therefore, if we can measure

Table 3.1 The approximate weight, volume and density of the main components of the adult body.

Component	Weight (kg)	Volume (l)	Density (kg/l)
Water	42.0	42.3	0.993
Protein	12.0	8.96	1.34
Mineral	4.0	1.33	3.00
Fat-free mass	58.0	52.6	1.1
Fat	12.0	13.3	0.90
Whole body	70.0	65.9	1.06

the density of the whole body (D), we can calculate the proportion of fat, as shown in Equation (2.1) below:

$$\text{Proportion of fat} = \frac{(4.96)}{D} - 4.50 \qquad (2.1)$$

3.1.2 Total body water

Fat is triacylglycerol, it contains no water. The average mixture of the fat-free tissues in the body, or fat-free mass (FFM), contains 73% water. If we measure total body water (TBW) by dilution of a tracer dose of labelled water, then we can calculate FFM by dividing TBW by 0.73. Total body fat is calculated by subtracting FFM from body fat.

3.1.3 Total body potassium

All potassium, including that in the human body, contains 0.114% of a very long-lived radioactive isotope, ^{40}K, which emits a high-energy gamma ray. If the total gamma ray emission from a body is measured in a suitably screened highly sensitive counter, the potassium content of the body can be measured. In men the potassium content of the FFM is 66 mmol/kg and in women it is 60 mmol/kg. So by using the appropriate factor, the FFM and hence the fat mass of men and women can be calculated.

3.1.4 Combined methods versus BMI

It is obvious that each of the above methods assumes that the FFM has some constant characteristic density, water content or potassium content. If this assumption is wrong, the calculation of body fat will also be wrong. The commonest way in which the FFM departs from the assumed characteristics concerns its water content. In an oedematous subject, the water content of FFM is >0.73; therefore FFM is overestimated by TBW and fat is underestimated. However, in oedematous subjects, the potassium content of FFM is less than the assumed value. As a result, potassium measurements lead to an underestimation of FFM and an overestimation of fat. Thus, by measuring FFM by both water and potassium, and averaging the answers, a fairly reliable estimate of total body

fat is obtained, even in subjects with abnormalities in body water content. If a third method (density) is added, the mean estimate of all three becomes more reliable.

Figure 3.1 shows the relationship between body weight and body fat among 104 women aged 14–60 years, who covered the range from very thin to very fat. The estimate of body fat is based on the mean of measurements in each woman by density, water and potassium. The correlation coefficient of 0.96 indicates that 92% of the variation in body weight is explained by variation in body fat. The slope of the regression line indicates that the excess weight in the heavier women, compared with the lighter women, comprises about 75% fat and 25% fat-free tissue (Webster *et al.*, 1984).

3.1.5 Other laboratory methods and multiple compartment models

Total body fat can also be measured by neutron activation, by total body electrical conductivity (TOBEC) and by various multiple compartment models. Discussion of these is beyond the scope of

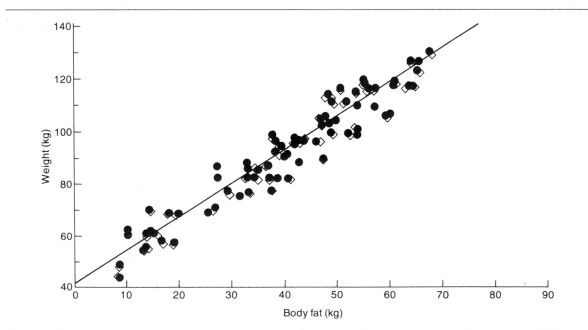

Fig. 3.1 The relationship between body weight and body fat among 104 women aged 14–60 years. n = 0.960, y = 41.4 + 1.27x

this chapter, but for further information see Sutcliffe (1996).

3.2 Methods for measuring the distribution of body fat

3.2.1 CAT and MRI scanning

An image of the cross-section of a human body can be constructed by computer, using data obtained by measuring the absorption of X-rays passed through the body, between a source and detector, which rotate around the axis of the body. In the resultant image, tissue with low absorption, such as fat, shows as a dark area and tissue with a high absorption, such as bone, as a white area. Intermediate tissue, such as muscle, is shown in a grey tone. Computer software is available that will calculate the area of fat as a percentage of the total area for each scan. If this is summed for slices through the whole body, an estimate of total body fat is obtained together with information about exactly where in the body this fat is located. MRI scanning obtains similar information, with no radiation load.

3.2.2 Dual-energy X-ray scanning

A longitudinal image of the body can be obtained by dual-energy X-ray scanning (DEXA). However, this does not provide reliable information about the distribution of fat in areas such as the abdomen.

These techniques represent the gold standard for measuring fat distribution, but they require expensive apparatus and are time-consuming for both subject and investigator. There is a need, therefore, for simpler techniques that can be used in field studies on large numbers of subjects.

3.3 Body fat techniques suitable for bedside use

3.3.1 Skinfolds

Measurement of the thickness of the layer of fat under the skin yields good estimates of total body fat in normal weight adults and children. Readings taken at four sites (biceps, triceps, subscapular and supra-iliac) yield good estimates of body fat in people who are not very obese (Womersley & Durnin, 1977). It is not suitable for severely obese

subjects and does not measure the important component of intra-abdominal fat.

3.3.2 Weight, height, and circumference of waist, hips and thighs

The ability of BMI to estimate total body fat has already been shown in Fig. 3.1. Recent publications indicate that the measure of obesity which best identifies health risks may vary according to the risk considered. For example, impaired glucose tolerance and diabetes are associated with both increased intra-abdominal fat and decreased muscle mass. In this case, the waist–hip ratio (WHR) is a good predictor of diabetes but, as decreased muscle mass is not a predictor of hypertension, the association between BMI and hypertension was stronger than between WHR and hypertension (Sakurai *et al.*, 1995).

It is emerging that waist circumference, alone, may prove to be a good measure of intra-abdominal fat (Han *et al.*, 1997a). It is little influenced by height or age and a reduction in waist circumference is associated with improvement in cardiovascular risk factors (Han *et al.*, 1997b). It is suggested that where waist circumference is > 94 cm in men or > 80 cm in women, no further weight should be gained. Weight reduction is required where waist circumference is > 102 cm in men and > 88 cm in women (Lean *et al.*, 1995, 1998).

3.3.3 Bio-electrical impedance

If an alternating current is passed between electrodes attached to the hand and foot, the impedance of the body reflects the relative amounts of conducting material (i.e. intra- and extra-cellular water) compared to insulating material (i.e. fat). However, there are many confounding factors, such as the cross-sectional area of the limbs which, for a given body composition, will affect the measured impedance (Heitmann, 1994).

Recently, attention has turned to the potential of multiple frequency bio-electrical impedance because, on theoretical grounds, intra- and extra-cellular water should offer different impedances at different electrical frequencies. It appears that this approach offers only marginal advantages in the measurement of total body water, except in situations where there are abnormalities in fluid distribution (Cornish *et al.,* 1996).

3.3.4 Near-infrared reactance

If monochromatic light in the near-infrared is shone into subcutaneous tissue, the reflected signal indicates the proportion of fat or lean tissue under the skin. This technique has been adopted commercially, using a simple infrared source combined with anthropometric data that together yield an estimate of body composition. The ability of this method to measure body composition arises, almost entirely, from the anthropometric data entered by the operator (Hortobagyi *et al.,* 1992).

3.4 Measurement of fat cell size and number

In normal subjects, it is possible to obtain a sample of about 20 mg of subcutaneous fat by needle biopsy at sites such as the abdominal wall or buttock. Hirsch and Gallian (1968) were the first to demonstrate that this sample can be used to estimate the size and number of fat cells in the whole body. Their technique involved fixing the sample in osmium tetroxide, gently breaking up the fixed tissue, passing it through sieves to remove strands of connective tissue and very small particles of debris, and counting the intermediate-sized particles in a coulter counter. Using this technique it was found that very fat subjects had very large fat cells and adults who had lost a large amount of fat had very small fat cells. Hirsch (1975) proposed the hypothesis 'that obesity may be accompanied by an excessive number of adipocytes, possibly brought about by excess feeding in infancy and childhood, and that the excessive number of adipocytes remains constant and in some way causes a drive for maintaining the obese state'.

This ingenious procedure gave birth to a whole new field of investigation of the morphology and biochemical characteristics of adipose tissue, but it was not satisfactory as a method for measuring fat cell size and number. The size of the mesh of the sieves arbitrarily set upper and lower limits to the size of the particles that were deemed to be 'fat cells'. Bray (1970) and Sjöström (1976) showed that, if a sample of adipose tissue was examined histologically, cells could be found that contained very little fat, which would be missed by the Hirsch technique. However, Björntorp *et al.* (1975) used a histological technique to measure fat cell size in 28 obese women. Initially, the women had 38 kg of fat and, on average, lost 15 kg of weight (of which 13 kg was fat) over a period of 26 weeks. Samples were taken before weight loss from gluteal, femoral and abdominal sites. The average fat cell size was $0.78 \pm 0.02 \,\mu g$. And the estimated fat cell number was 4.9×10^{10}. After weight loss, the average fat cell weight decreased by $0.24 \,\mu g$ but the fat cell number decreased by only 0.2×10^{10}. The authors concluded 'that when the fat cell size in different regions of an individual are known, as well as the total fat cell number, the success of an energy-reduced dietary regimen can be approximately predicted both in terms of remaining total body fat and in regional fat depot decrease'.

Many important implications arose from the view that the number of fat cells in the body is determined by the nature of nutrition in infancy and childhood and that when (some time before puberty) the number of fat cells in a region is fixed, this will in turn fix the amount and distribution of body fat. It seemed sensible to put emphasis on preventing obesity in children, to restrict their fat cell number and to protect them from adult obesity. Indeed, plastic surgeons offered to excise excess fat cells in adults from selected sites, claiming that in this way they could offer a permanent cure from excessive fat deposition in that region. More recent research has undermined the importance of apparent fat cell number, as calculated by dividing estimated total body fat by average fat cell size in samples of subcutaneous adipose tissue. Although some investigators found an association between the degree of hyperplasia in fat cells and resistance to treatment (Krotkiewski *et al.,* 1977), others did not confirm this finding (Ashwell *et al.,* 1978). It became evident that there are 'pre-adipocytes' in human subcutaneous tissue, which can be seen to differentiate into mature fat cells in tissue culture (Roncari *et al.,* 1986). This process of recruitment of adipocytes seems to be under multifactorial control (Löffler *et al.,* 1994). It is, therefore, no longer possible to defend the view that the number of mature adipocytes available can ever limit accumulation of fat at a given site, or in the whole body. This is because, under conditions of prolonged positive energy balance, more adipocytes will be recruited from the pre-adipocyte pool.

It has been suggested that liposuction, which removes fat cells from under the skin, provides a permanent cure (at least locally) for excess fat deposition. However, this is not supported by acceptable evidence. The treatment of obesity by liposuction and by apronectomy is discussed in Section 23.2.

It has also become clear that adipocytes at different sites have different functions and effects. Femoral fat depots in women, for example, seem to have a special role as an energy reserve to support lactation (Rebuffé-Scrive *et al.*, 1985). Further, as has already been mentioned, excessive amounts of intra-abdominal adipocytes have more serious metabolic consequences than a similar amount of adipose tissue in a subcutaneous site. Knowledge of the actual fat cell number in a person at any particular moment would not, therefore, be helpful in predicting health risks or response to treatment.

3.5 Brown adipose tissue

Brown adipose tissue (BAT) is highly vascular (hence its colour) and has a specialised function in generating heat that is required to maintain the body temperature of small mammals when the ambient temperature is low (Himms-Hagen, 1984). It has been shown that a failure of this thermogenic capacity in brown adipose tissue is the explanation for obesity in certain strains of rodent (Stock & Rothwell, 1982). The molecular biology of these defects is considered further in Section 8.1.2. It remains controversial as to whether a defect of thermogenesis has any part to play in the aetiology of human obesity.

3.6 Summary

- All methods for measuring the amount of fat and fat-free tissue in living subjects are limited by errors of two types. First, the assumption that fat-free tissue has a specific characteristic (e.g. its density, water content or potassium content) and, second, the measurement error in assessing the density, water or potassium content of the subject. With improving technology the measurement error is becoming quite small;

therefore, the main factor limiting accuracy is the validity of the assumptions underlying the measurement.

- In subjects with very abnormal body composition (e.g. in severe obesity), the density, water content and potassium content of fat-free tissue differs from that present in normal subjects. Fat-free tissue in obese people has a lower concentration of potassium but a higher content of water than that in normal subjects. Thus, the most accurate estimates of body composition are obtained by using several methods, that use different assumptions, and combining the results.

- In clinical practice, estimates of fatness are needed to assess the degree of obesity in a given person. Simple measures such as BMI serve well in such cases. However, it is more difficult to measure change in body composition with treatment. The same amount of weight loss (and hence decrease in BMI), brought about by two different treatments may signify different proportions of loss of fat, lean tissue and water. At present there are no methods that will reliably measure loss of fat in an individual with an accuracy of better than 1 kg.

- Many of the health hazards associated with obesity are particularly related to intra-abdominal fat (Section 2.5). Scanning techniques can measure intra-abdominal fat for research purposes (Section 3.2), but these are too expensive in terms of time and money for use in field studies. The minimum set of measurements that should be made in any person to define obesity status are: weight, height and waist circumference. However, small reductions in weight do not necessarily indicate loss of fat. Neither do small reductions in waist circumference necessarily indicate loss of intra-abdominal fat.

- Commercial instruments are available, based on electrical impedance or near-infrared reactance, which provide computer printouts of many parameters of body composition and energy requirements. However, these are subject to the errors mentioned above and manufacturers may make exaggerated claims for the accuracy of their instruments.

- Measurements of fat cell size and number have not proved useful in guiding the treatment or prognosis of obesity.

- It is not clear that brown fat has any relevance to human obesity.

4
Epidemiology of Obesity in the UK

Obesity is known to be more common in some populations than in others. However, accurate comparisons of the prevalence in different populations are very difficult because of differences between studies in sampling and in the obesity criteria used, and also because of secular trends in the prevalence of obesity within populations. Obesity is most common in western countries, such as the USA and Canada, and is low in China and Japan. Within Europe, prevalence tends to be lowest in Scandinavian countries and highest in eastern European countries, with the UK around the middle of the range (WHO MONICA Project, 1988; Gurney & Gorstein, 1988; Laurier *et al.*, 1992; Hodge & Zimmet, 1994).

The UK is fortunate in having data available from many studies which can be used to ascertain the relationships between obesity and factors such as age, gender, social class, smoking, region and ethnic group. These are listed in Table 4.1.

Table 4.1 Studies providing data on body fatness.

Study	Geographical area	Subjects
Adults:		
Khosla & Lowe, 1971	Port Talbot, S. Wales	10,482 male steelworkers aged 20–64 years
Khosla & Lowe, 1972	Port Talbot & Ebbw Vale, S. Wales	17,836 male steelworkers aged 20–64 years
Dept. Health & Social Security, 1972	England & Scotland	879 men & women aged ≥ 65 years
Ashwell *et al.*, 1978	London, England	1921 working men & women aged 18–64 years
Dept. Health & Social Security, 1979	England & Scotland	365 men & women aged ≥ 69 years
Rose & Marmot, 1981	Whitehall, London, England	18,403 male civil servants aged 40–64 years
Bingham *et al.*, 1981	Cambridgeshire, England	63 men & women aged ≥ 20 years
Shaper *et al.*, 1981	Great Britain	7735 men aged 40–59 years
Burr *et al.*, 1982a	S. Wales	1500 men & women aged ≥ 65 years
Burr *et al.*, 1982b	S. Wales	8 year follow-up of 830 men & women aged ≥ 65 years
Yarnell *et al.*, 1982	Caerphilly, S. Wales	819 women aged 18–69 years
Yarnell *et al.*, 1983	Caerphilly, S. Wales	711 men aged 30–69 years
Knight, 1984	Great Britain	men & women aged 16–64 years
Fehily *et al.*, 1984	Caerphilly, S. Wales	493 men aged 45–59 years
Fehily & Bird, 1986	Caerphilly, S. Wales	97 women aged 40–59 years
Barasi *et al.*, 1985	Llantwit Major, S. Wales	101 women aged ≥ 18 years
Braddon *et al.*, 1986 & Wadsworth, personal communication, 1997	Great Britain	3322 men & women; longitudinal study: birth to 43 years
Cox *et al.*, 1987	Great Britain	9003 men & women aged ≥ 18 years
Fulton *et al.*, 1988	Scotland	162 men aged 45–54 years

Contd.

Table 4.1 Continued.

Miller *et al.*, 1988	London, England	163 men aged 45–54 years
Barker *et al.*, 1989	N. Ireland	616 men & women aged 16–64 years
Gregory *et al.*, 1990	Great Britain	2197 men & women aged 16–64 years
Fehily *et al.*, 1990	4 areas of the UK	977 men aged 45–64 years
Wannamethee & Shaper, 1990	Great Britain	5 year follow-up of 7735 men aged 40–59 years
Marmot *et al.*, 1991	Whitehall, London, England	10,314 male & female civil servants aged 35–55 years
McKeigue *et al.*, 1991	South London	3754 men & women aged 40–69 years (industrial workforces + GP lists)
Bolton-Smith *et al.*, 1991 & Bolton-Smith *et al.*, 1993	Scotland	10,359 men & women aged 40–59 years
MRC Epidemiology Unit, 1991 & Sweetnam, personal communication, 1996	Caerphilly, S. Wales	5 & 10 year follow-up of 2512 men aged 45–59 years
Fehily *et al.*, 1992	Mid Glamorgan	371 men & women aged 20–23 years
Knight *et al.*, 1992 & Smith *et al.*, 1993	Bradford, W. Yorkshire	266 male textile workers aged 20–65 years
Scottish Office Home & Health Dept., 1993	Scotland	men & women aged 40–75 years 3 year follow-up of boys & girls aged 15 years
Cox, 1993	Great Britain	7 year follow-up of 9003 men & women aged $\geq$ 18 years
White *et al.*, 1993	England	3242 men & women aged $\geq$ 16 years
Breeze *et al.*, 1994	England	4018 men & women aged $\geq$ 16 years
Bennett *et al.*, 1995	England	16,569 men & women aged $\geq$ 16 years
Colhoun & Prescott-Clarke, 1996	England	15,809 men & women aged $\geq$ 16 years
Chaturvedi *et al.*, 1996	London, England	277 male & female diabetics
Children:		
Dept. Health & Social Security, 1975	Great Britain	1881 boys & girls aged 6 months–$4\frac{1}{2}$ years
Fox *et al.*, 1981	England	cross-sectional: 4045 boys and girls aged 2–4 years longitudinal: 4206 boys and girls from birth to 5 years
Holland *et al.*, 1981	England & Scotland	5 year follow-up of 19,300 boys and girls aged 5–11 years
Dept. Health, 1989	Great Britain	2697 boys & girls aged 10/11 years and 14/15 years
Adamson *et al.*, 1992	Northumbria, England	379 boys & girls aged 11–12 years
Gregory *et al.*, 1995	Great Britain	2101 children aged $1\frac{1}{2}$ years
Hughes *et al.*, 1997	England & Scotland	annual/biennial surveys: approximately 9000 boys & girls aged 5–10 years from 1974–1994

Subjects are community samples unless otherwise stated.

4.1 Age

4.1.1 Cross-sectional studies

In the *Health Survey for England 1996* (Prescott-Clarke & Primatesta, 1998), BMI was found to increase with age in both men and women up to 64 years of age, and to decrease slightly in older age groups (Fig. 4.1). The mean BMI of the age group

55–64 years was 27.6 in men and 27.7 in women; this compared to a BMI of 23.4 in men and 23.5 in women, in the age group 16–24 years. This trend of increasing BMI from young adulthood through to middle age, with a decrease among elderly people, has also been observed in many previous cross-sectional surveys of wide age-range population samples conducted in the UK.

Trends in waist–hip ratio (WHR) with age have

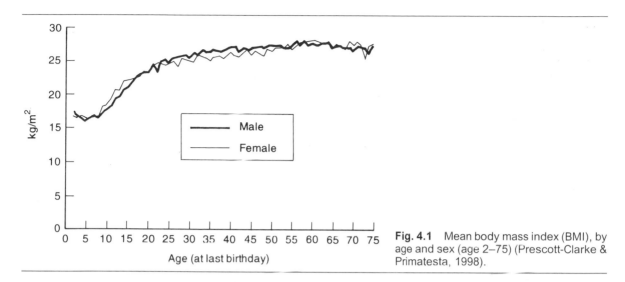

Fig. 4.1 Mean body mass index (BMI), by age and sex (age 2–75) (Prescott-Clarke & Primatesta, 1998).

only been reported in a few recent studies, but these were similar to trends in BMI. WHR was not recorded in the *Health Survey for England 1996* (Prescott-Clarke & Primatesta, 1998). However, in the *Health Survey for England 1994* (Colhoun & Prescott-Clarke, 1996) which did record WHR, although there was a slight decline in the mean WHR in the oldest age group (75 years and over) in men, this was not the case for women (Fig. 4.2).

Those aged 65–74 years had a mean WHR which was higher by about 11% (0.118 in men and 0.082 in women) than that for those aged 16–24 years. Trends in obesity with age during childhood and adolescence are discussed in Sections 7.3 and 7.4.

The interpretation of data from cross-sectional surveys presents a number of difficulties. For example, are the observed trends with age simply an indication that people born in successive periods

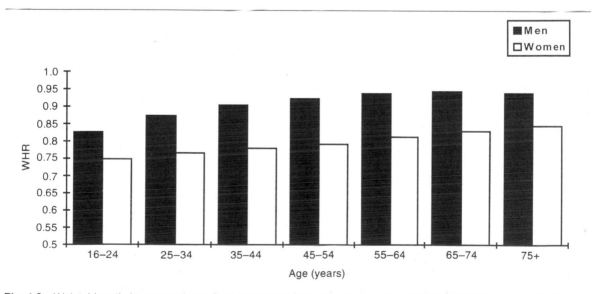

Fig. 4.2 Waist–hip ratio by age and sex. Standard error of the mean ranges from 0.001 to 0.003 (data from: Colhoun & Prescott-Clarke, 1996.

are heavier as adults (a cohort effect)? Is the higher BMI in middle age caused by the reduction in height that occurs with advancing age? Is the reduction in mean BMI among elderly people simply an indication that many of the fatter individuals have died? Data from longitudinal studies are needed to answer these questions.

4.1.2 Longitudinal studies

There have been few longitudinal community studies in the UK, particularly of children and young adults. Braddon *et al.* (1986) reported a 36-year follow-up of all babies born in Great Britain during one week in 1946. The subjects in this study experienced food rationing during their first eight years of life. The prevalence of obesity varied with age, it rose during childhood, reaching a peak at age 11 years. Prevalence then fell until age 20 years but subsequently rose to a much higher level at age 36 years. When re-surveyed at age 43 years, the prevalence of obesity was higher than at age 36 years (M. Wadsworth, personal communication 1997). At age 36 years, 3.4% of men and 4.8% of women had a BMI of more than 30; at age 43 years the proportions had increased to 9.3% and 12.5% respectively.

Longitudinal data for boys and girls from Scotland, initially aged 15 years, showed that the prevalence of obesity increased over a 3-year follow-up, from 0.9%–2.1% in boys and from 1.6–5.7% in girls (Scottish Office Home & Health Department, 1993).

Data from the Caerphilly Prospective Study, concerning men initially aged 45–59 years, are presented in Table 4.2 (MRC Epidemiology Unit, 1991; P. Sweetnam, personal communication 1996). These data show that, in each of the three age groups, BMI increased over the 10-year follow-up. Height was measured once only, when each man was first seen. Thus, the longitudinal increase in BMI with age must be due to increasing weight, and not decreasing height. One other possibility is that the changes in mean BMI may be caused by selective mortality (e.g. the thinnest people having died). However, this is unlikely since the mean baseline BMIs of those who died during the follow-up and those who survived are very similar (P. Sweetnam, personal communication 1996). The data in Table 4.2 also show evidence of a secular trend. For example, men aged 55–59 years in 1989–1993 had a mean BMI that was greater by 1, compared with the mean BMI of men aged 55–59 years in 1979–1983. Secular trends are discussed in detail in Section 4.8. Two other longitudinal studies have also shown an increase in weight in young and middle-aged adults (Wannamethee & Shaper, 1990; Cox, 1993).

In a study of elderly men and women, Burr *et al.* (1982b) reported loss of weight in both sexes over an 8-year follow-up (Table 4.3). Mean weight loss was least in the youngest age group (those originally aged 65–69 years), being only 1.4 kg. In other age groups, mean weight loss ranged from 2.3 kg–9.8 kg. The survivors had fairly similar weights, and showed similar rates of decline to those that would be anticipated from cross-sectional data. Among

Table 4.2 BMI by age and phase in the Caerphilly prospective study (data provided by Mr Peter Sweetnam, MRC Epidemiology Unit (South Wales).

Age (years)	Phase I: N	1979–83 Mean (SD)	Phase II: N	1984–88 Mean (SD)	Phase III: N	1989–93 Mean (SD)
45–49	815	26.19 (3.56)	–	–	–	–
50–54	795	26.32 (3.67)	828	26.53 (3.64)	–	–
55–59	860	25.99 (3.66)	753	26.55 (3.65)	703	26.96 (3.80)
60–64	–	–	786	26.23 (3.65)	632	26.83 (3.63)
65–69	–	–	–	–	609	26.47 (3.73)
All	2470	26.16 (3.63)	2362	26.44 (3.65)	1944	26.76 (3.33)

Phase I: all men aged 45–59 years within a defined geographical area.
Phase II: survivors from phase I plus 447 men of the same age range who had moved into the area.
Phase III: survivors from phase II.

Table 4.3 Changes in weight (kg) after 8 years in elderly men and women (reproduced with permission from: Burr *et al.*, 1982b).

Original age group (years)	Men		Women	
	N	Mean change (SD)	N	Mean change (SD)
65–69	21	–1.39 (6.28)	30	–1.35 (6.67)
70–74	15	–3.35 (5.61)	19	–2.31 (8.27)
75–79	26	–3.25 (6.25)	76	–4.69 (7.69)
80–84	5	–9.80 (8.84)	22	–4.20 (7.09)
85 +	0	–	6	4.20 (4.55)

those aged 70 years and over at baseline, those who died during the follow-up tended to have a lower initial BMI than those who survived. This was true even after excluding deaths occurring during the first year of follow-up. Thus, the decline in body weight among elderly people appears to be related to a loss of weight by individuals rather than to any survival advantages of less obese people.

Thus, data available from longitudinal studies support the findings of cross-sectional surveys, indicating that the trend in BMI with age is not a cohort effect.

4.2 Gender

In the *Health Survey for England 1996*, among those aged 16–64, mean BMI for men was 26.2 and for women it was 25.8. Other surveys of adults have also shown that mean BMI is not substantially different in men and women. Similarly, surveys of children have found little difference in mean BMI between boys and girls (Department of Health, 1989; Adamson *et al.*, 1992).

Despite the fact that mean BMI is similar in males and females, the proportion classified as obese has been consistently reported to be greater for women. However, in the *Health Survey for England 1996* (Prescott-Clarke & Primatesta), the difference between men and women is less than in previous surveys: 16% of men and 17% of women aged 16–64 had a BMI >30 (although overall, 16% of men and 18% of women had a BMI >30). In the *Health Survey for England 1994*, mean WHR was higher in men than in women, 0.902 in men and 0.791 in women. This was true for all age groups (Fig. 4.2).

4.3 Social class and education

4.3.1 Social class

In the UK, the relationship between BMI and social class varies with sex. In women, BMI has typically been reported to be higher in manual classes than in non-manual classes. However, in men the relationship is less consistent between studies (Table 4.4). In the Whitehall study of male civil servants, mean BMI was highest in the lowest employment grade (Rose & Marmot, 1981). In the Whitehall II study, which surveyed both men and women, there was also an inverse association between BMI and job status but, especially in men, the differences were small (Marmot *et al.*, 1991).

In the *Health Survey for England 1996*, the prevalence of obesity in men, and of being overweight in women, tended to be higher in manual (IIIM, IV, V) than non-manual (I, II, IIINM) social classes. The situation was reversed for prevalence of overweight in men. There was a clear social class gradient for obesity in women, with those in the manual classes almost twice as likely to be obese, compared with those in the non-manual classes. The presence of a desirable BMI (20–25) in women increased from social class V and IV to I, but there was no clear pattern in BMI in men (Fig. 4.5). In the Department of Health survey *The Diets of British Schoolchildren*, there was no correlation between BMI and social class (Department of Health, 1989).

In the *MRC National Survey of Health and Development* (1946 birth cohort), Braddon *et al.* (1986) reported a higher prevalence of obesity among manual classes than among non-manual classes, for both men and women, when the cohort

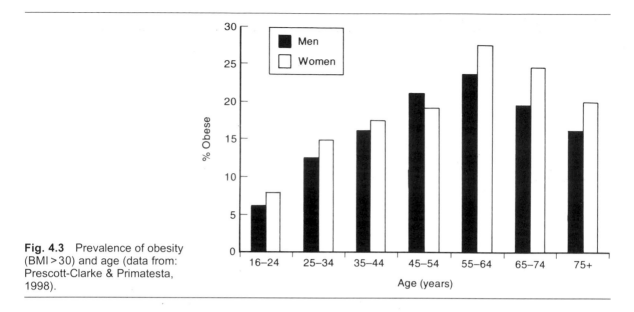

Fig. 4.3 Prevalence of obesity (BMI > 30) and age (data from: Prescott-Clarke & Primatesta, 1998).

was aged 36 years. Data at age 43 years also showed evidence of increasing prevalence of obesity with decreasing social class, the association being more marked among women than among men (M. Wadsworth, personal communication 1997). Of the women in social classes I and II, 9.4% were obese compared with 19.7% in social classes IV and V. For men, the proportions were 8.6% and 10%,

respectively. In both the Whitehall and Whitehall II studies, obesity was more prevalent in those with lower status jobs, especially in the clerical grade.

In the *Health Survey for England 1994*, social class was significantly associated with WHR in both sexes, when adjustments were made for age. Among men, WHR increased from social class I to IIIM and then remained fairly constant in social

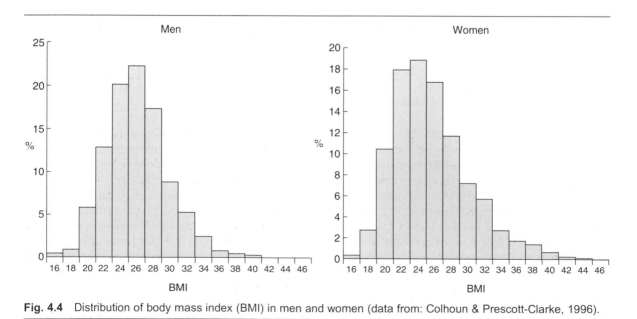

Fig. 4.4 Distribution of body mass index (BMI) in men and women (data from: Colhoun & Prescott-Clarke, 1996).

Table 4.4   Mean BMI and social class.

Study	I	II	IIINM	IIIM	IV	V
			Social Class			
Men:						
Bingham *et al.*, 1981			NM: 24.6	M: 25.4		
Fehily *et al.*, 1984	26.0	25.6	26.2	25.8	26.5	28.2
Braddon *et al.*, 1986 & Wadsworth, personal communication, 1997:						
Cohort at age 36 years	23.8	24.3	24.5	24.9	24.4	25.2
Cohort at age 43 years	24.8	25.3	25.5	25.7	25.2	25.6
Cox *et al.*, 1987			NM: 24.8	M: 24.8		
Fulton *et al.*, 1988:						
Non-smokers			25.5	26.1		
Smokers			25.7	25.8		
Barker *et al.*, 1989			25.4	24.9		
Gregory *et al.*, 1990	I & II: 24.7		25.1	25.2	IV & V: 24.8	
Bolton-Smith *et al.*, 1991	25.3	26.0	26.1	26.3	26.1	26.0
Colhoun & Prescott-Clarke, 1996	25.8	26.1	26.1	26.3	25.8	25.8
Women:						
Braddon *et al.*, 1986 & Wadsworth, personal communication, 1997:						
Cohort at age 36 years	23.1	22.6	22.9	23.8	24.5	25.3
Cohort at age 43 years	24.7	24.1	24.6	25.3	26.2	26.3
Cox *et al.*, 1987			NM: 23.8	M: 24.8		
Barker *et al.*, 1989			23.9	25.7		
Gregory *et al.*, 1990	I & II: 23.8		24.5	24.9	IV & V: 25.8	
Bolton-Smith *et al.*, 1991	24.2	24.9	25.3	26.0	26.3	27.0
Colhoun & Prescott-Clarke, 1996	24.8	25.4	25.5	26.1	26.5	26.7

NM = Non-manual; M = Manual

classes IV and V. Men in social class IIIM had a mean WHR that was 0.016 higher, than those in social class I, when adjustment was made for age. Among women, WHR increased steadily from social class I to V, with those in social class V having a mean WHR that was 0.027 higher, than those in social class I, adjusted for age. When the association between WHR and social class was adjusted for BMI in addition to age, the magnitude of the association was reduced, particularly in women, but remained statistically significant. When further adjusted for other potential confounders (smoking, alcohol consumption and physical activity), the estimated differences between social classes were not reduced. Therefore, these variables did not explain the social class differentials in WHR.

In the *MRC National Survey of Health and Development*, the relationship between social mobility (change in social class from childhood through to adulthood) and obesity was investigated (Braddon *et al.*, 1986). A change in social class in adult life, relative to that of their parents, was important in women but not in men. In employed women, the prevalence of obesity at 36 years of age, was significantly lower in those who moved from manual classes in childhood to non-manual classes

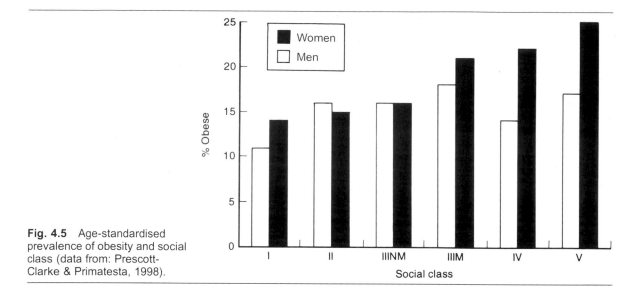

Fig. 4.5 Age-standardised prevalence of obesity and social class (data from: Prescott-Clarke & Primatesta, 1998).

in adulthood compared with those women who remained in manual classes. Data for the cohort at age 43 years showed a similar pattern (Table 4.5): 20.5% of women who remained in manual classes were obese compared with only 11.2% of those who moved from manual to non-manual classes. Thus, women who changed social class tended to show the prevalence of obesity of the class they joined.

4.3.2 Education

Few studies have investigated relationships between educational attainment and BMI. In the *Health Survey for England 1994*, a significant inverse association was reported for women, but not for men, after adjustment for age. Among

women with no formal qualifications, BMI was on average higher by 1.3 (5%) than among those with A-levels or higher qualifications. WHR was higher among both men and women with no formal qualifications, than among those with A-levels or higher qualifications, by 0.02 (2–3%), after adjustment for age.

In the *MRC National Survey of Health and Development*, BMI was significantly associated with educational achievement, in both men and women, when the cohort was surveyed at age 36 years (Braddon *et al.*, 1986), and again at age 43 years (M. Wadsworth, personal communication 1997). The highest prevalence of obesity was found in the least qualified. At age 43 years, 11% of men with qualifications up to and including O-levels had a BMI of more than 30, compared with only 5% of men with a degree qualification. Among women, these proportions were 15% and 4% respectively.

4.4 Smoking

Smoking is more common in manual classes than in non-manual classes. Therefore, smokers might be expected to be heavier than non-smokers. However, a number of studies have shown that cigarette smokers weigh less than non-smokers and are less likely to be overweight than non-smokers (Khosla & Lowe, 1971, 1972; Fehily *et al.*, 1984; Cox *et al.*, 1987; Bolton-Smith *et al.*, 1993; Colhoun & Pre-

Table 4.5 Social mobility* and prevalence of obesity. MRC National Survey of Health & Development, 1946 birth cohort at age 43 years (data provided by Dr Michael Wadsworth, University College London Medical School).

Social mobility	Men (%)	Women (%)
Always Non-Manual	6.9	6.1
Falling	7.6	10.3
Always Manual	10.1	20.5
Rising	12.2	11.2

* 'Social Mobility' comprises a comparison of father's social class when the cohort member was aged 15 years with the cohort member's own social class at age 43 years.

scott-Clarke, 1996). Others have reported a lower BMI and skinfold thickness among smokers only in social classes IV and V (Ashwell *et al.*, 1978), a lower BMI among male smokers but not female smokers (Gregory *et al.*, 1990), or no difference in the mean BMI and skinfold thickness measurements of smokers compared with non-smokers (Fulton *et al.*, 1988; Barker *et al.*, 1989).

Data from the *Health Survey for England 1994* are presented in Fig. 4.6 (unadjusted for confounding factors). In a multiple regression analysis that adjusted for age, alcohol consumption and physical activity, both male and female smokers had a lower mean BMI than never-smokers (by 1–4%). Figure 4.6 shows that the lowest BMI was found in moderate cigarette smokers. This is consistent with data from previous studies (Khosla & Lowe, 1971; Fehily *et al.*, 1984). The reason for the lowest BMI in moderate smokers is not clear.

Ex-smokers have been found to have a higher BMI than current smokers, by 2–6% (Ashwell *et al.*, 1978; Fehily *et al.*, 1984; Cox *et al.*, 1987; Barker *et al.*, 1989; Bolton-Smith *et al.*, 1993; Colhoun & Prescott-Clarke, 1996). Compared with never-smokers, the BMI of ex-smokers was reported to be similar (Fehily *et al.*, 1984) or slightly higher (Ashwell *et al.*, 1978; Barker *et al.*, 1989; Colhoun & Prescott-Clarke, 1996). Bolton-Smith *et al.* (1993) reported that BMI tended to increase with duration of ex-smoking. Data from these cross-sectional studies are consistent with data from longitudinal studies, showing weight gain following smoking cessation (Gordon *et al.*, 1975; Blitzer *et al.*, 1977; Williamson *et al.*, 1991). The amount of weight gained following cessation of smoking has been reported to vary with gender and race. A longitudinal study by Williamson *et al.* (1991), showed that the amount of weight gained was greater in women than in men and that black people who gave up smoking were more likely to gain weight than white people.

Data on WHR suggest that smokers, despite being leaner than non-smokers, have more central obesity than non-smokers (Colhoun & Prescott-Clarke, 1996). The higher WHR among smokers was found to be dose-dependent, being greatest in those smoking 20 or more cigarettes per day, and was independent of BMI. The magnitude of the difference was greater in women than in men. Among women who smoked 20 or more cigarettes per day, mean WHR was 0.026 (3%) higher than in

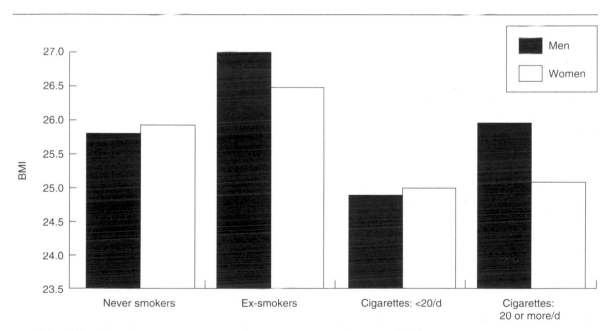

Fig. 4.6 BMI and smoking habit (data from: Colhoun & Prescott-Clarke, 1996). Standard error of the mean ranges from 0.09 to 0.25.

never-smokers. In both sexes, ex-smokers also had a higher mean WHR compared with never-smokers, but only by about 1% (0.005 for men and 0.006 for women).

4.5 Region

The *Health Survey for England 1996* showed no clear regional variation in the prevalence of overweight and obesity. Among men, the lowest prevalence of overweight was in West Midlands (39%) and the highest was in North Thames and Northern & Yorkshire (45%). In contrast, for women the prevalence of being overweight was highest in West Midlands (36%) and lowest in North Thames (31%). The level of obesity in men ranged from 13% in North Thames to 18% in Trent and West Midlands. In women, the level of obesity ranged from 17% in North and South Thames to 20% in Trent (Fig. 4.7).

In the *British Regional Heart Study* (Shaper *et al.*, 1981), a survey of men aged 40 to 59 years in 24 towns, the lowest BMI was reported for Guildford (Surrey). However, other towns in the south did not have lower BMIs than those in the midlands and north. In the *Dietary and Nutritional Survey of British Adults* (Gregory *et al.*, 1990), Scottish men and women were found to be shorter, on average, and had a lower mean BMI than people in other parts of Great Britain. In Northern Ireland (Barker *et al.*, 1989), mean BMIs for men and for women were identical to those reported for British adults. A survey comparing middle-aged men in Speedwell (Bristol), Caerphilly, Edinburgh and Northern Ireland found that differences in BMI between the four areas were small: 25.7, 26.2, 25.8 and 25.6, respectively (Fehily *et al.*, 1990).

In the *Health Survey for England 1994*, mean WHR among men ranged from 0.896 in North Thames to 0.911 in Trent. Among women, mean WHR ranged from 0.782 in South Thames to 0.795 in Trent. On adjustment for differences in age structure between regions, there was a statistically significant association between WHR and region in both men and women. In general, WHR tended to be higher in the regions in the north, than in the regions in the south, in both sexes.

4.6 Ethnic group

There have been few studies of relationships between obesity and ethnic group in the UK. In a study comparing European, Indian and West Indian (predominantly African descent) men living in London, Miller *et al.* (1988) found that the mean

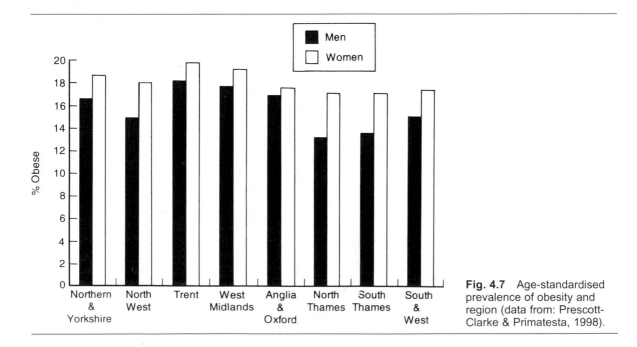

Fig. 4.7 Age-standardised prevalence of obesity and region (data from: Prescott-Clarke & Primatesta, 1998).

BMI of Indian men was similar to that of West Indian men and lower than that of European men (by 1.6). Skinfold thickness, however, was similar in Indians and Europeans, and least in West Indians (by 11mm). Other studies in Britain have reported that the average BMI in Asian men (Bangladeshi, Indian and Pakistani origin) and the mean for African Caribbean men are not significantly different from the mean BMI of European men (McKeigue *et al.*, 1991; Smith *et al.*, 1993). South Asian women have been reported to have a higher mean BMI than European women, by 1.8 (McKeigue *et al.*, 1991). Chaturvedi *et al.* (1996) compared African Caribbean men and women with Europeans, all of whom had NIDDM and were attending diabetic clinics in London. Mean BMI was slightly lower in the African Caribbeans (by 1.2 in men and 0.3 in women), although the difference was not statistically significant. Asian men and women have been reported to have a greater degree of central adiposity than Europeans (McKeigue *et al.*, 1991; Knight *et al.*, 1992).

The mean BMI among middle-aged people from the Indian subcontinent, living in West London, has been reported to be higher than that of their siblings living in India, by 3.9 and 4.7 for men and women, respectively (Bhatnagar *et al.*, 1995). Within India, average BMI has been reported to be lower in rural than in urban populations, by 3 (Snehalatha *et al.*, 1994).

Wilks *et al.* (1996) reported BMI data for black people aged 25–74 years living in Africa, the Caribbean and the USA (Table 4.6). Since these people are from the same genetic stock, any differences in obesity prevalence are likely to be related to environmental influences. Among both men and women, mean BMI was lowest in Nigeria and highest in the USA (by 5.4 for men and 8.2 for women). BMI was slightly higher in urban Cameroon, than rural Cameroon (by 2 for men and 3.5 for women). WHR were, however, similar in all groups.

4.7 Vegetarianism

Many studies have shown that vegetarians have a lower mean BMI than omnivores (Burr *et al.*, 1981; Thorogood *et al.*, 1987; Thorogood, 1995). The reason for the lower BMI is not clear. However, the diet and lifestyle of vegetarians differ in many ways from those of omnivores. Apart from avoiding meat, vegetarians tend to consume more vegetables, fruits and nuts, are more likely to be in non-manual jobs, are less likely to smoke, tend to drink less alcohol, and may also take more exercise.

4.8 Secular trends

Surveys of nationally representative population samples of adults indicate that mean BMI has increased since 1980 (Fig. 4.8). Among both men

Table 4.6 Mean BMI and WHR (sd) among blacks in Africa, the Caribbean and the USA (adapted from Wilkes *et al.*, 1996).

Site	N	BMI	WHR
Men			
Nigeria	1171	21.7 (3.6)	0.88 (0.06)
Cameroon (rural)	745	23.5 (3.1)	0.89 (0.05)
Cameroon (urban)	612	25.1 (3.6)	0.86 (0.06)
Jamaica	340	23.4 (4.0)	0.84 (0.07)
St Lucia	491	24.3 (3.7)	0.87 (0.06)
Barbados	330	25.9 (4.3)	0.88 (0.07)
USA (Maywood, Chicago)	708	27.1 (5.5)	0.89 (0.07)
Women			
Nigeria	1338	22.6 (4.7)	0.79 (0.06)
Cameroon (rural)	722	23.5 (4.3)	0.87 (0.06)
Cameroon (urban)	749	27.0 (4.7)	0.81 (0.07)
Jamaica	480	27.8 (6.5)	0.80 (0.07)
St Lucia	598	27.3 (6.2)	0.82 (0.07)
Barbados	483	29.4 (6.4)	0.82 (0.07)
USA (Maywood, Chicago)	810	30.8 (7.7)	0.82 (0.08)

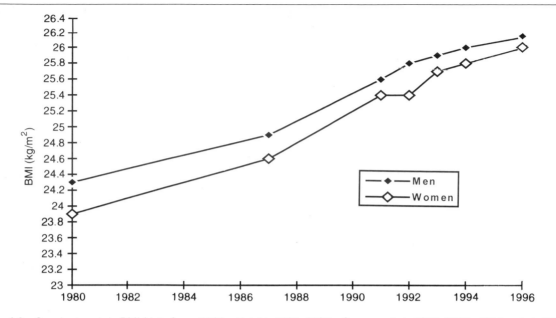

Fig. 4.8 Secular trends in BMI (data from: 1980 – Knight, 1984; 1987 – Gregory *et al.*, 1990; 1991 – White *et al.*, 1993; 1992 – Breeze *et al.*, 1994; 1993 – Bennett *et al.*, 1995; 1994 – Colhoun & Prescott-Clarke, 1996; 1996 – Prescott-Clarke & Primatesta, 1998).

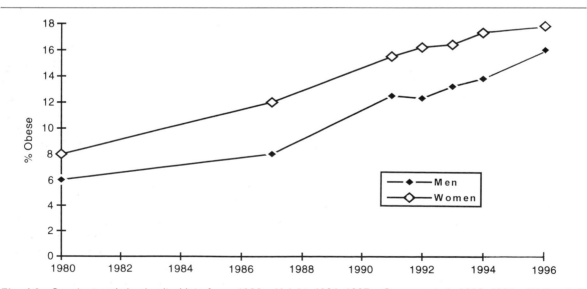

Fig. 4.9 Secular trends in obesity (data from: 1980 – Knight, 1984; 1987 – Gregory *et al.*, 1990; 1991 – White *et al.*, 1993; 1992 – Breeze *et al.*, 1994; 1993 – Bennett *et al.*, 1995; 1994 – Colhoun & Prescott-Clarke, 1996; 1996 – Prescott-Clarke & Primatesta, 1998).

and women, mean BMI increased by 1.9 between 1980 and 1996. There do not appear to have been comparable surveys of adults prior to 1980 and thus it is difficult to assess trends in BMI before that date.

Data also indicate that the prevalence of obesity is increasing (Fig. 4.9). In 1980, 6% of men and 8% of women were reported to be obese (Knight, 1984). This compares with data from the *Health Survey for England 1996,* showing that 16% of men and 18% of women were obese. The prevalence of obesity has, therefore, more than doubled in only 16 years.

During the period from 1993–1996, mean BMI and the prevalence of obesity increased for most age groups and for both sexes each year. BMI increased by about 0.4 in men and 0.3 in women during this 4-year period. There was more of an increase in the prevalence of obesity in men than in women between 1993 and 1996. Overall, prevalence of obesity increased by 3.2% in men, compared to 2.0% in women. This increase was greater in men aged 45 years and over and in women aged 25–34, and 55 and over, than those in other age groups.

There have been very few surveys of obesity among children that enable secular trends to be ascertained for this age group. Hughes *et al.* (1997) reported trends in growth in England and Scotland between 1972 and 1994, for children aged 5–10 years. Over this period, triceps skinfold measurement increased by almost 8% in 7-year-old English boys and by 7% in 7-year-old English girls. In Scotland, triceps skinfold measurement increased by nearly 10% in 7-year-old boys, and by 11% in 7-year-old girls. Weight for height index showed a similar trend. Adamson *et al.* (1992) compared children in Northumbria aged 11–12 years, surveyed in 1990 with those surveyed in 1980. Mean BMI was reported to have increased by 0.41 in boys and by 0.30 in girls over the 10-year period. In 1990, 4% of children had a BMI of 25 or more, compared with only 2% in 1980. Thus, the prevalence of obesity appears to be increasing in children, as well as in adults.

The UK is not alone in showing an increase in the prevalence of obesity. It has also increased in many other countries, for example, the USA (Kuczmarski

et al., 1994), Germany (Hoffmeister *et al.,* 1994), Sweden (Kuskowska-Wolka & Bergstrom, 1993a, b) and Denmark (Sorensen & Price, 1990) (Table 4.7). It is also increasing in countries that currently have a low prevalence, e.g. China and Japan.

4.9 Summary

- BMI increases with age in both men and women, up to about 64 years and then decreases slightly in older age groups.

- Mean BMI of women is similar to that of men, but the prevalence of obesity is slightly greater in women.

- In the UK, the relationship between BMI and social class varies with gender. In women, BMI has typically been reported to be higher in manual classes than in non-manual classes. However, in men the relationship is less consistent between studies. An inverse association has been reported between BMI and educational attainment, and this relationship is also more marked among women than among men.

- Cigarette smokers tend to have a lower BMI than non-smokers, but they have a greater degree of central adiposity than non-smokers. Ex-smokers tend to be heavier than current smokers.

- Regional variations in BMI are small.

- Mean BMI of Asian men in Britain is not significantly different from that of European men, although Asians have a greater degree of central adiposity. Mean BMI of African Caribbean men and women is slightly lower than that of European men and women, but the difference is not statistically significant.

- Vegetarians have a lower mean BMI than omnivores, but the reason for this is unclear.

- The prevalence of obesity is increasing in the UK and in many other countries. Between 1980 and 1996, the prevalence of obesity has more than doubled in the UK over the past 16 years, increasing from 6–16% in men and from 8–18% in women.

Obesity

Table 4.7 Recent trends in obesity prevalence in some European countries and the United States (from: Seidell, 1997).

Country	Obesity definition (BMI cut-off point)	Year	Ages	Men %	Women %
England	30	1980	16–64	6.0	8.0
		1986/7		7.0	12.0
		1991		13.0	15.0
		1993		13.0	16.0
Sweden	men: 30	1980/1	16–84	4.9	8.7
	women: 28.6	1988/9		5.3	9.1
Finland	30	1978/9	20–75	10.0	10.0
		1985/7		12.0	10.0
		1991/3		14.0	11.0
Germany	30	1985	25–69	15.1	16.5
		1988		14.7	17.2
		1990		17.2	19.3
East Germany	30	1985	25–65	13.7	22.2
		1989		13.4	20.6
		1992		20.5	26.6
Netherlands	30	1987	20–59	6.0	8.5
		1988		6.3	7.6
		1989		6.2	7.4
		1990		7.4	9.0
		1991		7.5	8.8
		1992		7.5	9.3
		1993		7.1	9.1
		1994		8.8	9.4
		1995		8.4	8.3
United States	30	1960	20–74	10.0	15.0
		1973		11.6	16.1
		1978		12.0	14.8
		1991		19.7	24.7

5
Aetiology of Obesity I: Introduction

Obesity is a complex syndrome with multifactorial origins. Its aetiology can range from the purely molecular (e.g. Prader–Willi and other obesity syndromes) to the purely behavioural (e.g. Sumo wrestlers). Most cases of obesity probably cluster towards the middle of this spectrum and can best be described as the outcome of an adverse 'obesogenic' environment, working on a susceptible genotype. The genetic susceptibility can potentially be mediated through defects in numerous different homeostatic mechanisms, ranging from the metabolic (e.g. control of fuel selection and disposal) to the psychological (e.g. Binge Eating Disorder). The environmental factors range from macro-environmental influences on food supply and lifestyle to micro-environmental effects of individual behaviour choices. This diversity of aetiological factors makes obesity one of the most complex and challenging of all chronic diseases. Chapters 5–15 attempt to summarise current knowledge on the causes of obesity. Although the shorthand term 'obesity' will be used throughout the chapters on aetiology, it is important to bear in mind that there are many different types of obesity with sometimes distinct and overlapping aetiologies.

5.1 The energy balance equation

One of the few statements about obesity that can be made with absolute certainty is that obesity can only occur when energy intake remains higher than energy expenditure, for an extended period of time. This is usually stated as a chronic displacement of the energy balance equation:

Energy intake – Energy expenditure
= Change in body energy stores

This is the incontrovertible foundation stone upon which any theories of obesity must be built. All putative mechanisms must ultimately act through increasing energy intake, decreasing energy expenditure, or both. Where changes in intake, or expenditure, are imposed by external environmental pressure, then individual susceptibility may be attributable to a failure in the normal homeostatic controls that regulate the above equation.

5.2 Hyperplastic versus hypertrophic obesity

Normal adults possess about 5×10^{10} mature fat cells (adipocytes) (Section 3.4). Changes in fat balance are usually accommodated through expansion (hypertrophy) or contraction of the existing quota of fat cells. This is a readily reversible process that is in a constant state of flux from meal to meal and from periods of relative excess to periods of shortage. The rate of flux of triacylglycerol across the fat cell membrane and the net balance are regulated by the relative activities of capillary lipoprotein lipase (LPL), which sequesters fat from the blood stream, and hormone-sensitive lipase, which liberates free fatty acids from stored fat. The process is under a complex series of minute-by-minute (activation/inhibition) and longer-term (transcriptional) controls, which are influenced primarily by insulin and catecholamines with broader modulation by cortisol and sex hormones, among others (Newsholme & Leech,

1983). Within the body, there are regional differences in the hormone sensitivity of fat cells leading to the suggestion that different depots have specific functions. For instance, the femoral and gluteal deposits in women are believed to serve a specific role in subsidising lactation (Rebuffé-Scrive *et al.*, 1985, 1987).

The size of fat depots is also influenced by the number of fat cells present (Section 3.4). Early work in this field suggested that a person's quota of fat cells was established in infancy and remained virtually immutable thereafter, leading to suggestions that obesity was programmed in early infancy (Section 7.2.6). It is now known that this is not the case and that fat cell number increases (hyperplasia) when the existing fat cells are full. The exact mechanisms controlling the formation and transformation of pre-adipocytes and their commitment to becoming mature adipocytes are still under investigation, but are known to involve a nuclear receptor PPARγ2, which is activated by prostaglandins and free fatty acids (Prins & O'Rahilly, 1997). This raises the possibility that hyperplasia might be induced by factors other than the state of fullness of existing adipocytes. These might include certain dietary components or drugs, and it is already known that glucose-sensitising agents (thiazolidinediones) act as a powerful *in vitro* ligand for PPARγ2 and might, therefore, stimulate hyperplasia *in vivo* (Prins & O'Rahilly, 1997).

Although it is difficult to accurately measure changes in fat cell number in very overweight people, it is generally believed that once new fat cells are formed they remain for many years. In fact, it has recently been demonstrated that adipocytes are capable of apoptosis, i.e. programmed cell death (Prins & O'Rahilly, 1997), but the significance of this finding in terms of the possible regression of fat cell number has yet to be clarified.

The anatomical purpose of adipocytes is to contain fat and it is, therefore, possible that a large number of fat cells in a depot may predispose an individual to easy fat gain and obesity. This suggests one possible mechanism to explain the high incidence of post-weight-loss relapse and the refractoriness of extreme obesity. It also emphasises the need to control the early stages of weight gain, in order to avoid the ratchet effect created by the (irreversible) creation of new adipocytes.

Careful consideration of the hypertrophic and hyperplastic aspects of obesity reveals important lessons for our understanding of energy balance in general. It is clear that fat depots exert a considerable autonomy in the control of their own size. This could be mediated by many factors, such as different levels of expression of LPL (sometimes described as the 'gating enzyme'), different regional sensitivity of hormone sensitive lipase, different levels of vascularisation, perhaps different expression of leptin, or different fat cell numbers (Section 6.5). These variations are, at least partly, under genetic control (Chapter 6) and may manifest as quite pronounced pathologies. In this respect the gross disparity between upper body wasting and lower body obesity in severe cases of lipodystrophy remind us of the importance of the self-determination of fat depot size. We cannot reasonably describe the phenomenon in terms of a differential state of energy balance in two regions of the same body; an observation of considerable significance when reviewing energy balance (Chapter 8).

5.3 Summary

- Obesity is a complex syndrome with multifactorial origins.

- Obesity arises as the outcome of an adverse environment working on a susceptible genotype. Susceptibility may be mediated through a wide range of metabolic and behavioural traits.

- Obesity can only occur when energy intake remains higher than energy expenditure, for an extended period of time. This is an incontrovertible cornerstone on which all explanations must be based.

- Early stages of fat storage involve expansion of existing adipocytes (hypertrophy). Later stages involve the recruitment of new adipocytes (hyperplasia). Current evidence suggests that hyperplasia is difficult to reverse once it has occurred, thus emphasising the need for preventive strategies.

6
Aetiology of Obesity II: Genetics

6.1 Overview

Obesity cannot be regarded as a single disorder, but as a group of heterogeneous disorders. The obesity phenotype is a multifactorial trait determined by genetic and non-genetic affectors. The regional distribution of fat is a reflection of this heterogeneity. It has become obvious that the obese genotype is not of the simple Mendelian kind. The segregation of genes is not easily distinguished and the influence of the genotype on aetiology is generally attenuated, or exacerbated, by non-genetic factors. Thus, the variation in body fat may be attributable to a complex inter-working of genetic, nutritional, energy expenditure, psychological and social variables. In such a complex situation, the study of the genetics of the trait must rely primarily on data from relatives by descent, or adoption.

6.2 Estimates of heritability

Heritability is the proportion of the total variation of a character that is attributable to genetic, as opposed to environmental, factors. Most studies have used BMI as an indicator of fatness. It must be recognised that the set of genes and environmental factors, which influence the general degree of obesity, may be different from those influencing various aspects of the regional distribution of fat.

Several large-scale family studies, in different ethnic populations, have shown a familial correlation in the degree of obesity, with a parent to offspring correlation of about 0.2 and a correlation around 0.25 for brothers or sisters (siblings) of the same gender (Bouchard & Perusse 1988; Friedlander *et al.*, 1988). Statistical modelling of such

data suggests that about half of the phenotypic variance is explained by the non-shared environmental influences (Tambe *et al.*, 1991). The fundamental weaknesses of using family studies to assess the genetic effects are the confounding influences of genes and the environment. This problem is addressed by studies of twins living together and twins living apart.

6.2.1 Twin studies

The assessment of genetic effects in twin studies is based on the difference in resemblance of monozygotic and dizygotic pairs, which share all the genes or, on average, half the genes respectively (Stunkard *et al.*, 1990). Such studies show a much higher correlation of the obesity measures among the monozygotic pairs, than among the dizygotic pairs, which provides strong evidence for a genetic influence. Genetic influences appear to account for 50–70% of the difference in BMI in later life in both monozygotic and dizygotic twins brought up apart, whereas the childhood environment had little or no influence. Allison *et al.* (1996) have estimated the heritability of BMI for three groups of twins (American, Finnish and Japanese twin pairs) and calculated this to be between 0.50 and 0.70. They concluded that 50% of the total variance found in BMI resulted from genetic factors if other influences were excluded, while 70% of the variance in BMI, not accounted for by these other factors, was owing to genetic variation.

6.2.2 Adoption studies

The use of adoption studies, to assess the genetic

influences, is based on the assumption that genetic effects are fully expressed in individuals adopted away from the biological family early in life, to a genetically unrelated family, and that there are no effects on the adoptee of the biological family's environment. Such studies show a strong relationship between the BMI of the biological parents and adoptee, for the whole range of body fatness (from very thin to very fat). No relationship is shown, however, between the adoptive parents and the adoptee, in relation to a body weight class (Stunkard *et al.,* 1986, 1990; Sorensen *et al.,* 1989).

6.2.3 Heritability of body fat

A study of families living in Quebec, in Canada, has provided useful information about the inheritance of the distribution of fat in particular regions of the body (Borecki *et al.,* 1995). Measures of fat mass and percentage body fat (using underwater weighing) suggest that there is a significant familial influence on the pattern of fat distribution, and that adjusting for total body fat results in an increase in this familiality. Estimates of the familial influence vary, from between 18–50%. This implies that for a given level of fatness, some individuals store more fat on the trunk or abdominal area, while others store primarily in the lower body. Nevertheless, evidence suggests that several genes, in combination with environmental factors, determine the phenotype of total body fatness.

6.3 Type of gene effects

An important concept, in relation to genetic influences in obesity, is that of susceptibility genes. A susceptibility gene is defined as one that increases susceptibility, or risk, for the disease but is not necessary for disease expression. An allele at a susceptibility gene may make it more likely that the carrier will become affected (predisposition), but the presence of that allele is not sufficient, by itself, to explain the occurrence of the disease. In other words, possession of such genes does not predestine an individual to become obese, but merely lowers the threshold for the development of the condition.

Obesity appears to be a polygenic disorder, with a non-Mendelian pattern of transmission. The findings from some of the family, twin and adoption studies suggest that a considerable proportion of the genetic variance is a major gene effect. In other words, only a single gene appears to determine obesity, rather than a combination of several genes. This explains the greater correlations between full siblings than between parents and offspring, even though they are assumed to share the same number of genes. It also explains the twofold greater correlation between monozygotic twins, compared to dizygotic twins. Thus, genetic interaction plays a role, both at the same loci, where the effect of some alleles may depend on which allele is present on the counterpart of the locus (dominance), and at different loci. This occurs in such a way that the effects of the alleles at one locus may depend on which alleles are present on another locus (epistasis).

The studies of regional distribution of body fat suggest that between individuals there are two or three different component distributions of fat (commingling analysis) where each component represents sub-populations with different allelic distribution on a locus with a major effect (Rice *et al.,* 1992). Analysis of large family studies suggests the tendency to store fat, as either deep or subcutaneous tissue, may be genetically determined, with both polygenic and major genetic components.

6.4 Environmental effects

The striking increase in the prevalence of obesity in the UK during the past decade confirms just how important the environment is as a determinant of obesity. Similarly, numerous studies cite a worldwide increase in obesity prevalence, with some reporting an apparent corresponding increase in the percentage of fat taken in the diet (Lissner & Heitmann, 1995). However, none of these studies distinguish between increasing incidence and changes in its persistence. Increased persistence may result from continuing exposure to a type of environment associated with obesity, coupled with improved survival. The study by Bouchard *et al.* (1990), of the response of monozygotic twins to enforced positive and negative energy balance over 12 weeks, demonstrates considerable within-pair differences in weight gain and alterations in the amount of visceral fat. This suggests that differences within the twin pairs in the environment they have been exposed to previously may determine their response to predetermined changes in energy intake or output. The nature of such environment influences is unknown. Nevertheless, even greater between-pair differences in response were seen, which are likely to be attributable to genetic differences. These findings underline the importance of considering possible interactions between genes and the environment, and the current poor understanding about such interactions. It would appear that obesity is more likely to occur in those who are genetically predisposed, but are also exposed to particular environment influences. Clinical manifestations of obesity are influenced over the lifetime of a person by a variety of interactions between the genes and the environment. These effects result from the fact that sensitivity to aspects of the environment, or lifestyle differences, vary from individual to individual because of genetic individuality. Few studies have attempted to address this, because of the difficulty in classifying particular genotypes and identifying the specific environmental factors.

6.5 Obesity genes

The search for obesity genes requires a multifaceted approach, involving the following investigative methods:

- the study of animal models and extrapolation to human homologous regions;
- the study of potential candidate genes for obesity;
- the study of human obesity syndromes that are inherited in a Mendelian fashion;
- a genome-wide search using microsatellite markers covering the human genome.

6.5.1 Animal models

Rodent models of obesity, whether produced by lesions of the ventromedial nucleus or homozygous *ob*, *db* and *fa* genes, are all characterised by hyperinsulinaemia and insulin resistance. The *ob* gene has been shown to be positioned on chromosome 6, close to a restriction fragment polymorphism (RFLP) marker (Friedman *et al.*, 1991; Bahary *et al.*, 1993). The gene has been localised to a 650 kb region, and of 6 genes isolated within this region one was found to be exclusively expressed in adipose tissue in normal mice. Northern blots of adipose tissue RNA, from a strain of mutated mice, showed an approximately twentyfold increase in the level of *ob* RNA, which suggests that the gene product is non-functional. Sequence data demonstrated a premature stop codon, which results in the translation of a truncated protein. Direct sequence comparison of mouse and human *ob* genes reveals an 84% overall homology. The derived protein has been named 'leptin', from the Greek word *leptos*, meaning thin (Zhang *et al.*, 1994). The increased level of *ob* RNA, in the *ob/ob* mutant strain of mouse, suggests that this gene may signal the size of the adipose tissue mass. It also implies that leptin may act on the central nervous system (CNS) to inhibit food intake and to regulate energy expenditure. Daily intraperitoneal injections of recombinant leptin, given to mice with a mutation in their *ob* gene, leads to reductions in body weight, percentage body fat, food intake, and serum glucose and insulin (Pelleymounter *et al.*, 1995). Leptin, introduced into the lateral or third ventricle of the brain, is effective at low doses in reducing body weight, indicating a likely central effect (Campfield *et al.*, 1995). A possible explanation for this central action is that leptin reduces the concentration of neuropeptide Y (NPY), a peptide which stimulates food intake (Stephens *et al.*, 1995). In contrast, the administration of leptin to *db/db* mice (diabetic mice which have high levels of circulating leptin protein) has no effect on appetite, body weight, percentage fat or metabolism. This suggests that the mutation in *db/db* mice renders them resistant to leptin, and that the *db* gene codes for the leptin receptor, or some part of the post-receptor pathway. The leptin receptor has now been cloned and, as predicted, is a membrane spanning receptor, which has many features of the class 1 cytokine receptor family (Tartaglia *et al.*, 1995). Recent mapping evidence places the mouse receptor gene on chromosome 4, in the same position as the *db* gene (Chua *et al.*, 1996). Mutations have now been observed in mRNA from *db* mice, which gives rise to a non-functioning receptor protein that probably lacks signalling ability.

6.5.2 Leptin in the human situation

In man, the precise role of leptin remains uncertain; leptin receptors are present in brain, haemopoetic stem cells, early fetal liver and placenta (Cioffi *et al.*, 1996). Recently, two severely obese children from related parents (consanguineous pedigree), have been reported to have very low levels of serum leptin, despite a markedly elevated fat mass. In both children, a homozygous frame-shift mutation was found, involving the deletion of a single guanine nucleotide in codon 133 of the gene for leptin (Montague *et al.*, 1997a). The severe obesity found in these congenitally leptin deficient subjects provides genetic evidence that leptin may contribute to the regulation of energy balance in man. However, the evidence to date about leptin in humans with 'spontaneous' obesity suggests that it is a fat 'messenger', rather than a fat 'controller'. Circulating leptin levels are positively correlated with measures of obesity, including BMI and percentage body fat, and are elevated in obesity (Considine *et al.*, 1995). Serum leptin in women suffering from various forms of eating disorders (anorexia nervosa, bulimia nervosa and non-specific types) are reduced, the level being unrelated to the specific pathology but correlated with the individual's BMI (Ferron *et al.*, 1997). Progressive weight loss in response to a reduced energy intake is accompanied by a decline in circulating leptin levels and adipose tissue mRNA. However, plasma levels rise again, once isocaloric diets are initiated to maintain reduced body weight (Maffei *et al.*, 1995). In addition, the expression of leptin mRNA in adipose tissue, is greater in obese than in lean individuals (Lonnqvist *et al.*, 1995). It has been proposed that human obesity results, as in the *db/db* mouse, from leptin resistance, which becomes more pronounced with progressive degrees of obesity. Caro *et al.* (1996) propose that this leptin resistance results from reduced levels of leptin transport into the cerebrospinal-fluid (CSF).

Recent studies have demonstrated higher expression of leptin mRNA in subcutaneous adipocytes than in intra-abdominal fat stores and that this finding is exaggerated in female subjects (Montague *et al.*, 1997b). A site-specific difference in adipocyte exposure to neural, endocrine or paracrine regulators could be the explanation. This raises questions about the different biological function of subcutaneous and intra-abdominal fat depots, and points to a possible role for leptin in determining regional fat distribution.

6.5.3 Melanocortin receptors

The signalling mechanisms beyond the leptin receptor are as yet poorly understood. The agouti yellow mouse becomes obese in adulthood as a result of decreased adrenergic tone. This is the consequence of antagonism of α-melanocytic stimulating hormone (α-MSH), the role of which is to activate melanocortin receptors (MCR). A study of 289 siblings, from 124 nuclear families in Quebec, has shown a relationship between polymorphisms of the melanocortin receptors: MC4R and MC5R. MC5R appears to be linked to increased BMI, fatness and resting metabolic rate, while MC4R seems to be linked with BMI and fatness. This supports a linkage between these polymorphisms and an obesity phenotype (Chagnon *et al.*, 1997).

6.5.4 Candidate gene approach

A candidate gene is defined as that part of the DNA molecule that directs the synthesis of a specific polypeptide chain closely associated with a particular disease. Several candidate genes have been associated with obesity or its metabolic complications.

β₃-adrenergic receptor

The adrenergic system plays a major part in controlling energy expenditure. β_3-adrenergic receptors are the principal receptor mediating catecholamine-stimulated thermogenesis in brown adipose tissue, but are also abundant in subcutaneous and abdominal white adipose tissue (Emorine *et al.*, 1989; Krief *et al.*, 1993). The β_3-adrenergic receptor molecule crosses the cell membrane seven times, it is coupled to guanine-nucleotide-binding (G) proteins and is localised in adipose tissue. Studies of the white and brown adipose tissue of genetically obese mice and rats have shown decreased expression of β_3-adrenergic receptors, but no change in β_1- or β_2-adrenergic receptors. In humans, reduced β_3-adrenergic activity in visceral fat may enhance lipogenesis and increased fat deposition. A mutation in the β_3-adrenergic receptor gene has been described whereby thymidine is replaced by cytosine at nucleotide position 190. This change causes a tryptophan (TGG) to arginine (CGG) substitution at position 64 (Trp64Arg). The amino acid is situated in the first three intracellular loops of the receptor. Preliminary reports suggest the possibility of Trp64Arg mutation being a candidate for a genetic alteration leading to obesity (Walston *et al.*, 1995; Widén *et al.*, 1995; Clément *et al.*, 1995). However, these results have not been substantiated by more recent studies (Gagnon *et al.*, 1996).

Uncoupling protein genes

The uncoupling proteins (UCPs) operate within the inner mitochondrial membrane as transporters. They dissipate the proton gradient, releasing stored energy as heat. Several UCPs have been identified including UCP1 (expressed in brown fat), UCP2 (widely expressed) and UCP3 (mainly expressed in skeletal muscle). Variants of the UCP genes may be involved in the aetiology of obesity via an effect on thermogenesis. In the mouse, UCP2 has been mapped to chromosome 7 and closely linked to the tubby mouse mutation; this mutation is known to be responsible for the adult-onset obesity. In humans, UCP2 has been mapped to chromosome 11q13. Recently, markers around this locus have been shown to be linked with measurements of resting metabolic rate (RMR). This suggests a possible biochemical mechanism involved in regulating RMR (Bouchard *et al.*, 1997).

Other possible candidate genes

The search for molecular markers, or genetic polymorphisms, is involving several candidates that are either associated or linked with obesity or related metabolic syndromes. Examples of the contribution of genetic individuality to such metabolic syndromes are: the reported genetic polymorphisms associated with insulin resistance, with the glucocorticoid receptor, and with apolipoprotein B, D and E genes (Beales & Kopelman, 1996).

6.5.5 Human obesity syndromes

Obesity is the consistent feature in many single gene disorders, of which the Prader–Willi syndrome (PWS) is typical (Hall & Smith, 1972). Table 6.1 details the characteristic clinical findings of the condition. The majority of PWS cases occur

Table 6.1 Clinical features of the Prader–Willi syndrome.

Short stature
Upper body obesity
Small hands and feet
Mental retardation of variable degree
Hypogonadism and testicular abnormalities usually
  resulting in sterility

sporadically, but familial inheritance is described and can be regarded as autosomal dominant. PWS is caused by a deletion of the paternal segment of 15q11.2-q12, with this loss occurring through two separate mechanisms. The first mechanism is the local deletion of the paternally derived segment, the second mechanism is the loss of the entire chromosome 15 with presence of two maternal homologues, uniparental maternal disomy (Nicholls *et al.*, 1989). The incidence of PWS is approximately 1 in 25000, with deletions accounting for 70–80% of cases of PWS. A second, but less common disorder, is the Bardet–Biedel syndrome (BBS) (Kwitek-Black *et al.*, 1993; Leppert *et al.*, 1994). Linkage studies have identified several loci for this syndrome (chromosome 16q21, 11q13, 3p13 and 15q22), which confirms the heterogeneity of the syndrome. An investigation of PWS, BBS and three other previously mapped genetic disorders of obesity in families in whom obesity was clearly segregating, revealed no evidence for linkage between obesity and the five disease loci (Reed *et al.*, 1995).

6.5.6 Genome-wide search

With the advent of marker libraries covering the entire human genome, it is possible to perform a random gene-wide search for candidate genes contributing to obesity by studying large single pedigrees (consanguineous), nuclear families or affected pedigree members (e.g. sibling pairs, grandparent, grandchild pairs). Such studies will include classical linkage analysis, affected pedigree member linkage analysis (sibling pairs, identity-by-descent [IBD] and identity by state [IBS]) or linkage disequilibrium analysis. The main limitation of classical linkage analysis is that the model of inheritance must be specified and, furthermore, family collection is time-consuming and costly. The

IBD method is likely to be the most powerful when, as is usually the case for obesity, both parents are alive. Calculations suggest a study of 200–400 sibling-pairs will achieve 90% power. This is based on the finding that the risk ratio of obesity for an offspring of an affected individual, compared with the general population, is in the order of 2–4 (Feingold *et al.*, 1993; Risch, 1990). This confirms a requirement to study a substantial number of related obese subjects to ensure that any genetic association is genuine, and not a spurious finding resulting from inadvertently selected individuals. Allison & Faith (1997) have published a simplified model of inheritance, artificially defined cut-offs of 'low environmental risk' for obesity and relative body weight scores for defining obesity. The resulting statistics help the understanding of how heritability is estimated.

6.6 Summary

- Obesity cannot be regarded as a single disorder but a group of heterogeneous disorders.

- The variations seen in the distribution of body fat are attributable to a complex inter-working of genetic, nutritional, energy expenditure, psychological and social variables.

- Studies, which have included twins, adoptees and families, confirm a strong genetic influence on fatness and the distribution of fat tissue.

- The rapid increase in the prevalence of obesity, in a genetically stable population, confirms the important influence of the environment. Nevertheless, it is difficult to isolate the effects of the environment from genetic influences, and a better understanding is needed about gene-environmental interactions.

- The recent advances in knowledge of the genetic basis of obesity in rodent models are providing a useful insight into the human situation.

- A number of candidate genes have been reported in association with human obesity. The advent of marker libraries, covering the entire human genome, will facilitate gene-wide searches for candidate genes contributing to obesity.

- It will be essential that the biochemical mechanisms, metabolic significance and possible social interaction be addressed for any gene identified as potentially predisposing to obesity.

7
Aetiology of Obesity III: Critical Periods for the Development of Obesity

7.1 Introduction

Much of the obesity that is contributing to the current epidemic in affluent nations represents a very gradual adult-onset weight gain, which is the outcome of many years of slightly positive energy balance, interspersed by occasional periods of restraint or weight loss. In Australia, it has been estimated that this weight gain averages 1 g per day for the adult population (Australasian Society for the Study of Obesity, 1995).

However, in some people obesity develops much more rapidly. This suggests a more pathologic cause or the presence of a critical physiological phase, in which energy balance is more easily perturbed and after which the effects seem to be difficult to reverse. These putative critical periods include: fetal growth, infancy and childhood, adolescence, reproduction (pregnancy and lactation) and middle age, especially the menopause in women. It will be clear from the following sections that the significance of these critical periods is not universally accepted. Furthermore, even where there is evidence of a discrete susceptibility, this usually applies only to a small fraction of people. A critical period of growth is a developmental stage in which long-term growth may be substantially altered by events that occur in a relatively short period of time (Dietz, 1996a).

7.2 *In utero*

The term 'programming', has been used to describe the situation 'when an early stimulus or insult, operating at a critical or sensitive period, results in a permanent or long-term change in the structure or function of the organism' (Lucas, 1991). This stimulus, or insult, may affect the development or the function of a particular organ or tissue. These effects may be immediate or may not become apparent for some time. McCance and Widdowson considered and demonstrated some of the possible consequences of disturbing the 'harmony of growth' (McCance & Widdowson, 1974; Widdowson & McCance, 1975). In his theory of 'fuel mediated teratogenesis', Freinkel *et al.* (1985) proposed that exposure to inappropriately high levels of nutrients *in utero* may programme long-term structure and function by modifying phenotypic gene expression of cells that are terminally differentiated during intrauterine development. Barker's 'fetal origins of adult disease' hypothesis proposes that an adverse nutritional environment *in utero* causes defects in the development, structure and function of organs, leading to a programmed susceptibility, which interacts with later diet and environmental stresses to cause overt disease many decades later (Barker, 1995).

There are two potentially critical periods for the development of obesity *in utero*. In early gestation, when the hypothalamic centres are most susceptible, exposure to over- or under-nutrition may affect regulation of appetite and growth, and hence predispose to later obesity. In late gestation, when differentiation and hyperplasia of adipocytes occurs, and the fetus accumulates fat, differential effects may protect against, or promote, later obesity. Exposure to under-nutrition may reduce adipocyte replication, while exposure to over-nutrition may cause adipocyte hyperplasia (Brook, 1972; McCance & Widdowson, 1974; Widdowson & McCance, 1975; Garn & Cole, 1980; Dietz, 1994, 1996.

7.2.1 Fetal growth, nutrient supply and body composition

In early- to mid-gestation, fetal growth is primarily a result of an increase in cell numbers under genetic control. In the third trimester, fetal growth is primarily the result of increasing cell size and fat deposition, and nutrient supply is the dominant factor. Glucose crosses the placenta from mother to fetus, by facilitated diffusion, and amino acids traverse by active transport. Esterified lipids cannot cross the placenta, but free fatty acids (FFA) cross readily. Although both the fetus and placenta can synthesise FFA, the majority is maternally derived, and lipids acquired by the fetus result from passive transfer of FFA between the maternal and fetal circulations (Stacey, 1991).

In normal pregnancies, maternal insulin does not cross the placenta. Secretion of fetal insulin, an important anabolic hormone, is limited. Although fetal insulin is present from about 8–10 weeks gestation, it is relatively dormant until about 20 weeks, when the fetal response to glucose develops. Insulin receptors become maximal at 19–25 weeks and an increased affinity occurs in late gestation. Since fetal glucose passively tracks the maternal glucose level, the latter dictates the sensitivity of fetal beta-cells. Both glucose and amino acids stimulate fetal insulin secretion, which promotes growth in insulin-sensitive tissues. In pregnancies complicated by diabetes, fetal development occurs in a relatively insulin enriched environment. The higher levels of maternal circulating amino acids and glucose lead to the increased transplacental flux of nutrients, and impose increased amounts of fuels on the fetus. This over-nutrition triggers hyperplasia and hypertrophy of fetal islets, the groups of cells that produce insulin, leading to fetal hyper-insulinaemia and increased anabolism (Klopper, 1991; Langer, 1991; Hollingsworth, 1992).

At term, a normal healthy newborn infant, born to a mother with an uncomplicated pregnancy, typically weighs about 3.4 kg, of which about 440 g is fat. Fat accumulation is minimal in the first half of pregnancy, but increases to account for 30% of total weight gain from 38 weeks. At birth, neonatal fat mass comprises about 14% of total body weight; lean body mass represents, on average, 86% of birthweight and accounts for 83% of the variance. It has been suggested that lean body mass is relatively stable *in utero*, compared with alterations in the maternal metabolic milieu. In contrast, fetal fat mass accumulation may be more sensitive to factors that affect fetal growth (Zeigler *et al.*, 1976; Hytten, 1991; Catalano *et al.*, 1992).

Mothers with diabetes have a two to sixfold increase in the rate of 'large for gestational age' (LGA) babies. The typical infant born to a diabetic mother is of high birthweight and macrosomic (birthweight > 90th or 95th percentile, or birthweight > 4 kg). The macrosomia occurs because of excess fat deposition, and hyperplasia and hypertrophy of bones and viscera. Central obesity of the neonate is a common cause of complications during labour, particularly shoulder dystocia.

7.2.2 Studies of *in utero* determinants of obesity

In humans, studies of *in utero* determinants of obesity fall into four categories:

- effects of fetal over-nutrition;
- effects of fetal under-nutrition;
- relationship between fetal and maternal adiposity;
- tracking of weight/adiposity from birth into adulthood.

The definitive studies would be those which prospectively follow subjects from, or prior to, birth through to late adulthood. But these, by their nature, are very difficult and time-consuming to conduct. Therefore, with few exceptions, although the determinants of obesity in newborns are being elucidated, studies of the influences on the longer-term development of obesity are less clear. Pima Indians are probably the most intensively studied people with respect to longitudinal follow-up and development of obesity. However, this population is one in which the prevalence of both obesity and non-insulin-dependent diabetes mellitus (NIDDM), with its consequent gestational effects, are among the highest in the world. The findings may, therefore, be atypical.

7.2.3 The effects of fetal over-nutrition

i Obesity in offspring resulting from diabetic pregnancies

Infants born to poorly controlled diabetic mothers with hyperglycaemia form the population in which most work has been conducted with respect to *in utero* influences of obesity. Over the past 20 years, there has been a dramatic reduction in the rates of stillbirth, congenital malformations and perinatal mortality associated with diabetic pregnancies. However, the incidence of macrosomia has remained unchanged. A number of studies have shown that, compared to normal pregnancies, babies of diabetic mothers are more likely to be large for gestational age. They are both heavier and fatter, as assessed by thickness of skinfolds and anthropometry, regardless of gestational age or maternal obesity (Pettitt *et al.*, 1983; Freinkel *et al.*, 1985; West & Brans, 1986; Hollingsworth, 1992; Vohr *et al.*, 1995).

ii Relationship between birthweight and adiposity and maternal glucose metabolism in non-diabetic pregnancies

Increased birthweight and adiposity is not only a consequence of frank diabetes during pregnancy. A number of studies have also found a progressive increase in both birthweight and obesity as glucose tolerance decreases. Even minor abnormalities are sufficient to increase the risk of increased newborn weight and adiposity (Freinkel *et al.*, 1985; Pettitt *et al.*, 1985; Leikin *et al.*, 1987). Furthermore, even in women with normal pregnancies, variations in glucose metabolism, considered to be within the normal range, have been shown to be positively associated with infant weight and adiposity (Langhoff-Roos *et al.*, 1988). The activity of fetal beta-cells (the insulin producing cells), as assessed by amniotic fluid or cord insulin or C peptide, was found to be correlated with birthweight in infants born to women with, and women without disturbances of carbohydrate metabolism during gestation (Dornhorst *et al.*, 1994).

7.2.4 The effects of fetal under-nutrition

i The 'infant and fetal origins of adult's disease' hypothesis

Recent epidemiological studies, particularly in the UK, have led to the hypothesis that adverse nutritional experiences *in utero* have a powerful influence on the development of diseases in adulthood (Goldberg & Prentice, 1994; Barker, 1995). Many of the studies have focused on the relationships between various measures at birth (weight, length, circumferences) and heart disease and diabetes in adulthood. To date, there have been no reports of effects of size at birth and subsequent incidence of obesity, although one study has demonstrated an inverse relationship between birthweight and abdominal fatness (WHR), later in life, in adult men (Law *et al.*, 1992). Data from the San Antonio Heart Study have also demonstrated inverse relationships between central obesity (assessed as the ratio of subscapular to triceps skinfold thicknesses) and birthweight (Valdez *et al.*, 1994). Since obesity is an important determinant of the diseases predicted by fetal and infant growth rates, the programming of obesity will certainly have been examined, and the absence of published reports suggests that the effects are weak (Dutch famine data below).

ii The Dutch famine

During the winter of 1944–1945, the cities of north west Holland were blockaded. This meant that the population was subjected to famine conditions for 9 months, until the advance of the Allied forces lifted the blockade. Data from cohorts born around the time of the Dutch famine have provided some of the most convincing evidence that both early and late gestation are critical periods for the subsequent development of obesity. Ravelli *et al.* (1976) compared groups of young men whose mothers were not exposed to famine during pregnancy (controls) with groups whose mothers were exposed at different stages of pregnancy. Compared to the control group, the prevalence of obesity was significantly higher in those whose exposure to famine coincided with the first two trimesters of pregnancy (2.77% and 1.45%, respectively). Prevalence of obesity was significantly lower in those whose exposure to famine was in the third trimester, or shortly after birth (0.82% and 1.32%, respectively). These findings are consistent with an appetite rebound after the famine, when the mothers who were exposed to famine in the first two trimesters were able to eat more normally at the end of pregnancy. The availability of nutrients was, therefore, affected at a critical time for fat accumulation. In offspring exposed to famine in the third trimester, adipocyte numbers and fat accumulation appear to have been irrecoverably reduced.

7.2.5 Relationships between maternal and fetal adiposity

It is well established that maternal nutritional status before and during gestation is related to fetal size. Although diabetes is associated with a much higher risk of macrosomia, diabetic pregnancies account for the minority of LGA infants. The majority are associated with maternal obesity and high gestational weight gains, both conditions likely to be associated with increased materno-fetal transfer of fuels and, therefore, increased fetal beta-cell activity and fetal growth.

Positive relationships have been found between maternal BMI and neonatal adiposity (Neggers *et al.*, 1995; Vohr *et al.*, 1995) and between maternal weight and infant birthweight (Maresh *et al.*, 1989). In treated gestational diabetic mothers, birthweight was found to be more a function of maternal weight than a function of the severity of diabetes before onset of treatment (Maresh *et al.*, 1989).

Silliman & Kretchmer (1995) used TOBEC (Section 3.1.5) to measure adipose tissue in mothers and their infants. Compared to those of lean women, infants born to obese mothers were significantly heavier and longer. At birth, infant adiposity was significantly and positively related to maternal adiposity. However, at six weeks postpartum, maternal adiposity was no longer a predictor of infant fatness and there were no differences in weight, length or skinfold thickness between infants of lean and obese women.

Brown *et al.* (1996) found that maternal WHR was related to infant birthweight, length and head circumference. The interaction of maternal WHR was graded according to BMI. The authors suggested that the metabolic and hormonal effects of central body fat stores influenced fetal growth. Central fat storage is associated with higher circulating levels of FFA, insulin resistance and higher fasting glucose levels, all of which affect the availability of energy and nutrients to the fetus.

7.2.6 The tracking of obesity: do large fat neonates become obese adults?

Charney *et al.* (1976) found that adults aged 20- to 30-years-old, whose weights were in excess of the 75th and 90th percentiles at birth and in early infancy, were more than twice as likely to be obese than those who were of average or low weight. Seidman *et al.* (1991) found a strong correlation between birthweight and BMI in young men and women and that the proportion of those classified as overweight, or severely overweight, increased as birthweight increased. In contrast, Björntorp *et al.* (1974) studied young adults all of high birthweight, who had been born to mothers with poorly controlled diabetes during pregnancy. The group was not obese compared to controls, and there was no difference in body fat content, average cell size or number of adipocytes and no correlation between birthweight and fat cell number.

Metzger *et al.* (1990) found that the concentration of insulin in amniotic fluid (reflecting fetal insulin) of infants born to diabetic mothers, predicted obesity in children at 6 years of age born to diabetic mothers. Significant correlations remained after correction for maternal obesity and macrosomia at birth. Silverman *et al.* (1991) also reported that fatness at birth and amniotic fluid insulin concentration correlated with obesity at six years. However, after six years, when there was a general increase in the prevalence of obesity, the relationship between neonatal fatness and childhood obesity was no longer significant.

In the studies of Pima Indians, mentioned previously (Section 7.2.2), offspring are being followed up and data have been reported for 5- to 9-year-old, 10- to 14-year-old and 15- to 19-year-old cohorts (Pettitt *et al.*, 1983, 1985, 1987, 1993). The percentage of those classified as obese increased with age, as is well established with this population. Within each age group, the percentages of those classified as above their ideal body weight (15–20%) or as obese (10–20%) were similar in the non-diabetic and impaired glucose tolerance (IGT) groups, although the proportion who were over-weight and obese in the IGT group were slightly higher. In contrast, 30–50% of people with insulin-dependent diabetes (IDDM) were above their ideal body weight and 40–60% were obese. Furthermore, even in those of normal birthweight, in each age group, significantly more subjects with IDDM were obese compared to those born to women with IGT or normal women. In diabetic pregnant women, infant birthweight was predictive of later weight at age 5–9 years and 10–14 years. Birthweight was not predictive of subsequent obesity at any age in off-spring of normal and pre-diabetic women. These data indicate that maternal diabetes during preg-nancy has a specific effect on obesity in the off-spring, not only at birth but also up to at least 19 years of age. Pettitt concluded that the presence of diabetes during pregnancy exerts an influence on the development of obesity in offspring, which is stronger than that related to either birthweight or maternal obesity, and that high birthweight is not a necessary prerequisite for later development of obesity in individuals with IDDM.

Finally, Allison *et al.* (1995) analysed long-itudinal data from monozygotic and dizygotic twins and examined relationships between birthweight and self-reported adult weight, height and BMI. They observed that intrauterine effects on birth-weight did not have an enduring effect into adult-hood. However, adult height was influenced and they concluded that in well-nourished women, the third trimester was a critical period for develop-ment of height.

7.3 Infancy and childhood

7.3.1 Patterns of fat deposition

The natural pattern of adiposity during childhood is a period of rapid fat deposition during the third trimester of pregnancy and the early months of postnatal life, peaking at about nine months and then going into reverse for several years. During this period, there is a net loss of adipose tissue despite the increasing size of the child. A second stage of fat deposition starts at about six years and continues into adulthood. This pattern of an initial rise, followed by a fall and a second rise, can be seen in growth standards for triceps and subscapular

skinfolds (Tanner & Whitehouse, 1975) and BMI (Cole *et al.*, 1995).

The amount of fat in an individual is the product of the number of fat cells and the mean size of the cells (Hirsch, 1975; Sections 3.4 and 5.2). The rapid deposition of fat in late gestation and infancy was seen, during the 1970s, as a critical period for the development of obesity, with excess numbers of adipocytes (hypercellularity) coupled with later growth in cell size leading to adult obesity. It was believed that the number of fat cells might be influenced by the infant's environment, particularly the diet, and that high-energy artificial milk for-mulae might, therefore, pose a risk for later obesity (James, 1976). However, the theory was not widely supported and little evidence has emerged since then to substantiate the theory (Gurr *et al.*, 1982).

7.3.2 Tracking of obesity from childhood to adulthood

A history of obesity during infancy tends not to be a strong predictor of obesity later in childhood (Poskitt & Cole, 1977), although some authors have shown a relationship (Rolland-Cachera *et al.*, 1987). There is a stronger link between obesity in child-hood, particularly adolescence (Section 7.4), and obesity as an adult (Power *et al.*, 1998), although this applies only to a minority of obese people. The vast majority of obese adults were not obese as children. In this context, it is noteworthy that results from the 1958 Birth Cohort suggest that obesity is more likely to track from childhood to adulthood in lower social class children than in the high social classes, where much childhood obesity resolves by adulthood (Power *et al.*, 1998).

The timing of the second rise in adiposity (termed the 'adipocity rebound') has been shown to relate to adult fatness, with an earlier rebound being associated with greater fatness in later life (Rolland-Cachera *et al.*, 1984; 1987 [Fig. 7.1]). This may reflect physiological differences around the age of 5–7 years, or it may simply mean that during a period of generally increasing fatness, those that start earlier tend to end up fatter.

7.4 Adolescence

Adolescence is the period of growth and develop-ment that links childhood and adulthood. A good

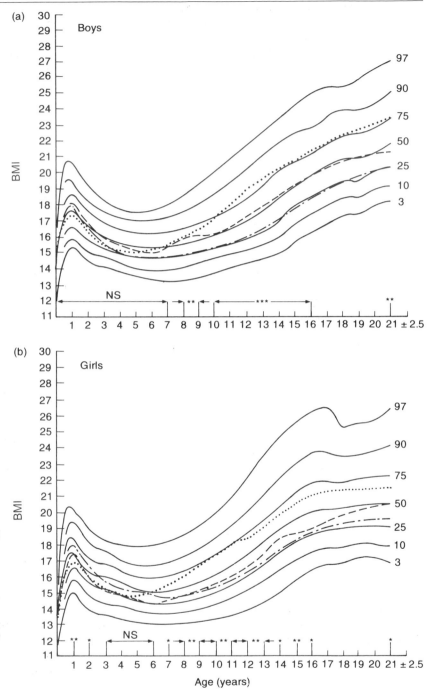

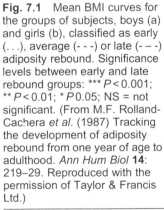

Fig. 7.1 Mean BMI curves for the groups of subjects, boys (a) and girls (b), classified as early (. . .), average (- - -) or late (- – -) adiposity rebound. Significance levels between early and late rebound groups: *** $P < 0.001$; ** $P < 0.01$; * $P\,0.05$; NS = not significant. (From M.F. Rolland-Cachera *et al.* (1987) Tracking the development of adiposity rebound from one year of age to adulthood. *Ann Hum Biol* **14**: 219–29. Reproduced with the permission of Taylor & Francis Ltd.)

knowledge of the abnormal patterns associated with this period of this growth and development is a prerequisite to any understanding of the normal pattern of adolescent obesity (Johnson, 1985). In relation to the question of adolescence as a critical period for the development of obesity, there are several reasons why males and females should be considered separately, including such pertinent issues as sex differences in maturational timing, body composition and health consequences of obesity during adolescence. The start of adolescence is characterised by the pubertal growth spurt, which represents the most rapid growth after infancy that the human being experiences, while a slower period of growth occurs during later adolescence after the menarche or adrenarche is reached (Tanner, 1962). Females mature earlier than males and generally experience the growth spurts about two years before males. Most females enter puberty before they reach 10 years of age, are peripubertal between 10 and 14 years and reach late adolescence by 15 years; while males most usually enter puberty under 12 years of age, are peripubertal from 12–17 years and reach later adolescence by 18 years or older. In addition to these sex differences, maturational timing also varies within each sex. Inception of the growth spurt may occur between the ages of 9 and 13 years in girls and between the ages of 11 and 15 years in boys, depending on whether they are early or late maturers. In terms of body composition, female adolescence is characterised by an increase in adiposity. This is in contrast to males who, during adolescence, actually experience some depletion in their fat stores and tend to gain more height, weight and lean body mass. Cross-sectional data on the subcutaneous fat stores (using triceps skinfold thickness) of white Americans participating in the Ten States Nutrition Survey (Garn & Clark, 1976) clearly demonstrate these sex differences in adiposity during adolescence (Fig. 7.2). These sex differences in fatness trends may explain why adolescence has been described as a critical period for the development of obesity, particularly in females (Dietz, 1994).

7.4.1 The importance of growth and maturational timing

Two recent papers from the Amsterdam Growth and Health Study demonstrate that the timing of

biological maturation during adolescence may be important in the development of obesity in both sexes, and may influence the development of abdominal body fat distribution in females. In this 15-year follow-up study, the effects of both rapid and slow biological maturation on the development of obesity was investigated in boys (n = 79) and girls (n = 98). The subjects initially were a mean age of 13 years and were each measured 6 times, up to a mean age of 27 years. During this period, BMI and the sum of skinfold thickness for individuals who matured rapidly during adolescence, were significantly higher than for slowly maturing individuals (based on skeletal age in both sexes, age at peak height velocity in boys and age at menarche in girls). This is shown in Figs 7.3, 7.4, 7.5 and 7.6 (van Lethe *et al.*, 1996a). Furthermore, girls who experienced menarche relatively early (lowest tertile for age at menarche i.e. before age 12.9 years) had higher mean trunk-oriented skinfold ratios than those who experienced menarche relatively late (highest tertile i.e. after 13.9 years). These differences persisted throughout the follow-up period (van Lethe *et al.*, 1996b). This association of abdominal body fat distribution and early menarche in girls, from adolescence into adulthood, still existed after taking into account the differences in level of body fatness between the two groups (van Lethe *et al.*, 1996b).

The high degree of agreement between the three indices of biological maturation used in this study reduces the chances of misclassification of early and late maturers, and thereby strengthens the significance of the findings (van Lethe *et al.*, 1996a). It is well established that early maturing male and female adolescents tend to be fatter (Tanner, 1962), and the link between this early/rapid maturity and the development of chronic obesity has been suggested by previous studies. Using data on almost 17 000 adult white women, Garn *et al.* (1986) found that women who matured early (menarche at age 11 years or younger) were slightly shorter and significantly fatter than those maturing later (menarche at age 14 years or later). Furthermore, these differences in fatness were found to increase with age. By age 30 years, 26% of the early maturers were obese compared with less than 15% of the late maturers, thus indicating that maturational timing probably has a greater long-term effect on the level of fatness than the level of

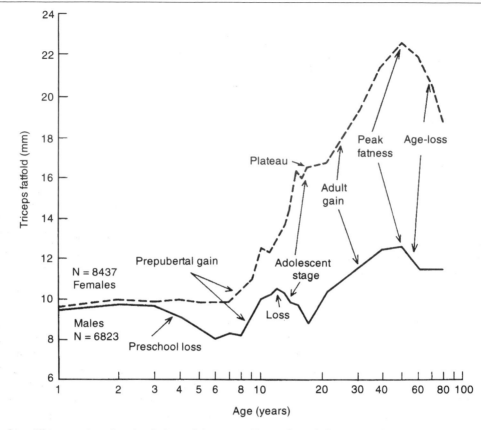

Fig. 7.2 Sex differences in adiposity during adolescence (from: Garn & Clark, 1976). Reproduced with permission from *Paediatrics* **57** 443–56.

fatness has on maturational timing (Garn *et al.*, 1986).

In these studies, differences in obesity and body fat distribution between rapidly and slowly maturing adolescents persisted well into adulthood (when the process of biological maturity was complete). (Garn *et al.*, 1986; van Lethe *et al.*, 1996a,b). This suggests that, instead of a causal relationship, another factor, which in addition to being associated with timing of maturity was also responsible for these differences in body fatness. Using nutrient intake data (Post & Kemper, 1993) and physical activity data (Verschuur & Kemper, 1985) from the Amsterdam Growth and Health Study, Van Lethe *et al.* (1996a) suggest that although greater total energy intakes by rapidly maturing adolescents may partly explain their higher levels of body fatness, data on the tracking of these energy intake differ-

ences (Post & Welton, 1995), make it unlikely that persistent high energy intake was the main cause of the greater obesity of the rapidly maturing individuals. Other possible explanations worthy of further exploration include: increased hormonal activity associated with the promotion of fat accumulation in females, and genetic differences in rapid and slow maturers with respect to vulnerability to obesity (van Lethe *et al.*, 1996a).

7.4.2 Fatness during adolescence as a predictor of chronic obesity

Apart from the intricate relationship between level of body fatness, maturational timing and the development of obesity, it is important to consider how well fatness during adolescence predicts

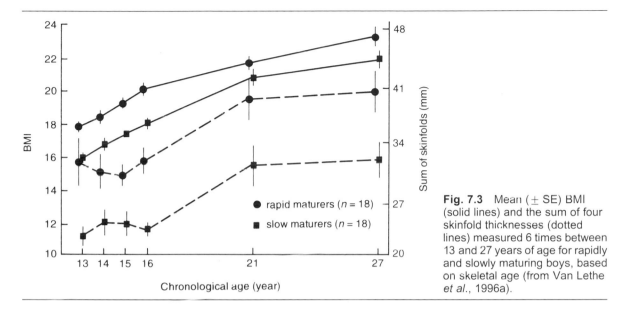

Fig. 7.3 Mean ($\pm$ SE) BMI (solid lines) and the sum of four skinfold thicknesses (dotted lines) measured 6 times between 13 and 27 years of age for rapidly and slowly maturing boys, based on skeletal age (from Van Lethe *et al.*, 1996a).

obesity. Recent studies, including a nationally representative cohort study of over 10 000 Americans, suggest that fewer females compared with males (66% versus 70–78%, respectively) who were overweight during adolescence remain overweight as adults (Gortmaker *et al.*, 1993; Guo *et al.*, 1994). In support of this, a recent examination of the tracking of BMI over a 50-year period in a longitudinal study (n = 67 boys and n = 67 girls) reported that the prediction of ponderosity in middle age, from BMIs during childhood and adolescence, may be more reliable for males than for females (Casey *et al.*, 1992). Overall, the tracking of body size from childhood to middle age was found to be poor for females, improving slightly after adolescence. It has been suggested that these sex differences may be related to the marked increase in adiposity experienced by girls during adolescence (Fig. 7.2),

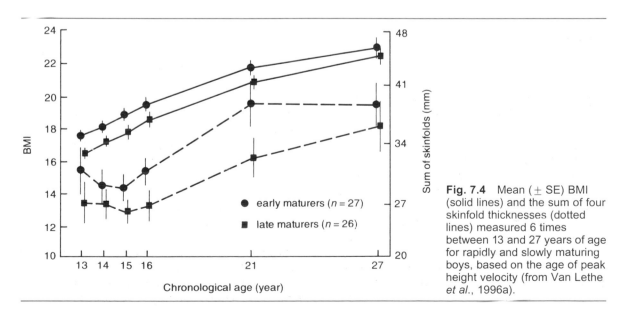

Fig. 7.4 Mean ($\pm$ SE) BMI (solid lines) and the sum of four skinfold thicknesses (dotted lines) measured 6 times between 13 and 27 years of age for rapidly and slowly maturing boys, based on the age of peak height velocity (from Van Lethe *et al.*, 1996a).

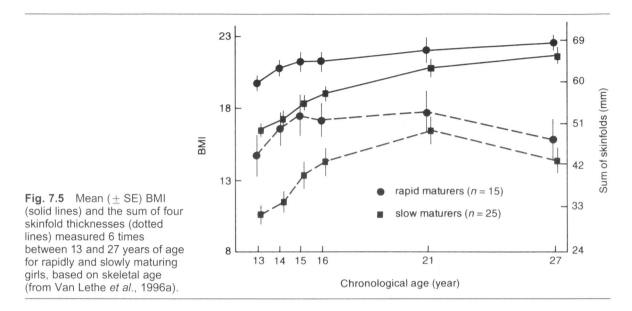

Fig. 7.5 Mean (± SE) BMI (solid lines) and the sum of four skinfold thicknesses (dotted lines) measured 6 times between 13 and 27 years of age for rapidly and slowly maturing girls, based on skeletal age (from Van Lethe *et al.*, 1996a).

which may weaken the effect of body size during this period of growth on that in middle age. From an earlier analysis of data from six American longitudinal studies, however, Cronk *et al.* (1982) concluded that influences beginning after adolescence have a greater effect on body fatness during adulthood, in both males and females. Further support for the hypothesis that early adulthood may be a more critical period than adolescence, for the

development of chronic obesity in both sexes, is evident from the findings of Braddon *et al.* (1986), who tested the predictive value of childhood obesity on body weight in adult life. Using a large UK national cohort of children (n = 3322) who were studied from birth to 36 years, these workers found that only 21% of 36-year-old obese people were obese during childhood/adolescence (Braddon *et al.*, 1986).

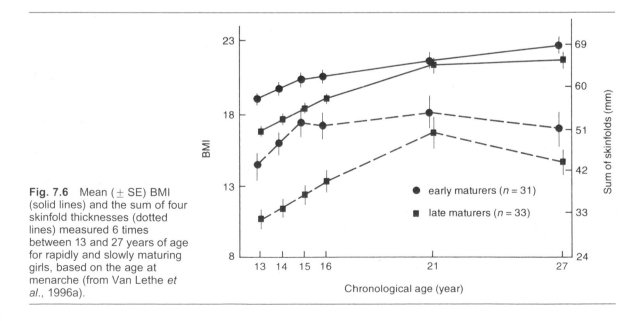

Fig. 7.6 Mean (± SE) BMI (solid lines) and the sum of four skinfold thicknesses (dotted lines) measured 6 times between 13 and 27 years of age for rapidly and slowly maturing girls, based on the age at menarche (from Van Lethe *et al.*, 1996a).

7.5 Reproduction

The reproductive cycle poses three risk periods for the development of obesity: pregnancy, lactation, and a longer, less clearly defined, post-partum period. 'Maternal obesity' was first described over 40 years ago (Sheldon, 1949; Richardson, 1952). Anecdotally, many overweight and obese women claim that the onset of their weight problems was coincident with their having children and that they became fatter after each child was born. Some studies have shown that parous women have cumulative increments in body weight after successive pregnancies (Beazley & Swinhoe 1979; Samra *et al.*, 1988; Rossner, 1995). Records from obesity clinics in Australia and Sweden, indicate that 50–80% of female patients cite pregnancy as the reason for their obesity (Bradley, 1985; Ohlin & Rossner, 1990).

7.5.1 Pregnancy

In normal healthy well-nourished women, the gestational weight gain associated with the best pregnancy outcome is around 12.5 kg. It is assumed that approximately one-quarter of this increment is fat deposition in maternal adipose tissue; the remainder comprises the products of conception and hypertrophy of maternal tissues (Hytten, 1991).

Data from groups of well-nourished women, of normal pre-pregnant BMI, with uncomplicated pregnancies resulting in normal birthweight babies, indicate that mean gestational weight gains in Europe, North America and Australia are between 11 and 16 kg. The variability in gestational weight gain is very large, indicated by standard deviations that are typically 3–4 kg. In those studies that have reported the ranges of weight gained by individuals, the greatest increments ranged from 18–33 kg.

Longitudinal studies of maternal fat stores, in which whole body methods (underwater weighing, total body water, MRI) were used to assess changes during pregnancy, have shown mean increases of between 2.0–5.8 kg (Forsum *et al.*, 1988; van Raaij *et al.*, 1989; Goldberg *et al.*, 1993; Sohlstrom & Forsum 1995). As with weight gains, intra-individual variability in body fat gain is also very large, with the greatest increases ranging from 8–12 kg.

Over a certain limit, especially in overweight women, excess maternal weight gain has no significant effect on fetal weight; the extra fat is deposited in maternal adipose tissue stores (Langhoff-Roos *et al.*, 1987; Lawrence *et al.*, 1991). Furthermore, there is evidence to show that excess fat is more likely to be deposited centrally, where it carries greater health risks (Smith *et al.*, 1994; Sohlstrom & Forsum 1995).

Concern has been expressed about the potential impact of excessive gestational weight gains on the rising prevalence of obesity (Abrams 1993; Keppel & Taffel 1993; Manson *et al.*, 1994). Many studies have shown that postpartum weight retention is significantly and positively correlated with gestational weight gains (Fig. 7.7). Once again, the variability is very large. Mean weight changes one year postpartum, relative to pre-pregnant weight, range between –1 and +8 kg in these studies, with associated standard deviations of a similar magnitude (Greene *et al.*, 1988; Ohlin & Rossner, 1990; Parham *et al.*, 1990; Schauberger *et al.*, 1992; Keppel & Taffel 1993; Parker & Abrams 1993; Scholl *et al.*, 1995). The combined evidence from all of these studies supports the view that excess fat gain often occurs during pregnancy (sometimes to a remarkable degree) and that most of it is retained post-partum.

Studies in the literature about postpartum obesity vary widely with respect to study design, original purpose, choice of control group (if any) and methods used. Postpartum periods range from a few weeks to 10 years. Data is often obtained retrospectively, by examination of hospital notes or asking women to recall their weight at certain ages or on particular occasions.

Since 1994, data relating to reproductive history and weight changes from four large cohort studies, which were originally designed to investigate general changes in health indices, have been published (Smith *et al.*, 1994; Williamson *et al.*, 1994; Troisi *et al.*, 1995; Björkelund *et al.*, 1996; Wolfe *et al.*, 1997). The subject numbers are very large and although the studies do suggest positive relationships between parity and obesity, again effects tend to be small when data are adjusted for the confounding variables of age and social status. Furthermore, the adjustments made may not always be the most appropriate because information relating to pregnancy and lactation was not obtained.

There are many confounding variables, which should be taken into account when considering the

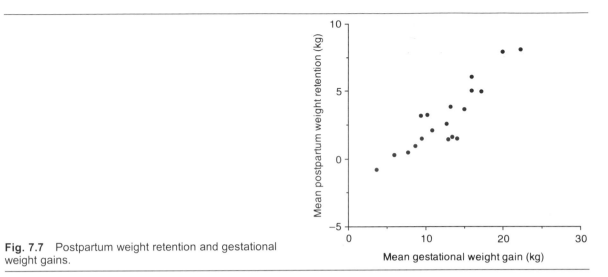

Fig. 7.7 Postpartum weight retention and gestational weight gains.

relationship between parity and weight gain. A major confounder, particularly in studies of long duration, is age since weight tends to increase with age, as does parity. In some studies, significant relationships between parity and weight gain are lost after adjustment for age (Rookus *et al.*, 1987; Brown *et al.*, 1992). Parity is also associated with factors known to be associated with higher rates of obesity, e.g. socio-economic status, social class and ethnicity. Lifestyle factors, such as occupation, leisure time activities and smoking, also have to be taken into consideration (Lederman, 1993). The effect of socio-demographic and behavioural factors leads to much greater parity-associated weight increases in some sub-groups than others (Wolfe *et al.*, 1997). A recent systematic review of post-partum obesity discarded most pertinent studies, on the grounds of inadequate controls (Harris & Ellison, 1997). It concluded that pregnancy was not a major risk period for populations as a whole, but that in certain individual cases it could certainly be blamed for precipitating obesity (Figs 7.8 and 7.9).

There has been considerable interest in the question of whether postpartum obesity may be caused by the induction of energy-sparing metabolic adjustments during pregnancy, which fail to switch off after delivery. It has been concluded,

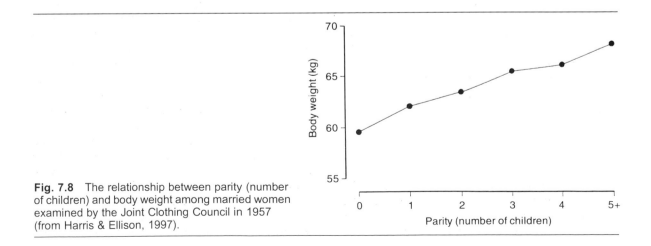

Fig. 7.8 The relationship between parity (number of children) and body weight among married women examined by the Joint Clothing Council in 1957 (from Harris & Ellison, 1997).

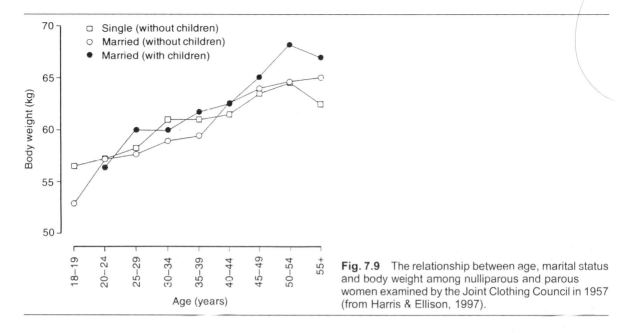

Fig. 7.9 The relationship between age, marital status and body weight among nulliparous and parous women examined by the Joint Clothing Council in 1957 (from Harris & Ellison, 1997).

however, that there is little evidence to support this hypothesis (Prentice *et al.*, 1996). In fact, it tends to be the fatter, better nourished women whose metabolic rates rise most during pregnancy (Poppitt *et al.*, 1994). Thin, under-nourished women display energy-sparing changes in metabolism (Poppitt *et al.*, 1994).

Although there is not a detailed literature to support the contention, many observers believe that excessive fat gains in pregnancy occur as a result of changes in lifestyle, activity and employment. Excessive fat gain may also occur in formerly restrained eaters, who relapse in response to the excuse to 'eat for two', or because of so-called 'motivational collapse', when they are confronted by the inevitable weight gain of pregnancy (Leifer, 1977; Clissold *et al.*, 1991). There is a need for more research to understand the behavioural changes associated with pregnancy and motherhood.

7.5.2 Lactation

The fat deposited during pregnancy is assumed to be an energy store that can be mobilised to buffer the extra energy costs of lactation. However, significant weight and fat losses are not an obligatory feature of lactation, especially in well-nourished or affluent women, who are able to increase energy intake and/or decrease physical activity (Prentice *et al.*, 1996). Two studies have reported increases in body fat during the first three months of lactation (Forsum *et al.*, 1989; Goldberg *et al.*, 1991). Rookus *et al.* (1987) have suggested that some differences in post-partum weight changes between lactating and non-lactating women may be because the latter actively attempt to lose weight after pregnancy. In contrast, lactating women are advised not to lose weight by restricting energy intake or exercising too vigorously, in order to avoid compromising their health and the quantity and quality of their milk. However, in studies of well-nourished lactating women whose babies were exclusively breast-fed, neither exercise (Dewey *et al.*, 1994) nor weight loss programmes (Dusdieker *et al.*, 1994) adversely affected milk output or infant growth. Exercising women compensated for the imposed increase in energy expenditure by spontaneously increasing their energy intake and by reducing other forms of physical activity. Janney *et al.* (1997) have concluded that, although lactation influences the pattern of post-partum weight retention, the effect is limited. Therefore, minimal emphasis should be placed on lactation as a means of weight control.

7.5.3 The postpartum period

Schauberger *et al.* (1992) analysed the factors that affected weight loss in the first year postpartum. They found no difference in weight changes associated with self-reported exercise levels, but the earlier women returned to work outside the home, the greater their weight loss at six months. This may have been because of increased energy expenditure and more restricted access to food. Women, who did not resume paid employment, remained, on average, 2 kg above their pre-pregnant weight. In the Stockholm Pregnancy and Weight Development Study, Ohlin & Rossner (1994, 1996) found that postpartum weight retention was greater in women who increased their total energy intake during and after pregnancy, increased the frequency of snacking after pregnancy and had more irregular eating patterns. They also found that weight retention was negatively correlated with the degree of physical activity postpartum. Significant postpartum differences in weight retention between black and white women have been found by Boardley *et al.* (1995). In black women, they found

that total energy intake and percentage of energy from fat were significantly higher and prenatal and postnatal physical activity levels were significantly lower. Janney *et al.* (1997) found that women, who breast-fed, retained less weight over time than those who did not and, in addition, that older women and unmarried women retained greater weight postpartum.

Issues relating to weight control and weight loss during reproduction are discussed in Section 17.2.4.

7.6 Middle age and menopause

Obesity develops gradually over many years. It is, therefore, hardly surprising that the peak prevalence is only reached in middle age. Figure 7.10 illustrates the age trend for obesity in the *Health Survey of England 1996* (Prescott-Clarke & Primatesta, 1998). In both men and women, the prevalence of clinical obesity (BMI > 30) increased by over threefold, from young adulthood to middle age. The figures for overweight (BMI > 25) are perhaps even more striking, with only 26% of men

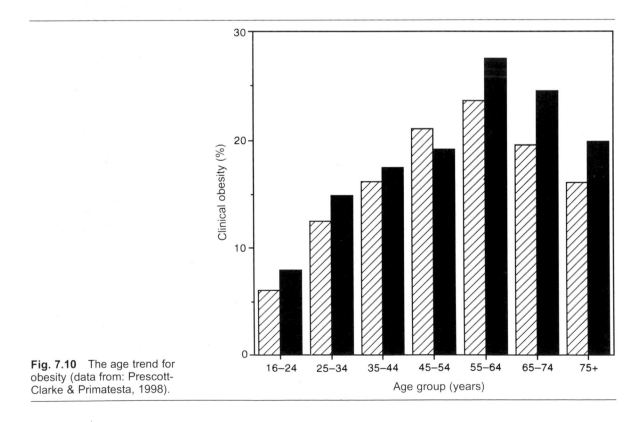

Fig. 7.10 The age trend for obesity (data from: Prescott-Clarke & Primatesta, 1998).

and 32% of women avoiding excess weight gain during middle age. The fact that the prevalence of obesity appears to decline over the age of 64 years, in this analysis, should be interpreted with some caution, as the data are cross-sectional and may not accurately reflect longitudinal changes within individuals. It may, however, be significant that many people increase their levels of physical activity at retirement age, when they have more time for active leisure pursuits (Patrick *et al.*, 1986).

This age-related increase in obesity, during young adulthood and middle age, is not only a consequence of a slowly accumulating excess of fat. It is also likely to be promoted by the fact that most people reduce the frequency, duration and intensity of physical activity very considerably as they age (McGandy *et al.*, 1966; Cunningham *et al.*, 1969; Shock, 1972; Prentice, 1992). Section 15.2 summarises the evidence that decreases in physical activity result in weight gain. This increase in body weight is compounded by the fact that metabolic rate declines as muscle and metabolically active organ mass is replaced by fat during the ageing process in affluent sedentary societies. There is no evidence that metabolic rate declines when expressed per unit of active cell mass (Shock, 1972).

Menopause is often believed to cause weight gain, though there is little secure evidence to describe it as a particular risk period. However, menopause is associated with a change in fat distribution, from a gynoid-type to an android-type pattern, with an increased waist–hip ratio owing to a greater deposition of visceral fat (Björntorp, 1996). Several lines of evidence suggest that this is a specific effect of the change in oestrogen:androgen balance. For instance, it is prevented by hormone replacement therapy (Haarbo *et al.*, 1995), it is associated with changes in lipoprotein lipase (LPL) activity in gluteal adipocytes (Rebuffé-Scrive *et al.*, 1987) and, in women being prepared for sex-change operations, the long-term administration of androgens leads to increased accumulation of visceral fat (Elbers *et al.*, 1995).

7.7 Summary

- Maternal obesity and high rates of gestational weight gain tend to produce larger, fatter babies.

- High circulating maternal fuel levels (caused by IDDM, NIDDM, gestational diabetes, or even quite mild IGT) also lead to larger, fatter babies.

- There remains controversy as to whether these fatter babies are more likely to be obese in later life. The requisite longitudinal studies with adequate controls for genetic and familial influences have yet to be performed.

- There is evidence from Pima Indians that alterations in the maternal glucose/insulin axis may predispose babies to later obesity, irrespective of their birthweight.

- There is little evidence that intra-uterine growth retardation leads to later obesity.

- It is possible that fetal programming represents an important aetiological factor in some individuals and that the failure to detect clear relationships is owing to the dilution effect caused by the high prevalence of non-specific lifestyle obesity.

- There are two potentially critical periods for the development of obesity during infancy and childhood.

- Early infancy (as a continuation of late intra-uterine life) is a key period for alterations in body fat, but obesity at this time has poor prognostic value for later obesity.

- The age of adiposity rebound is the other critical period, although this association may be epidemiological rather than physiological.

- The importance of reproductive cycles as risk periods for future obesity remains controversial, in spite of much research. On balance, pregnancy seems to be a critical phase in small numbers of women, but does not have much impact on the average age-related weight gain of whole populations of women.

- Excessive gestational weight and fat gains in a single pregnancy place the mother at immediate risk of postpartum overweight or obesity.

- Body weight and adiposity may be 'ratcheted' up with each successive pregnancy, if retained weight is not lost between reproductive cycles.

- There is evidence to suggest that pregnancy is associated with the development of increased central adiposity.

- Pregnancy *per se* is not the only cause of excess weight gain associated with parity. Some women gain weight postpartum, indicating that there are other factors; including lactation, diet and activity, that are related to child-rearing rather than childbearing.

- Fat loss is not an obligatory component of lactation; some women may increase their body fat.

- Behavioural and environmental factors may have an important modulating role on postpartum weight changes and can be significant determinants of weight gain during a reproductive cycle.

- Advice that focuses on the impact of gestational weight gain or postpartum lifestyle and cultural factors may help in the prevention of obesity in women.

- In spite of these associations, it must be stressed that most obese adults were not obese as children and adolescents.

- The prevalence of obesity increases greatly during adulthood, to reach a peak in late middle age.

- There is little evidence that the menopause represents a discrete risk period for extra weight gain, but the loss of oestrogen activity does cause a redistribution of fat towards the visceral region with a consequent increase in WHR.

8
Aetiology of Obesity IV: Metabolic Factors

The energy balance equation, and its central and immutable role in any theories concerning the aetiology of obesity, is discussed in Section 5.1. The following sections describe current knowledge about the possible role of metabolic and physiological factors in the development and maintenance of the obese state. Once again, it must be stressed that such factors may only play a role in certain discrete forms of obesity, or may play only a modulating role in the more recent and widespread problem of adult-onset 'lifestyle' obesity. The interplay between inherent physiological factors (whether they are genetically or phenotypically set) and the complex web of psycho-social and environmental influences, which impact on the problem, must be borne in mind at all times.

8.1 Energy expenditure

Energy expenditure is classically divided into three major components: basal metabolic rate, thermogenesis and activity (Fig. 8.1). Basal metabolic rate (BMR) represents the fundamental running costs of the organism, and includes such factors as respiration, circulation, cellular homeostasis (e.g. ionic pumping) and cellular repair (e.g. protein turnover).

Basal metabolic rate, which represents 60–75% of total energy expenditure in sedentary people, is measured under highly standardised conditions early in the morning, when the subject is at complete rest in a thermoneutral environment and at least 12 hours after the last meal. It is about 5–10% higher than minimal metabolic rate, which occurs

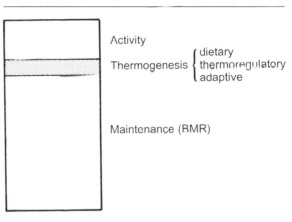

Fig. 8.1 Components of energy expenditure.

during deep sleep (Goldberg *et al.*, 1987). The widespread adherence to these conditions makes it possible to make robust comparisons between different studies and to develop standard predictive equations based on body weight and height (Schofield, 1985). The term resting metabolic rate (RMR) describes analogous measurements made within a shorter interval since the last meal.

The catch-all compartment 'thermogenesis' includes, firstly, any heat production specifically generated for the maintenance of body temperature (thermoregulatory thermogenesis). Secondly, the obligatory heat loss (inefficiency) associated with the absorption, transport and metabolism of recently ingested food (diet-induced thermogenesis, DIT), and finally, a component of heat production which switches on in order to dissipate

61

excess dietary energy as heat (adaptive thermo-genesis or luxus consumption). The first of these is usually of minor importance in humans, because our large body size and resultant low surface area:volume ratio means that normal metabolic processes usually produce enough heat to maintain thermoregulation. Also, we habitually adjust our microenvironment (with clothing and heating) to avoid cold stress. The second component, post-prandial thermogenesis (PPT), is mostly obligatory but does contain a so-called 'facultative' fraction, which is stimulated by sympathetic nervous activity and is non-obligatory (Acheson *et al.*, 1984). The final component, adaptive thermogenesis, is important in some animals but remains con-troversial in terms of its potential importance in the regulation of human energy balance (Section 8.1.2). Some investigators use the term DIT to describe this adaptive thermogenesis, while others use PPT and DIT interchangeably.

The component of energy expenditure allocated to physical activity is self-explanatory. It represents that sum of external Newtonian work performed by a person. In people of the same body weight, the efficiency of work output is somewhat influenced by factors such as fitness, but is actually surprisingly constant. Thus, the main determinant of the energy expended on physical activity is behavioural and relates to people's employment and their choices as to their leisure-time pursuits. As people gain weight, the energy cost of fixed tasks, especially weight-dependent ones, such as climbing stairs, rises in proportion to their mass.

In the 1970s, the perception that overweight and obese people ate similar, or smaller, amounts of food than their lean counterparts precipitated a world-wide search for metabolic, or behavioural, energy-sparing defects, in an attempt to explain this apparent paradox. For many years, such theories dominated obesity (Royal College of Physicians, 1983). The following sections summarise the ensu-ing findings and describe how extensive under-reporting of food intake, by obese and weight-conscious people, in fact, generated the initial paradox.

8.1.1 Basal metabolic rate

There is now universal agreement that BMR is correlated with body weight (Fig. 8.2) and is,

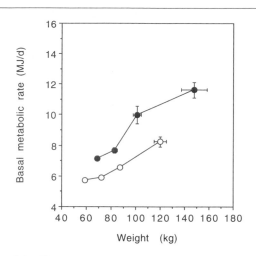

Fig. 8.2 The correlation between BMR and body weight in free-living subjects (from Prentice *et al.*, 1996). Open circles, women; closed circles, men; error bars = SE.

therefore, higher in obese than in non-obese people (Ravussin *et al.*, 1982; Garrow, 1987; Prentice *et al.*, 1989). The reason for this is that the weight gain associated with obesity does not consist only of metabolically inert fat (Forbes & Welle, 1983), a proportion of the additional weight, usually about 25%, is lean tissue. This comprises increases in heart and skeletal muscle, which are necessary for supporting the increased mass, and an enlargement of the digestive tract and liver, which is necessary for the processing of the increased energy flux. This increased mass of muscle and viscera (also termed fat-free mass, FFM) is metabolically active and, therefore, raises BMR.

The issue of whether the observed increase in BMR is entirely in line with the increase in lean tissue is slightly problematic for statistical reasons. Ravussin & Bogardus (1987) have pointed out that it is inappropriate simply to use FFM as the denominator, when adjusting for body size effects, because the FFM to BMR relationship has a non-zero intercept. When this is taken into account, there is little evidence of any constitutive differ-ences between lean and obese people. Garrow and Webster (1985) concluded that it is unlikely that pre-obese people display thrifty metabolisms that become normalised upon weight gain.

A longitudinal follow-up study in Pima Indians found that weight gain was higher in subjects who had a relatively low BMR at baseline (Ravussin *et al.*, 1988). However, this should only be extrapolated with caution, since the finding relates to a group who have very high rates of obesity for reasons other than a low metabolic rate (Ravussin *et al.*, 1993). Also, very few individuals from the total sample contributed to the association between low BMR and high weight gain.

8.1.2 Thermogenesis

Studies in young overfed rodents show that increases in metabolic rate can dissipate much of the extra energy consumed, thereby reducing or even completely inhibiting the deposition of excess body fat. This metabolic response means that they are energetically less efficient; i.e. a greater percentage of food energy is converted to heat through DIT. Genetically obese rats and mice eat more than their lean counterparts, but they are also energetically much more efficient than the lean animals. This means that the obese animals gain more body energy (i.e. fat) than the lean animals, even when they are fed exactly the same amount of food. Furthermore, the obese animals fail to increase DIT in response to overfeeding. The high efficiency, low DIT and excessive fat gains are seen at an age before the animals start to overeat, and show that the primary cause of obesity in these rodent models is a defect in thermogenesis. The excessive food intake is a secondary, but exacerbating, influence on the development of obesity.

The DIT seen in young overfed rodents is almost entirely owing to sympathetic activation of brown adipose tissue (BAT) thermogenesis. DIT can be blocked by inhibitors of sympathetic β-adrenoceptors (e.g. propranolol) and can be mimicked by sympathomimetics (e.g. noradrenaline, ephedrine). In this respect, the increased sympathetic activation of BAT thermogenesis by feeding is almost identical to that seen when animals are exposed to the cold and exhibit increased non-shivering thermogenesis (NST). All of these responses (including NST) are blunted or absent in the genetically-obese rodent models. Moreover, obesity can be induced in normal rodents, simply by interfering with the sympathetic activation of BAT, either by chemical sympathectomy or by genetic ablation of BAT. In either case, the animals increase body weight and fat stores without increasing food intake, thereby

demonstrating the crucial role of DIT, the sympathetic nervous system and BAT in controlling energy balance (for reviews of these animal studies, see Rothwell & Stock 1986; Trayhurn, 1986).

The above conclusions, derived from nearly two decades of detailed animal studies, have been included in this section because they provide unequivocal evidence for a biological body weight control system, operating through thermogenesis. This contrasts with the evidence for such a system operating in humans, which is weak and equivocal, and few would subscribe to the view that human obesity was a result of a thermogenic defect. At the same time, however, it should be remembered that reliable evidence for a pathophysiological defect in the control of energy intake in human obesity is also limited (Chapter 10). Given such uncertainty about possible defects in physiological control systems in human obesity, it would be unwise to discard any explanation for a physiological susceptibility to weight gain. It has been argued that increased food intake could be a secondary response to a decreased energy expenditure and obesity in humans (Trayhurn, 1996).

Most of the evidence implicating a metabolic or thermogenic component to human energy metabolism and obesity relies on establishing links between metabolism and the activity of the sympathetic nervous system (SNS). Table 8.1 provides a summary of the known connections between SNS activity and human energy expenditure. This logical and consistent sequence of established connections between SNS activity and energy expenditure in humans is precisely what one would predict, given the evidence from animal studies. However, all the animal studies have highlighted BAT as the primary thermogenic effector tissue, whereas, the amount and activity of BAT in adult humans is thought to be too small to be of any significance. Nevertheless, very little BAT (less than 40–50 g) will be required to produce a small (e.g. 10%), but significant, effect on daily energy expenditure and there are now some genetic correlations between obesity and aspects of BAT function in humans (Section 6.5). The first of these involves a receptor, the β₃-adrenoceptor, that is found in both white and brown adipose tissue, but its main thermogenic effects depend upon its presence in BAT. There is a mutation (Trp64Arg) in the human gene for this β₃-adrenoceptor. Although there is little difference in

Table 8.1 Evidence linking sympathetic activity with energy expenditure in humans.

1 Catecholamines stimulate metabolic rate.
2 β_3-adrenergic blockade decreases resting metabolic rate, fat oxidation and postprandial thermic responses.
3 Consuming food (particularly high-carbohydrate foods) increases SNS activity and resting metabolic rate.
4 Daily energy expenditure correlates with SNS activity.
5 Energy restriction and weight loss decreases SNS activity and resting metabolic rate.
6 SNS activity during food restriction predicts weight loss.
7 Sympathomimetics (e.g. ephedrine) potentiate weight loss.

the frequency of this mutation, between obese and normal weight subjects, or between normal subjects and those with NIDDM; those NIDDM or obese subjects with the mutation have an earlier onset of the condition. They are also more likely to have abdominal obesity, a lower resting metabolic rate and a greater capacity for weight gain (Walston *et al.*, 1995; Widén *et al.*, 1995; Clément *et al.*, 1995).

A further potential link with BAT thermogenesis has been established with the gene for uncoupling protein (UCP). UCP is a mitochondrial protein unique to BAT and is responsible for this tissue's remarkable capacity for heat production. Recent studies have shown that a UCP gene variant of the Bcl I restriction polymorphism is associated with a propensity to gain weight over a 12-year period (Oppert *et al.*, 1994). The same variant is associated with resistance to weight loss on a low energy diet (Fumeron *et al.*, 1996). Finally, an additive effect of an A > G (–3826) variant of the UCP gene and the Trp64Arg mutation in the 3-adrenoceptor gene (Section 6.5) is associated with greater weight gain in morbid obesity (Clément *et al.*, 1996).

These indirect, and often weak, links between SNS activity, thermogenesis, BAT-specific genes and susceptibility to weight gain require further, more rigorous investigation, but they do show that the well-established genetic component to obesity can be tied-in to aspects of metabolism relevant to energy balance regulation. The quantitative importance of these metabolic links in determining energy balance regulation and susceptibility to obesity in humans is unknown and is likely to be limited. There have been only a few direct experiments to test the ability, or the capacity, of normal adults to exhibit DIT when overfed. Some of the earlier experiments, particularly in young adults fed low-protein diets (Miller & Mumford, 1967; Miller *et al.*, 1967), produced results very similar to those seen in overfed young rodents, namely much lower

weight gains than predicted. However, later studies, carried out with more detailed and accurate measures of changes in body composition and energy expenditure (e.g. Diaz *et al.*, 1992), suggest that adaptive thermogenesis may play only a minor role in adjusting daily energy expenditure to meet increases in energy intake. This does not, however, explain the low weight gains seen in earlier studies, and a case could be made for undertaking further overfeeding studies using low-protein and other unconventional diets.

Even if the capacity for DIT in humans under normal conditions is small, this does not mean that it is unimportant. If it were limited to as little as 10–12% of energy turnover, the loss of this capacity would have a significant impact on energy balance regulation in the long term. It has to be remembered that the physiological controls operating on energy intake are also weak and not very precise. Covert increases in energy intake of more than 10% are required before these are compensated for in subsequent meals or snacks. Thus, it would seem quite reasonable to assume that a capacity to compensate for these errors in intake, by increasing or decreasing energy expenditure to the same extent (10–12%), would result in a more precise control of energy balance regulation because both sides of the energy balance equation would be controlled. Of course, the problem is that this physiological control over expenditure may be able to deal with only up to 10% of energy turnover. It is now clear that even larger increases in daily energy intake can go unnoticed and fail to produce compensatory decreases in the next day's intake (Johnstone *et al.*, 1996).

8.1.3 Physical activity

The activity component of energy expenditure is the most complex and variable. It consists of the integrated sum of all minor physical movements (sometimes described as fidgeting), together with all gross muscular work involved in moving the body or in performing physical work. These activities can be divided into weight-independent activity (e.g. swimming or cycling) and weight-dependent activity (e.g. walking up a slope). The energy cost of the latter is highly correlated with body weight and is, therefore, much higher in the obese (Prentice *et al.*, 1996). In order to visualise this, it is only necessary to note that a person, whose weight is, say, 40 kg heavier than ideal, is constantly carrying around the equivalent of two very heavy suitcases.

Activity can be further divided according to whether it is essentially obligatory (e.g. agricultural work by subsistence farmers) or discretionary (e.g. leisure time sports). In modern societies, where mechanisation is replacing most manual labour, leisure time physical activity is assuming a dominant role in determining energy expenditure (Livingstone *et al.*, 1991). Thus, behavioural and lifestyle choices play the major role in setting the level of energy expended on activity (Chapter 15).

Numerous individual studies (Prentice *et al.*, 1986) and several meta-analyses have shown that the total amount of energy expended on physical activity is generally higher in obese compared to lean people (Fig. 8.3). This contrasts markedly from descriptions of slothfulness in the obese. However, since this is largely owing to the fact that the obese have to expend much more energy in performing identical tasks, it begs the question as to whether overweight people choose to do fewer tasks and might have been less energetic in the pre-obese state. In attempting to answer this, many studies have plotted activity-related energy expenditure divided by body weight, against percent body fat (Bandini *et al.*, 1990; Schoeller & Fjeld, 1991; Rising *et al.*, 1994; Davies *et al.*, 1995). This yields a strong inverse correlation, suggesting that obesity is associated with slothfulness, but it has recently been pointed out that this is an artefact caused by the fact that using body weight as the denominator for activity represents a substantial over-correction (Prentice *et al.*, 1996). Use of the physical activity level index (PAL) partly, but not completely, overcomes this problem by adjusting total energy expenditure (TEE) by BMR. This is shown in Equation (8.1).

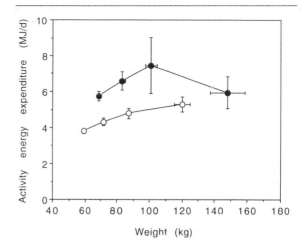

Fig. 8.3 Energy expenditure on physical activity in relation to body weight in free-living subjects (from Prentice *et al.*, 1996). Open circles, women; closed circles, men; error bars = SE.

$$PAL = \frac{TEE}{BMR} \qquad (8.1)$$

Figure 8.4 contains data from 319 doubly labelled water measures of TEE (Prentice *et al.*, 1996). It suggests that there is little evidence that the average obese person is less active than the average lean

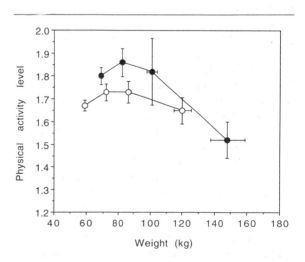

Fig. 8.4 Influence of body weight on total energy expenditure in free-living subjects (from Prentice *et al.*, 1996). Open circles, women; closed circles, men; error bars = SE.

person, until obesity becomes very severe and handicaps the sufferer, at which point there is a definite decline in PAL.

The issue of low levels of physical activity as a possible precipitator of obesity is a complex one. On the one hand, there seems abundant evidence that the general secular trend towards less active lifestyles in affluent countries is a major contributor to the burgeoning levels of obesity in the population as a whole (Prentice & Jebb, 1995; Chapter 15). But on the other hand, there is surprisingly little solid evidence to support the view that exceptional inactivity is a specific predictor of obesity at the individual level. There is an extensive historical literature covering attempts to assess activity levels and to relate these to subsequent weight gain. Ingenious methods were used, such as: time-lapse photography of girls at summer camps, covert observations of stair use versus escalators, use of movement sensors attached to chairs, pedometers, heart-rate monitors, and radar. These techniques suffered from a lack of accurate quantification and no clear consensus has emerged as to whether or not, pre-obese people tend to be particularly inactive.

More recently, it has been possible to accurately assess physical activity either by means of the doubly labelled water ($^2H_2^{18}O$) method, which measures total free-living energy expenditure, or in the artificial, but highly reproducible, conditions of a whole-body calorimeter (Prentice *et al.*, 1991a). Two detailed prospective studies have used these techniques to try to relate activity levels to future weight gain. In Pima Indians, Ravussin *et al.* (1993) noted that the energy expended on minor spontaneous physical movements (fidgeting), by subjects in a calorimeter, was significantly related within families and that a low level of fidgeting was a predictor of future weight gain. Once again, this finding should be extrapolated with some caution since the low level of fidgeting was not the primary cause of weight gain, but rather was an accelerating influence in a population already predisposed to obesity. The second study used doubly labelled water to assess energy expenditure in the 3-month-old babies of lean and obese parents (Roberts *et al.*, 1988). This study reported low levels of activity and thermogenesis (calculated as TEE minus BMR) in 6 babies who went on to become overweight at 1-year of age. This study suffers from a very small sample size and on-going attempts to replicate it are so far proving unsuccessful.

Larger scale cross-sectional and prospective epidemiological studies addressing the linkage between activity and obesity are discussed in Chapter 15.

8.1.4 Total energy expenditure

Summation of each of the above components gives total energy expenditure, which is ultimately the key variable on the output side of the energy balance equation. As in the case of physical activity, this can most accurately be measured using whole-body calorimetry or the doubly labelled water method.

Measurements made in a whole-body calorimeter do not represent real life, but have the great advantage that subjects can be asked to follow a strictly defined activity protocol. This permits investigation of the underlying physiological determinants of energy expenditure without interference from any behavioural 'noise' (Prentice *et al.*, 1991a). It also allows minute-by-minute measurements, which can discriminate diurnal patterns (e.g. sleep, BMR, arousal and exercise) and the different components of expenditure such as the post-prandial increment. Figure 8.5 shows a typical comparison of the energy expenditure of lean and obese subjects in a whole-body calorimeter (Prentice *et al.*, 1989). It is clear that the obese person has a much **higher** energy expenditure at all times of the day than the lean person, thus running quite contrary to the 'energy sparing defect' hypothesis. Figure 8.6 shows values for 24-hour energy expenditure in groups of women at three levels of fatness: ideal body weight (IBW); IBW + 50%; and IBW + 100%. Although there is a variance of about 8% in each group, it is evident that all of the overweight subjects have a much higher expenditure than the lean subjects. There are no cases of exceptionally low levels of expenditure, which could explain patients' claimed inability to lose weight on low energy diets. These findings have been replicated in research centres around the world and no single case of exceptionally low energy expenditure has yet been found (Ravussin *et al.*, 1982; Schutz *et al.*, 1982; Prentice *et al.*, 1986; Jequier, 1989; Prentice *et al.*, 1989).

Potential behavioural differences between lean

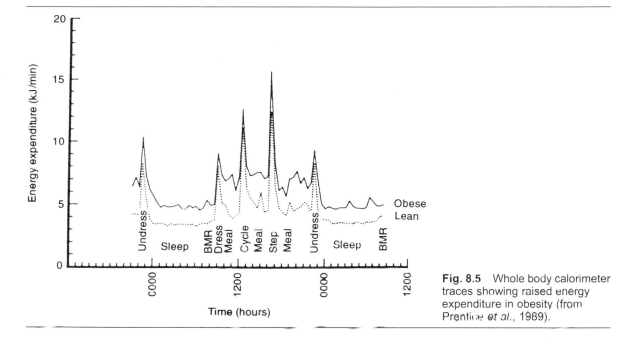

Fig. 8.5 Whole body calorimeter traces showing raised energy expenditure in obesity (from Prentice *et al.*, 1989).

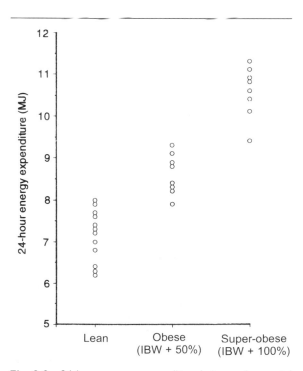

Fig. 8.6 24-hour energy expenditure in lean, obese and super-obese subjects (IBW = ideal body weight) (from Prentice *et al.*, 1989).

and obese subjects can be assessed using doubly-labelled water, which provides an accurate estimate of free-living TEE with minimal interference to the subject (IDECG, 1990). Figure 8.7 illustrates a compilation of results from 319 men and women, divided into 4 categories of BMI (Prentice *et al.*, 1996). It shows that TEE rises progressively, with increasing BMI, and reaches levels of over 13 MJ/d (>3000 kcal/d) in obese women and 18 MJ/d (>4000 kcal/d) in obese men. These are values derived from people with established obesity and reflect the high-energy cost of supporting and moving such high body weights. They do not indicate whether TEE was likely to have differed in the pre-obese state, except by inference; it being highly unlikely that people with abnormally low TEEs, prior to obesity, would actually increase their weight-adjusted TEE as they became fatter. One way around this problem is to measure TEE in post-obese people. Several studies have attempted this with rather mixed results. Astrup (1996) has performed a meta-analysis from which he concludes that TEE is very slightly lower in the post-obese (~5%). However, it must be remembered that weight-loss has a suppressive effect on metabolism (Prentice *et al.*, 1991b) and on physical activity (Prentice *et al.*, 1992), and that this might

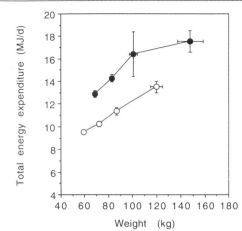

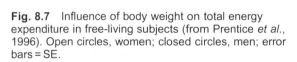

Fig. 8.7 Influence of body weight on total energy expenditure in free-living subjects (from Prentice *et al.*, 1996). Open circles, women; closed circles, men; error bars = SE.

still influence TEE in post-obese restrained subjects for long periods after weight loss.

8.2 Summary

- The main components of energy expenditure and their approximate proportions in sedentary people are basal metabolic rate (~65%), thermogenesis (~10%) and physical activity (~25%).

- Basal metabolic rate is generally **higher** in overweight and obese people because weight gain increases lean tissue mass (muscle and visceral organs) as well as fat. Cases of extraordinarily low BMR in obese patients have yet to be found.

- Small animals show clear differences in thermogenesis between lean and obese individuals. Some evidence suggests that obese humans have a lower diet-induced thermogenesis, but support is waning for the view that this is a likely causal factor.

- The energy expended on a fixed activity is always higher for people carrying extra weight. Combined with the raised BMR this means that obese people generally have much **higher** total energy expenditure than lean people.

- There is some evidence that low levels of spontaneous physical activity are a familial trait, which may predispose to obesity. This adds to the more general finding that low societal levels of activity are an important risk factor, which correlates well with the secular trend in obesity (Chapter 15).

9
Aetiology of Obesity V: Macronutrient Balance

In recent years, interest has developed concerning the question of whether, or not, it might be more useful to separate the classic energy balance equation into four component equations, separately representing each of the energy-giving macronutrients; fat, carbohydrate, protein and alcohol (Prentice, 1995a; Stubbs, 1995). As indicated below, this has an advantage in terms of understanding how the system is regulated, but can be confusing if not explained in sufficient depth. It is essential to understand the fact that viewing the problem from the macronutrient balance perspective does not invalidate any aspects of the basic energy balance equation which, as has been stated before, is the one absolutely secure cornerstone on which any theories about the aetiology of obesity must be built. A kilojoule is always a kilojoule, even though one derived from fat may have a different metabolic effect to one derived from carbohydrate.

9.1 Differences in macronutrient absorption

Many obese people claim that they do not overeat and that they must, therefore, be much more efficient at extracting energy from food. There is little support for this view, the main reason being that energy extraction from food is extremely efficient even in lean people. The classic studies of Atwater, resulting in the 'Atwater Factors' for converting the gross energy contents of foods into their metabolisable energies, and the later extension of these studies (Southgate & Durnin, 1970), show that

available carbohydrates are completely absorbed, that fat is 96–97% absorbed (except in pathological states) and that protein is over 90% absorbed. Resistant carbohydrates are less available but their intakes in western diets are very low. Thus, there is little room for improving on the digestion efficiencies of lean people and there is no clear evidence of any systematic differences between lean and obese subjects (Prentice, 1995b).

9.2 The macronutrient balance equation and oxidative hierarchy

Figure 9.1 presents a scheme of the energy balance equation divided into separate compartments and listed in a particular order according to the 'oxidative hierarchy' (see over). This scheme acknowledges that the original view, that all macronutrients form a readily inter-convertible energy currency within the body, was overly simplistic. Perhaps the key breakthrough in support of this more refined concept, was the finding that *de novo* fat synthesis is a relatively rare event in humans (Hachey *et al.*, 1989; Hellerstein *et al.*, 1991; Leitch & Jones, 1993) and that most deposited fat is, therefore, derived directly from dietary fat, under normal circumstances. This places a partial division between fats and carbohydrates, in the post-absorptive state, and demonstrates that the initial source of any dietary energy does have significance in terms of its metabolic fate.

The third column in Fig. 9.1 lists what are thought to be the key factors in determining how the body

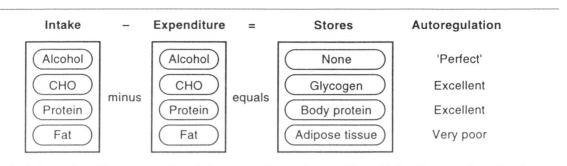

Fig. 9.1 Scheme describing macronutrient balance equations in terms of the oxidative hierarchy (from Prentice 1995a). Note that there is no particular significance to the order in which carbohydrate and protein are illustrated; both show good autoregulation. The key feature is that fat is at the bottom of the hierarchy.

regulates macronutrient balance, namely the storage capacity (Flatt, 1987a; Prentice 1995b). Alcohol comes at the top of the oxidative hierarchy because the body has no way of storing it and because it is a toxin that can only be eliminated by oxidation (Prentice, 1995a). When alcohol is ingested, it immediately stimulates alcohol oxidation and forces the suppression of oxidation of the other macronutrients (Shelmet *et al.*, 1988; Reinus *et al.*, 1989) because total energy expenditure is only marginally raised (Sonko *et al.*, 1994; Suter *et al.*, 1992). The body will clear alcohol within about six hours of ingesting a moderate load and the auto-regulation of alcohol 'balance' is therefore described as 'perfect'. Carbohydrate comes next in the hierarchy with a tight auto-regulatory linkage between levels of intake and oxidation made imperative through the body's small storage capacity for carbohydrate (as glycogen) and its need to always ensure an adequate supply of glucose in the bloodstream (Flatt, 1987a). Protein comes close to carbohydrate, again because the body has limited capacity for short-term storage of amino acids or protein, in any labile form. As with carbohydrate, this makes it imperative for the organism to maintain a close auto-regulation between intake and oxidation. The relative levels of carbohydrate and protein in this hierarchy are a matter of some debate (Stubbs, 1995; Jebb *et al.*, 1996), but this is not critical to the overall understanding of macro-nutrient regulation. Finally, fat comes firmly at the base of the oxidative hierarchy and stands quite distinct from the other macronutrients in so far as there is virtually no auto-regulatory drive from fat intake onto fat oxidation (Prentice, 1995b). The

teleological explanation for this is that fat has been selected as the most efficient means of storing energy, and humans have developed a virtually infinite capacity to expand adipose stores under conditions of excess intake. Thus, fat is the one macronutrient in which there is no imperative to regulate balance.

9.3 Short-term regulation of fat balance

The position of fat at the base of the oxidative hierarchy is critical to explaining why fat balance is often so poorly maintained in humans. Numerous experiments have demonstrated that human metabolism is highly competent at adjusting the metabolic fuel mix being oxidised; in order to bring alcohol, carbohydrate and protein utilisation rates into line with levels of ingestion (McNeill *et al.*, 1992; Shetty *et al.*, 1994; Prentice, 1995b). Total energy expenditure over a 24-hour period, i.e. total substrate oxidation, is little affected by the macro-nutrient mix ingested even over the maximum practical range of fat-to-carbohydrate ratios (Thomas *et al.*, 1992; Shetty *et al.*, 1994). Therefore, fat oxidation is determined totally by the levels of oxidation of the other fuels; when oxidation levels are high, fat utilisation is suppressed, and vice versa.

The above arguments explain why the short-term regulation of fat balance is poorly controlled. They are probably implicated in the fact that fat has a low satiety index (Weststrate, 1992) and also in the phenomenon of the hyperphagia associated with a high fat intake (Chapter 10).

9.4 Long-term regulation of fat balance

The extent to which body fat stores exert a longer-term influence on food intake and energy balance in humans remains unclear. Small animal experiments involving surgical removal of fat (lipectomy) show that compensatory responses result in surprisingly accurate regulation of total body fat and energy content (Chouverakis & Hojniki, 1974). Other experiments indicate that the overall state of energy balance can be re-set by hypothalamic lesions, but is rather accurately regulated at these 'pre-set' or 're-set' levels and will return there after any experimental perturbations, such as temporary food restriction or forced overfeeding by gavage (Rothwell & Stock, 1979). In addition, several well-known genetic abnormalities result in profound disturbances of energy balance (Chapter 6). Any genetic variants, with the capacity to suppress food intake, would tend to be rapidly lethal, and so the obesity variants predominate.

The exact molecular mechanisms underlying these defects are rapidly being uncovered. In this respect, the elucidation of the mechanisms involved in leptin signalling have generated renewed interest into the concept of an 'adipostat', which may control a set point of body weight (Rink, 1994; see also Chapter 10). In the case of leptin, the necessary components of at least one adipocyte detector-effector control pathway have been elucidated in animal models (Frühbeck *et al.*, 1998), and other energy homeostatic mechanisms may follow. For instance, it is now clear that adipose tissue can be considered to be an active endocrine organ releasing peptides capable of humoral signalling, which may impact on regulation of energy balance as well as influencing the pathophysiological sequelae of obesity (Hotamisligil & Spiegelman, 1994; Sniderman & Cianflone, 1994).

9.5 Summary

- The primary macronutrients (carbohydrate, fat, protein and alcohol) supply energy through separate, but interlocking, metabolic pathways. This has important implications for understanding how energy balance is regulated.

- The classic energy balance equation can usefully be broken down into separate equations describing the balance of each macronutrient. This reveals different control processes related to the body's storage capacity for each fuel.

- For alcohol, carbohydrate and protein there are efficient auto-regulatory processes, which automatically adjust oxidation rates to match intake. This process is almost totally absent for fat, giving it a special adipogenic potential.

- An 'oxidative hierarchy' exists, by which alcohol, carbohydrate and protein dominate oxidative pathways and readily suppress fat oxidation. In this way, they can lead to lipid storage through a fat sparing effect.

10
Aetiology of Obesity VI: Appetite Control, Physiological Factors

The central role of the hypothalamus in the regulation of mammalian feeding behaviours has been known for decades, together with many of the details of the neuronal networks responsible for afferent and efferent signalling. More recent discoveries have started to reveal how humoral factors such as insulin and glucagon, gut-derived peptides, melatonin, leptin and cytokines modulate hypothalamic function, and hence also control appetite and satiety (e.g. Clark *et al.*, 1984; Tartaglia *et al.*, 1995; Fan *et al.*, 1997; Huszar *et al.*, 1997). However, there is still much to be learnt about the finer details of the complex neuroendocrine controls of energy balance and, as yet, there are no clear leads linking specific defects in appetite control to the majority of human obesity cases. There are, however, clear mechanisms emerging in most of the monogenic animal models of obesity, and some very rare cases of the human analogues of these conditions have now been identified (Jackson *et al.*, 1997; Montague *et al.*, 1997a). Each of these monogenic rodent obesity cases has a clear defect in appetite control, which almost certainly represents the primary reason for the obesity. It is interesting, however, that defects in appetite regulation and in energy expenditure usually seem to go hand in hand, and in some cases the latter may appear first (Stock, 1999).

It is worth noting at the outset that one of the reasons that it has proved so difficult to establish a full picture of all of the neuroendocrine pathways involved in feeding control is because of the great complexity of the system. It involves numerous parallel mechanisms each of which may play a dominant part under different physiological conditions. It has also become clear that there are multiple redundancies within the system, such that if one pathway fails others can take over. This was graphically demonstrated by the fact that transgenic mice lacking neuropeptide Y (NPY) had entirely normal body weight and composition in spite of the fact that NPY is the most potent known appetite stimulant (Erickson *et al.*, 1996) and the virtual lack of effect of liver denervation on food intake, meal patterns or weight gain provides another example (Langhans & Scharrer, 1992). Under such conditions, it will be readily appreciated that it is difficult to track down what may be subtle differences in the susceptibility of individuals to the external (adipogenic) environment.

A detailed review of all the evidence linking the physiological regulation of human food intake to obesity would be beyond the scope of this chapter, and would be premature since there is no leading theory linking potential defects in the system to obesity. The following sections, therefore, provide a brief summary and some guidance on further reading. The regulatory systems are reviewed on a temporal basis from meal-to-meal, through day-to-day to long-term regulation of food intake.

10.1 Meal-to-meal regulation of food intake

10.1.1 Basic principles

Although the availability of food may often influence feeding behaviour, leading to opportunistic eating, many mammals have discrete meal-eating patterns that may vary in interval from a few minutes in some of the smallest rodents to several days in large carnivores. These behaviours are influenced by external cues, such as the light/dark cycle and day length. In traditional societies, humans generally have rather fixed meal times ranging from three to five meals daily (Langhans & Scharrer, 1992), though this is increasingly being substituted by a 'grazing' pattern of eating in modern societies.

Blundell has devised a formalised scheme (the satiety cascade reproduced in Fig. 10.1) to describe the various influences that may control the inter-meal interval and the amount of food consumed at a subsequent meal (Blundell & Halford, 1998). The sensations regulating feeding are divided into hunger (the drive to eat), appetite (the desire to eat particular foods), satiation (the feeling of fullness which terminates a meal) and satiety (the feeling of repletion that inhibits future hunger). These sensations can co-exist with varying intensity and in complex ways that are heavily influenced by factors in the external environment, such as the sight and smell of food, and the physical setting. There can frequently be paradoxical aspects to these sensations, such as the fact that 'appetisers' or 'aperitifs' may promote prospective appetite rather than inhibit it, and the fact that total satiation with one food (e.g. a main course) can be immediately followed by appetite for another (e.g. a dessert). This phenomenon is known as 'sensory-specific satiety' (Rolls *et al.*, 1981).

In humans, the underlying physiological controls described by Blundell's satiety cascade are deeply embedded beneath multiple levels of social conditioning. Animal experiments have often been used in an attempt to get clearer insights into the regulatory mechanisms. The fact that rats usually eat 8–12 meals per day, when food is freely available, gives some concern about the relevance of certain aspects of these studies, though they remain very useful in elucidating the detailed neuroendocrine pathways (Langhans & Scharrer, 1992).

10.1.2 Metabolite availability and oxidation

Langhans & Scharrer (1992) have extensively reviewed the topics covered in this section.

i Glucose

The primary function of eating is to replete the energy and nutrient stores used up since the last meal. It is, therefore, logical to expect that mechanisms will have evolved to monitor peripheral substrate stores (e.g. in liver, muscle and adipose tissue) and to send afferent signals to the hypothalamic control centre to modulate eating behaviour. Circulating metabolite levels in blood and plasma provide the simplest possible candidates for a signalling pathway. In the past, there has been considerable interest in glucose, free fatty acid and amino acid levels (Langhans & Scharrer, 1992 give a detailed review).

In the early 1950s, Mayer proposed the 'glucostatic' theory which postulated the existence of glucose-sensitive chemoreceptors to act as a stimulus for hunger or satiety (Mayer, 1953). In rats, there is evidence that a decrease in blood glucose level is among the physiological signals that triggers the onset of feeding (Louis-Sylvestre & LeMagnen, 1980), but attempts to detect a similar response in humans have often failed (e.g. Pollak *et al.*, 1989). This may be because it is difficult to measure metabolite levels frequently, at the same time as observing normal feeding behaviour. There is considerable evidence that intragastric administration of glucose suppresses food intake in rats (e.g. Booth & Jarman, 1976). Intravenous administration is less effective but the effect is potentiated by concomitant carbohydrate intake (Novin *et al.*, 1985). Simultaneous administration of insulin appears to increase the satiating power of glucose, suggesting a role for glucose utilisation in the effect (Even & Nicolaidis, 1986). The interplay of these effects has created recent interest in the relationship between the glycemic index of foods and their satiating power (Holt *et al.*, 1996).

A potential role for hepatic glucosensors in the control of eating has also been extensively studied since it was first proposed by Russek (1963) who reported that intraportal, but not intrajugular infusion of glucose suppressed eating. Although many subsequent studies have yielded equivocal results, the work of Tordoff & Friedman is generally accepted as conclusive support to the theory (Tordoff & Friedman, 1986; Langhans & Scharrer, 1992). It is suggested that intraportally infused glucose forms the basis for the acquisition of a

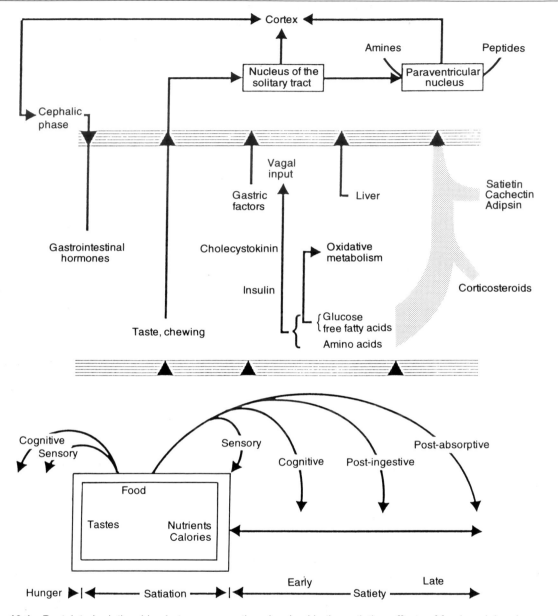

Fig. 10.1 Postulated relationships between operations involved in the satiating effects of food, peripheral psychological events and important appetite loci of the CNS (from Blundell & Halford, 1998).

learned eating behaviour, and it may be for this reason that hepatic vagotomy is without major effects on body weight (Langhans & Scharrer, 1992).

Friedman has proposed the theory that it is the oxidation rate of metabolites in the liver and other peripheral tissues that regulates hunger (Friedman & Tordoff, 1986; Friedman *et al.*, 1990; Friedman, 1997). Stubbs (1995) has advanced this theory to suggest that the position of macronutrients in the so-called 'oxidative hierarchy' (alcohol → carbohydrate → protein → fat) governs the satiating power. However, the evidence for this remains inconclusive. In all these discussions, it is worth re-emphasising that it is inappropriate to search for a single unifying theory of appetite control since there are several overlapping mechanisms.

ii Free fatty acids, triacylglycerols and glycerol

It has been suggested that circulating fuels, whose levels may reflect adiposity, could regulate food intake (Kennedy, 1953). Changes in plasma concentration and utilisation of free fatty acids and glycerol have, therefore, been implicated (LeMagnen, 1983, 1985). Langhans & Scharrer (1992) provide an extensive review of the evidence. They conclude that, although fatty acid oxidation contributes to the maintenance of postprandial satiety, it is as yet unproven that physiological fluctuations in fatty acid oxidation play a role in meal-to-meal control of eating.

Meal-derived or infused triacylglycerols have a rather weak satiating effect (Langhans & Scharrer, 1992). This is assumed to be because long-chain fats are channelled preferentially towards storage, rather than oxidation, as indicated both by their lack of effect on post-meal respiratory quotient (Flatt *et al.*, 1985) and by the observed meal-induced increase in lipoprotein lipase (West *et al.*, 1989).

Various other metabolic fuels have been proposed to signal hunger and satiety according to their circulating levels in plasma. Langhans & Scharrer (1992) found that glycerol, malate, D-3-hydroxybutyrate, lactate and pyruvate all reduced food intake after injection in rats, but dihydroxyacetone, oxaloacetate and acetoacetate failed to have an effect. The effects on food intake were greater than that required for caloric compensation for the injected energy, and hence the findings are interpreted as supporting theories which implicate the rate of energy production in the control of food intake (Friedman & Stricker, 1976; Nicolaidis & Rowland, 1976).

Glycerol has been another obvious candidate, as a possible metabolic regulator, because it is released from adipose tissue together with fatty acids. However, although an infused glycerol dose suppresses hunger, it usually does this at supraphysiological levels, and Ramirez & Friedman (1982) have excluded it as a metabolic signal. As

with infusion of other single metabolites, interpretation of the results is limited by the unphysiological nature of single fuel elevations.

iii Amino acids

Circulating amino acids have frequently been implicated in the control of appetite in both animals and man, as administration of balanced amino acid preparations suppresses food intake (Mellinkoff *et al.*, 1956). At high doses, this may occur as a result of an ammonia toxicity effect, but at lower doses there are other mechanisms involved (Simson & Booth, 1973).

Of particular prominence in the field of human obesity has been Wurtman's theory that the plasma ratio of tryptophan to large neutral amino acids controls carbohydrate and protein selection, by influencing levels of the brain neurotransmitter, serotonin (Fernstrom *et al.*, 1979). This theory remains controversial (Peters & Harper, 1981).

10.1.3 Neuroendocrine regulation of food intake

A detailed coverage of the rapidly developing discoveries in the field of neuroendocrine control of feeding is beyond the scope of this chapter and would be made rapidly obsolete by the pace of new discoveries. Liebowitz & Hoebel (1998) have written a detailed and well-referenced recent review of the background knowledge.

10.1.4 Gastric emptying and gastro-intestinal satiety signals

The rate of gastric emptying appears to be greater in obese people relative to lean controls, as is the volume of the stomach itself. Wisen & Hellstrom (1995) suggest that the larger gastric volume of obese people means that appropriate satiety signals are not triggered in response to gastric distension. Intestinal transit time is similar in lean and obese subjects. Sensitivity to cholecystokinin (CCK) is decreased in obesity, and plasma concentrations of somatostatin and neurotensin are lower in obese relative to lean controls. Wisen & Hellstrom suggest that these changes favour rapid intestinal absorption in obesity and decreased satiety in response to ingested food. It may be that these factors when combined with impaired post-absorptive processing of nutrients (e.g. insulin resistance) favour high levels of energy intake and the maintenance of the obese state. There is less evidence to suggest that these changes caused obesity in the first place.

There is very little evidence, therefore, that the obese state has been caused by defects in the physiological signals that influence appetite, except in a minority of extreme conditions (e.g. Prader–Willi syndrome). As Blundell has pointed out, many so-called satiety signals are mechanisms that have other primary functions, e.g. gastric emptying, nutrient oxidation. It is not, therefore, surprising to see a number of alterations in the functioning of these components of satiety, when body composition changes from the lean to the obese state. It is unclear whether these changes even represent physiological defects, as some changes may actually be adaptive responses to the obese state (e.g. insulin resistance). There is less evidence of physiological defects occurring in pre-obese subjects, which increase appetite (or weaken satiety) and subsequently promote the development of the obese state. This is not surprising because energy balance is determined by an on-going interaction between physiology and behaviour. This view suggests that certain behavioural changes which lead to the development of obesity (e.g. a change to a more sedentary lifestyle, selection of a high-fat diet) may also produce some of the physiological differences that are apparent between the lean and the obese. Some of these physiological changes that have occurred in the development of obesity may also promote its maintenance, e.g. increased rate of gastric emptying, adaptation to a high-fat diet and insulin resistance. Understanding these mechanisms and designing appropriate interventions may be of value in reversing the obese state.

10.1.5 Social influences on meal pattern in humans

The work of de Castro has illuminated many of the psycho-social correlates of feeding behaviour in man. By means of detailed analysis of the meal size and pattern in free-living individuals self-recording their intake, de Castro has documented the most important external influences. He uses the terms 'satiety quotient' and 'hunger quotient' to sum-marise the retrospective and prospective effects of individual meals on meal patterns (de Castro & de Castro, 1989; de Castro, 1990). Significant pre- and post-meal inverse correlations between meal size and interval reveal the expected underlying physiological regulation of eating, but this is easily disrupted by the external context of eating (Langhans & Scharrer, 1992).

De Castro's work demonstrates clear inter-individual differences in feeding behaviours. Studies in twins suggest that these have a strong genetic component which outweighs familial entrainment effects (de Castro, 1997). Nonetheless, the social setting in which food is consumed heavily influences most people. One of the most potent of these effects is a strong positive correlation between meal size and the number of people present, described by de Castro as 'social facilitation' of eating (de Castro, 1990). Religious and social convention (feasting and fasting) will also affect patterns of consumption, and some of these may ultimately contribute to long-term weight change. However, more potent effects (by virtue of their ever presence) can be achieved by modern food manufacturers and retailers, who have achieved high levels of sophistication in inducing people to eat when not hungry, and to over-consume at particular times. The role of television advertising of high-fat energy-dense convenience foods to young children, for example, has been highlighted as a particularly damaging practice (Dibb, 1993; Dibb & Castel, 1995). Chapter 14 discusses these issues further and addresses the role of palatability.

The macronutrient composition of individual meals can also influence consumption at a subsequent meal. These effects have been extensively studied, using experiments involving a covertly manipulated pre-load, followed by an *ad libitum* test meal at which voluntary intake is quantified (Rolls *et al.*, 1994). Such studies have generally shown that protein is the most satiating of the macronutrients, followed by carbohydrate and then fat, with the place of alcohol in this hierarchy still in dispute (Weststrate, 1991; Stubbs, 1995). A limited ability to auto-regulate future intake after varying fat pre-loads, especially in obese, post-obese and restrained women, has emerged as the most consistent finding (Rolls *et al.*, 1994). One of the problems with all such studies is that they are very dependent on the imposed interval between pre-load and test meal, and they are also conducted outside a normal social context.

10.2 Day-to-day regulation of food intake

Since there is no clear distinction between body weight regulation taking place over a number of days and over longer periods, this section should be read in conjunction with Section 10.3.

10.2.1 The glycogenostatic theory of appetite control

In recent years Flatt's glycogenostatic theory of weight regulation has dominated theories about day-to-day regulation (Flatt, 1987a,b). This works on the precept that the need to maintain an equilibrium in carbohydrate status will drive fuel selection and appetite, since labile carbohydrate stores are so much smaller than fat stores and will, therefore, suffer a proportionately greater perturbation whenever energy reserves are out of balance. Flatt's experiments in mice have shown that the previous day's carbohydrate imbalance is the most powerful predictor of prospective food intake (Flatt, 1987b). However, careful experiments using whole-body calorimetry to manipulate and monitor changes in glycogen status have shown that subsequent food intake was unaffected by

large imposed changes in glycogen status (Stubbs *et al.*, 1995b; Shetty *et al.*, 1994)

10.2.2 High-fat hyperphagia and passive over-consumption

One of the most consistently reproducible observations on human feeding behaviour involves the phenomenon of high-fat hyperphagia. Medium- to long-term experiments (ranging from 1 day to 11 weeks) have frequently shown that, if subjects are asked to eat freely from diets that have been covertly manipulated to have a range of fat contents, then they will over-consume energy at high-fat concentrations (Duncan *et al.*, 1987; Lissner *et al.*, 1987; Stubbs *et al.*, 1995a,b). Figure 10.2 illustrates this effect for a single representative subject fed ostensibly identical diets containing 20, 40 or 60% fat by energy, while confined to a whole-body calorimeter. This technique allows accurate measurements of fat balance (Stubbs *et al.*, 1995a). Figure 10.3 translates the group mean data from this study into overall energy imbalances (left-hand values) and shows analogous data from 14-day experiments conducted in free-living volunteers (right-hand values). The figure reveals an important interaction between dietary fat and physical inactivity because, although the treatment effect is similar across different fat levels, there is an offset in terms of absolute energy balance. In the confined

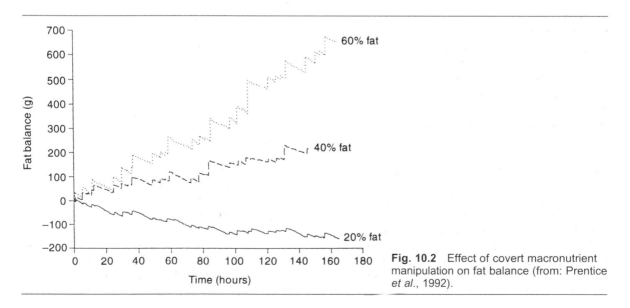

Fig. 10.2 Effect of covert macronutrient manipulation on fat balance (from: Prentice *et al.*, 1992).

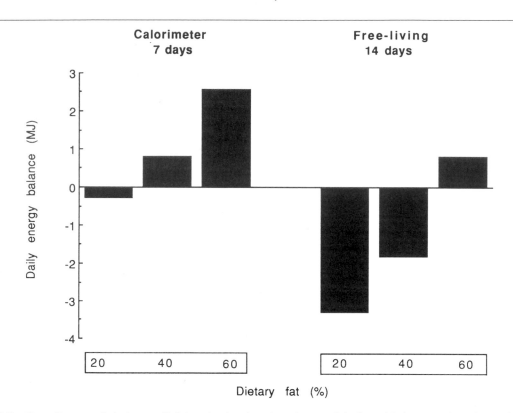

Fig. 10.3 Overall energy imbalances (left-hand values) and analogous data from 14 day experiments conducted on free-living volunteers (right-hand values) (from Prentice & Poppitt, 1996).

state the 40% diet induced a positive energy balance, whereas it did not in the free-living state.

The reason for high-fat hyperphagia is that the subjects in all these experiments tend to consume a weight of food that remains similar across treatments and has presumably been habitually entrained over many years. As a consequence of this failure to down-regulate the amount of food eaten in concordance with its energy density, there is an accidental over-consumption of fat and energy on the high-fat diets. For this reason, this situation has been termed 'passive over-consumption' (Blundell & Macdiarmid, 1997). Further experiments, in which the energy density of diets have been artificially maintained at a constant level, in spite of different fat levels (Stubbs, 1995; van Stratum *et al.*, 1978), have shown that high-fat hyperphagia is not a specific attribute of fat, but results from the normally high correlation between fat content and energy density of foods (Poppitt & Prentice, 1996).

10.3 Long-term body weight regulation

There has recently been renewed interest in the concept of lipostatic factors regulating the adipose tissue mass, with the unravelling of the leptin system (Zhang *et al.*, 1994) (see also Section 6.5.1 and 6.5.2). Leibel *et al.* (1995) noted that establishing a feedback link between adipose tissue and food intake required support for the concept that the anatomically dispersed fat depots are in some way integrated into a unitary adipose tissue mass. This is the case for myeloid tissues and also bone in the regulation of calcium status. It is not yet clear whether the same is true for fat mass, but it appears that it may be so. It is also of interest that leptin occurs at much higher levels in the plasma of obese subjects (Considine *et al.*, 1995). The same is true for insulin (Karam *et al.*, 1963; Bogardus *et al.*, 1985). As the higher level of plasma insulin in obese subjects is caused by insulin resistance, the concept of leptin resistance in obese subjects has been developed (Frederich *et al.*, 1995). Furthermore, it appears that high-fat diets (Storlien *et al.*, 1986), especially diets high in saturates (Storlien *et al.*, 1991), induce insulin resistance in rodents and possibly in humans (Borkman *et al.*, 1993). High-fat diets also appear to induce leptin resistance in rats (Frederich *et al.*, 1995). Clearly, then, by the time obesity has developed, both the leptin system and the entero-insular axis appear to have been perturbed. It may be that these changes or 'defects' are not causally involved in the development of the obese state, but that they are important for the maintenance of the obese state. It is interesting that a number of laboratory studies suggest that in the short- to medium-term there is little negative feedback from the fat mass in limiting an excess of energy intake. Indeed, in one human study where the potential for nutrient balance to feedback and influence subsequent days' energy balance was investigated, fat balance exerted the least potential negative feedback on subsequent energy intake (Stubbs *et al.*, 1995a).

10.3.1 Set point theory

Genetically pure laboratory rodents, fed a uniform laboratory 'chow', follow a predictable trajectory of body weight throughout life. If they are temporarily overfed, or underfed, they gain or lose weight but, when returned to *ad libitum* feeding, they will (after a week or so) return to the original trajectory. This establishes that, for this animal in these circumstances, there is a physiological 'set point' for body weight. The discovery of leptin (see Sections 6.5.1 and 6.5.2) provides a possible explanation of how this feedback regulation can be established.

Researchers into human obesity have suggested that a similar set point determines human body weight (Keesey, 1986). Leibel *et al.* (1995) reviewed changes in human energy expenditure associated with changes in body weight and comment 'Body weight in adults is remarkably stable over long periods of time'. Wilding (1997) claims that, normally, 'Body weight is very tightly regulated'.

Sound data in support of this contention are, however, not abundant. In the Nurses Health Study (Willett *et al.*, 1995), there were clearly more women whose weight changed by more than 5 kg over 14 years follow-up than those whose weight

changed by less than 5 kg, suggesting that changing more than 5 kg is 'normal'.

This finding is not explained by reported errors, or any peculiarity of nurses, because the early data from Framingham show a mean change (maximum–minimum) of 10 kg over the first 10 examinations (i.e. 18 years) for both men and women (Gordon & Kannel, 1973). The average weight of the subjects did not change much over the 18 years, because gainers and losers cancel each other out. Similar observations come from Finland (Rissanen *et al.*, 1991).

Regulation of body weight within limits of 10 kg is no better than could be achieved by cognitive control. An experimentally induced weight change of more than 5 kg cannot fail to be perceived by the subject, even if he is being weighed 'blind' (Garrow & Stalley 1975, 1977). It is, therefore, not necessary to postulate a physiological regulation of body weight to a 'set point' to explain the relative constancy of body weight in adults, nor is it necessary to postulate a defect in this 'set point' to explain human obesity.

Flatt prefers the concept of a 'settling point', in which body weight adjusts until energy intake and expenditure reach a dynamic equilibrium. The point at which this occurs will depend on numerous factors, including the subject's propensity to metabolise fat versus carbohydrate as the preferred fuel, the subject's level of exercise and their dietary habits. The key distinction between a 'set point' and a 'settling-point' is that the former envisages a system of sensor and effector mechanisms, which might be genetically determined.

10.4 Evidence from behavioural studies of physiological defects that might lead to obesity

Studies which have examined human feeding behaviour in the natural setting and in response to dietary manipulations have found little evidence that lean and obese people respond differently (Spitzer & Rodin, 1981). In a number of studies, however, obese people appear to eat less than their lean counterparts. This is thought to be because of the greater prevalence of dietary under-reporting that occurs in obese people when their feeding is being studied (see Chapter 12). Thomas *et al.* (1992) found that high-fat, energy-dense diets promote higher energy intakes relative to lower fat, less energy-dense diets in both lean and obese subjects. Hill & Blundell have also found that subjective sensations of hunger and fullness are very similar in lean and obese subjects, in response to similar nutrient loads. Furthermore, if the tendency of the obese to lower their energy intakes when studied is taken into account, the obese appear to respond similarly to the lean in a number of studies where the diet is manipulated (Wooley *et al.*, 1972, Spitzer & Rodin 1981; Durrant *et al.*, 1982; Duncan *et al.*, 1987, Thomas *et al.*, 1992). There are, however, some studies which suggest the lean regulate intake more accurately than the obese (e.g. Campbell *et al.*, 1971; Rolls *et al.*, 1994).

10.5 Summary

- Human energy balance is regulated primarily through the modulation of food intake.

- There is physiological control involving appetite, hunger, satiation and satiety, each of which has a different regulatory mechanism.

- These controls occur from meal-to-meal, day-to-day and over the longer term, and involve highly complex interactions between neural and hormonal regulatory systems.

- There is considerable overlap and redundancy between different neuroendocrine pathways modulating food intake.

- In humans, true physiological regulation of food intake is often deeply embedded within social and environmental influences, which can readily lead to dysregulation.

- The phenomenon of high-fat hyperphagia, also referred to as 'passive over-consumption' is readily reproducible in experimental settings and helps to explain the increasing prevalence of obesity.

- There is some evidence of an inability to accurately regulate food intake in obese people, but it is uncertain whether this is a *post hoc* effect.

- There is now evidence that the leptin system plays a role in signalling the size of the fat mass to the hypothalamus, thus providing the messenger of an adipostatic system. But the precise details of this system and its physiological significance in human weight control remain to be fully elucidated.

11
Aetiology of Obesity VII:
Endocrine Causes

Despite popular belief, there is little evidence that classical endocrine or hormonal disorders 'cause' obesity. In general, endocrine alterations in obesity are secondary as they can be induced by overfeeding and reversed by weight loss (Sims *et al.,* 1973). Even where an endocrine disorder is causally associated with obesity, the clinical presentation is usually related to specific consequences of the hormonal state rather than weight gain.

11.1 Genetic disorders linking obesity and endocrinopathies

A number of rare genetic syndromes in which obesity develops alongside endocrine alterations have been identified (Beales & Kopelman, 1996). The fact that the neural pathways that influence body weight and those controlling hypothalamic–pituitary function are closely adjacent to each other, may account for the frequent co-existence of obesity and endocrine abnormalities. The mechanistic associations are, however, unknown.

11.1.1 Prader–Willi syndrome

This rare disorder, incidence 1 in 25 000 of the population (Prader *et al.,* 1956), is associated with a partial deletion of the long arm of chromosome 15 (Ledbetter *et al.,* 1981). Despite neonatal hypotonia that results initially in feeding difficulties and failure to thrive, by the age of 2–3 years affected children develop a voracious appetite and insatiable food-seeking behaviours that result in weight gain and obesity. Cryptorchidism is common in

males, but there is also evidence that delayed puberty, in some cases, results from hypogonadotrophic hypogonadism. Fertility in both sexes is severely reduced. The hypogonadism may, in part, account for the finding of a relatively low lean body mass, a factor that contributes to a lowered absolute basal metabolic rate.

11.1.2 Bardet Biedl syndrome

This syndrome is an autosomal recessive condition, comprising mental retardation, retinitis pigmentosa, polydactyly, hypogonadotrophic hypogonadism and obesity, which develops from early childhood. It is less common than the Prader–Willi syndrome. Locus heterogeneity, and linkages to chromosomes 11, 15 and 16 have been demonstrated in different families.

11.1.3 Other genetic syndromes

Cohen's syndrome is an autosomal recessive condition manifesting in learning difficulties, a typical facial appearance, small hands and feet, short stature and truncal obesity. It is thought to be associated with a defect on chromosome 8. A number of other conditions associated with primary hypogonadism have also been described (Kopelman, 1994).

Newly described cases of rare endocrine causes of obesity are starting to emerge as a result of recent genetic studies. For instance, both leptin deficiency and leptin-receptor defects can cause severe obesity, but only a handful of cases have been described world-wide (Montague *et al.*, 1997a; Strobel *et al.*, 1998; Clément *et al.*, 1998).

11.2 Thyroid disease

Thyroid hormones increase cellular metabolic activity in a variety of ways (enhanced Na$^+$, K$^+$-ATPase pumping across cell membranes, increased mitochondrial oxidative phosphorylation, hepatic lipogenesis and sensitisation of brown adipose tissue to sympathetic nervous system stimulation have all been described). Thus, in conditions of thyroid underactivity, basal metabolic rate is reduced, potentially predisposing to positive energy balance and weight gain. Although the public and many doctors believe that thyroid underactivity is an important cause of obesity, there is little evidence to support this belief. Most studies investigating weight gain and hypothyroidism have relied upon self-reported weight before the occurrence of the disease, or, have focused on the response of weight to treatment (Plummer, 1940; Hoogwerf & Nuttall, 1984; Pears *et al.*, 1990). About 60% of patients with hypothyroidism report weight gain, but specific features of hypothyroidism such as coldness, lethargy, skin change and oedema are much more common (Larsen & Inggbar, 1992). One study of 88 patients with hypothyroidism showed a mean BMI of 28.8 (range 17.2–42.5) which is significantly greater than expected in the general population. However, treatment produced only modest weight loss (mean loss of 2.3 kg, 6 months after starting treatment) (Lessan & Finer, 1996). Since hypothyroidism and obesity are both common (prevalence of about 3% and 15%, respectively), the two conditions will by chance co-exist frequently. Hypothyroidism is not found among patients who attend hospital obesity clinics (Finer & Zarb, 1984). The symptoms and signs of hypothyroidism are distinct from those of simple obesity, and will usually prompt diagnosis.

11.3 Adrenocortical disease

Cushing's syndrome results from excess corticosteroid secretion from the adrenal gland resulting from primary adrenal disease, excessive stimulation from the pituitary or from ectopically secreted ACTH. Progressive central obesity is common (77–97% incidence), but has poor sensitivity as a diagnostic tool for adrenocorticol disease (Howlett *et al.*, 1985). The presence of thin skin, with abnormally little subcutaneous fat despite the degree of obesity, together with other specific features of Cushing's syndrome (bruising, myopathy, clinical depression), allows easy differentiation of the condition from 'simple' obesity.

11.4 Ovarian disease

Polycystic ovarian syndrome (PCOS) is the association of hyperandrogenism with chronic anovulation in women, without specific adrenal or pituitary disease. It is most commonly diagnosed on the basis of typical ultrasonic appearances of the ovary. Obesity is common, but not universal (Franks, 1995). Insulin resistance and hyperinsulinaemia are more common than in weight-matched controls, and their influence is independent of the effect of obesity. The mechanism for the association between obesity and PCOS is unclear.

11.5 Pancreatic endocrine disease

Spontaneous hyperinsulinisms, as a result of insulin-secreting tumours of the pancreas, are rare with an incidence of about one in one million people (Kalvie & White, 1972). Recurrent hypoglycaemia is the usual presenting symptom and this with the subsequent stimulus to appetite and the need to eat often results in weight gain.

11.6 Summary

- There are several clear endocrine abnormalities that cause obesity. However, they are very rare and, although they should be considered as part of the diagnostic process, they are an unlikely cause of obesity.

12
Aetiology of Obesity VIII: Psychological Factors

12.1 Behavioural aspects of food choice and eating patterns

Biological research identifies obesity as the consequence of a sustained positive energy balance and there is an increasing understanding of the underlying genetic and physiological processes. Psychological research is concerned with the association between behavioural, cognitive and emotional processes and obesity. These psychological processes themselves could be either genetic or environmental in origin. A number of different psychological models of the nature and causes of obesity have been put forward. They range from psychosomatic theories, which suggest that unconscious conflicts motivate the individual to overeat, to psycho-physiological theories, which propose that disturbances of the processes of appetite regulation are responsible for overeating. There have been few attempts to bring together and compare the different theories of obesity, despite the importance placed on psychological factors by the wider health community. In this chapter the principal psychological approaches to obesity are summarised and the association between psychological factors and obesity is discussed.

12.2 Psychological theories of eating disorders and obesity

12.2.1 Emotional disorders as a cause of obesity

The view that psychological or psychiatric disorders play a significant role in the aetiology of obesity is widespread, especially among non-psychologists. The main support for this idea comes from psychotherapeutic case studies, which give accounts of the emotional disorders of obese patients. However, case reports of patients who have been referred for psychotherapy are neither drawn from representative samples, nor use replicable methods. Larger-scale comparative studies, using objective measures of personality or psychiatric disorder, are necessary to provide a secure basis for generalisations about obesity. Community studies generally fail to find a higher prevalence of psychiatric disorders among obese than among normal weight adults (Wadden & Stunkard, 1987), although some disorders, particularly depression and anxiety, do appear to be over-represented among the sub-set of obese patients who also report binge eating (Specker *et al.*, 1994). Parallels with bulimia nervosa suggest that emotional disorders among obese binge eaters (aside from the binge eating itself) are probably secondary to the eating disorder. Preliminary evidence from clinical case series supports this view, indicating an improvement in emotional well-being following treatment for binge eating (Smith *et al.*, 1992).

The psychosomatic theory of obesity proposes that certain personality characteristics or dispositions are linked with obesity (Kaplan & Kaplan, 1957). These have ranged from psychodynamic theories of conflict and defence (Mills, 1994), to the suggestion of low self-control among obese people. Again, there has not been a great deal of research in this area, and many existing studies have methodological problems, such as biased selection of obese patients, small sample sizes, or non-validated measures. At present, there are no very convincing demonstrations of any particular personality type being associated with a greater risk of obesity (Friedman & Brownell, 1995). However, among certain sub-groups, such as the severely obese (Sullivan, 1993), and obese binge eaters (Telch & Agras, 1994), there do appear to be higher than normal levels of emotional distress and lower self-esteem. Again, there is some evidence that these characteristics improve following successful treatment (Larsen & Torgerson, 1989). In general, psychologists have neglected this area of research, and Friedman and Brownell (1995) have suggested that a new generation of studies is needed to establish the circumstances under which obesity can produce adverse psychological effects and the best means of prevention.

Although personality and emotional factors probably play only a minor role in the aetiology of obesity, they may be more important in relation to responses to treatment. Emotional distress is often cited by patients as an explanation of why they have failed to comply with treatment and studies of the relapse process suggest that low mood is related to dietary violations (Laporte, 1990). Other studies have found that a better treatment outcome is associated with higher self-control or self-efficacy (Berman *et al.*, 1993).

One aspect of emotional behaviour that is attracting attention from researchers from diverse backgrounds, is stress. Community studies have shown a link between stress and weight gain (Van Strien *et al.*, 1986a) and experimental research suggests that stress might be associated with consumption of higher fat foods (McCann *et al.*, 1990). There is also a growing interest in the role of the sympathetic nervous system in abdominal fat deposition. If cortisol plays a fundamental role in the regulation of abdominal fat stores, as has been suggested in some theories (Björntorp, 1996), then stress is implicated in the aetiology of some variants of obesity. As with emotional disorders, it is also possible that stress compromises treatment compliance, and therefore that stress management training could be a valuable adjunct to dietary advice in some cases.

12.2.2 Appetite/satiety disorders as a cause of obesity

The psychobiological approach has provided a very different theoretical perspective, proposing fundamental disturbances in the regulation of energy intake as the cause of obesity. In the 1960s, there was a plethora of studies on eating behaviour in the obese, suggesting variously that obese people ate too fast, didn't display normal satiety patterns (e.g. the progressive slowing of feeding rate over the course of a meal), or were too responsive to taste and smell. Schachter & Rodin developed the idea of 'externality' in the obese, proposing that obese people were unusually responsive to food cues and, therefore, ate more when the food was attractive or accessible (Schachter *et al.*, 1968). The other facet of the model was attenuated responsiveness to internally-generated satiety cues, such as stomach distension. Schachter argued that the eating behaviour of obese humans had many parallels with the eating behaviour of rats with a ventromedial hypothalamic lesion (Schachter & Rodin, 1974).

Externality theory lost favour over subsequent years, partly as a consequence of studies showing that even thin people were responsive to external cues, while neither fat nor thin people showed much capacity to regulate their intake in relation to internal cues (Rodin, 1980). In addition, research on 'restrained eating' suggested that externality was primarily related to higher levels of dietary restraint (see below) and as such was higher in the obese only because of their greater dietary restraint. In fact, there are inconsistent findings in the literature, some of which suggest that the concept of externality in the obese may have been abandoned prematurely. Rodin & Slochower (1976) assessed externality of children at a summer camp when they arrived and then related this to their weight gain over the 8-week camp. External eaters, both normal weight and overweight, gained significantly more weight than did non-external eaters. The development of psychometric measures of externality has meant that it is possible to carry out larger-scale studies of the relationship between externality, restraint and obesity. A prospective study of weight change during a depressive episode, showed an association between externality and weight gain (Weissenburger *et al.*, 1986), while data from a community sample showed externality to be correlated with BMI even after controlling for restraint (Van Strien *et al.*, 1985). The uncertainties in this literature suggest that it could be timely to re-explore the role of external cue responsiveness in obesity, both in terms of the risk of weight gain and the relationship to dieting.

At present, research on eating behaviour among obese people is more likely to be carried out by nutritionists than psychologists, so attention has turned to the macronutrient content of obese people's diets. There is evidence that obese people eat a diet with a higher fat content and, because fat is easily 'over-consumed', they are at risk of a positive energy balance. If fat consumption is a risk factor for obesity, this raises the question of why some individuals choose a higher fat diet. One possibility is that there is variation, perhaps genetically based, in preferences for high-fat foods, which underlies the behavioural differences. There is some evidence that obese adults prefer a higher level of fat in foods (Drewnowski & Holden-Wiltse, 1992) and also some recent work suggesting that the children of overweight parents (who stand a high chance of becoming overweight themselves) show a greater preference for fatty foods (Fisher & Birch, 1995). These observations may be related to external responsiveness, in that fatty foods are also usually more palatable, and a stronger response to palatability is one feature of externality.

12.2.3 The role of dietary restraint in the understanding of obesity

Restraint theory (see also Section 14.1.ii) revolutionised psychological thinking on obesity, by suggesting that abnormalities of eating behaviour in the obese were caused by restrained eating, and were not necessarily a cause of obesity. In its most extreme form, restraint theory has been extended to argue that dieting could promote later weight gain and therefore could even be contributing to the rise in obesity. The first suggestion that dieting could be implicated in the eating pathology of obesity came from Nisbett's idea that obese dieters, as a consequence of their successful weight control, were below their individual set point for weight, although they might still be heavier than the medical or social ideal weight (Nisbett, 1968). Herman & Mack (1975) then suggested that the crucial determinant of regulatory disturbances was not the

discrepancy from set point, but the attempts to control (restrain) food intake and, thus, abnormal eating behaviour would be shown by all restrained eaters at any weight. They developed a measure of dietary restraint and demonstrated that normal weight women scoring high on restraint showed 'counter-regulation', i.e. they ate more following a large than a small pre-load. In another study, weight and restraint were directly compared as predictors of counter-regulation (Hibscher & Herman, 1977) and restraint was found to be more significant than overweight. Data on control of eating in everyday life also showed that restrained eaters reported more food craving and binge eating (Wardle & Beinart, 1981), while clinical data from eating disorder patients suggested that development of binge eating was almost invariably preceded by dieting (Wardle & Beinart, 1981). However, there has been a heated debate about the measurement of restraint, which may have important implications for work on obesity and dieting. In Herman's original scale to assess restrained eating (the 'Restraint Questionnaire', RQ), there were some items related to food restriction, but others related to disinhibition of eating, e.g. 'I eat sensibly in front of others and splurge alone'. It has been argued that some of the observed correlations between RQ scores and disinhibited behaviour could be related to the disinhibitory items on the scale and not the restrictive items. The newer scales (e.g. Stunkard & Messick, 1985; Van Strien *et al.*, 1986b) separate items concerned with control, from those to do with loss of control, and studies which use these scales typically do not find such striking associations between restraint and disinhibition.

Whatever the relationship between restraint and disinhibition, this whole area of work has called into question the value of dieting. It has even raised the spectre that the vogue for dieting is the cause of the epidemic of eating disorders among young women. These ideas have spawned a vigorous 'anti-dieting' movement and there are now many (therapy) programmes dedicated to 'undieting'. Both the poor outcomes of dietary treatments and some of the observations on the epidemiology of weight and dieting support this view (Garner & Wooley, 1991). Population levels of dieting have increased substantially over the past few decades, yet obesity prevalence has also risen. Women in Western countries diet much more than men, but they are no less likely to develop obesity and more likely to develop binge eating or anorexia. Even more worryingly, prospective studies suggest that dieting at the time of the baseline assessment is, at least among women, associated with **greater** weight gain over the follow-up period (French *et al.*, 1994). Against this view is the fact that successful dieters do exist, that good behavioural programmes do produce sustained, albeit modest, weight loss, and that during the course of a well-supported weight loss programme, most participants report better not worse, self-control over eating (Harvey *et al.*, 1993). There is also a higher prevalence of dieting and lower levels of obesity among higher social status groups, which could be interpreted as pointing to the effectiveness of dieting (Sobal & Stunkard, 1989). It would, therefore, appear that restraint does **not** cause eating problems in all people and in all circumstances. Nevertheless, identifying who is adversely affected by restraint, how they are affected and how the effects can be minimised, is an important area for research.

12.3 Psychological disturbances in obesity

12.3.1 Binge eating disorder

Stunkard (1959) identified binge eating as one of eating patterns observed in obese patients, but it received little attention until recently. In the 4th revision of the *American Psychiatric Association's Diagnostic and Statistical Manual (DSMIV)*, binge eating disorder (BED) was identified as a specific disorder for the first time. It is categorised as one of the 'Eating disorders not otherwise classified', and therefore, is diagnosed only when anorexia nervosa and bulimia nervosa have been excluded. According to this definition, binge eating is defined as eating objectively large amounts of food with a subjective sense of loss of control, at least twice a week. A diagnosis of BED also requires that the binge eating problem has been present for at least 6 months and causes marked distress (Brody *et al.*, 1994). Community surveys identify a BED prevalence of 2.5% of adult women and 1.1% of adult men and it is associated with, but not exclusive to, obesity (Spitzer *et al.*, 1992). The prevalence of BED among obese patients attending clinics is even higher, at 20–30% (Spitzer *et al.*, 1992).

As yet, there have been few studies of the epidemiology and natural history of BED. Observations from one small-scale study of women receiving treatment for BED, showed the onset of binge eating was reported to have been in the late teens and to have predated the onset of obesity or dieting (Mussell, 1995). Another study identified the onset of dieting in BED patients (15.0 years) to have been later than the onset of binge eating (14.2 years), contrasting with the reverse pattern for patients with bulimia (dieting at 16.2 years, binge eating at 19.8 years) (Raymond *et al.*, 1995). The question of the timing of onset of dieting and binge eating is particularly significant, because the literature on bulimia nervosa, which provides one of the closest parallels, identifies dieting as a major aetiological feature in binge eating. In a survey of clinic attendees who were obese and who reported binge eating at least once a week, many denied ever having dieted (Wilson & Fairburn, 1993). Also, obese binge eaters have been shown to have lower dietary restraint scores than patients with bulimia nervosa (Fichter *et al.*, 1993). Likewise in Spitzer's community samples (Spitzer *et al.*, 1992, 1993), which of course have comparatively few cases, 50% had never dieted or been overweight. However, among the obese clinic samples, dieting and weight variation was higher in those with, than without, BED. These observations suggest that careful exploration of the role of restraint in the aetiology of binge eating among obese people is required, and caution should be exercised in recommending strict dieting to obese patients with BED, until we have a better understanding of its effects.

An alternative aetiological theory links binge eating with emotional distress. As discussed above, studies of psychopathology indicate higher levels of both personality disorders and depressive disorders among obese binge eaters than among obese non-binge eaters (Specker *et al.*, 1994). It is not certain whether the emotional problems precede or follow binge eating, although one study suggested that binge eating preceded the onset of depressive disorder (Mussell, 1995). Again, parallels with bulimia nervosa suggest that depression is more likely to be secondary to the eating disorder, and so treatment of the emotional disorder is unlikely, in itself, to resolve the eating/weight problem.

Treatment of bulimia has emphasised strategies to reduce restraint, improve body image, and control exposure to binge cues. This may provide a model for the treatment of BED, although no clear predictions can be made concerning the effects on body weight. Porzelius *et al.* (1995) reported both a significant reduction in binge eating and short-term weight loss, using cognitive behaviour therapy (CBT) for binge eating, but Agras *et al.* (1994) found a reduction in binge frequency accompanied by a slight weight gain in the CBT group.

12.3.2 Emotional eating

Emotional eating deserves a mention in its own right, in that significant numbers of obese patients who do not report frank binge eating, nevertheless report being more likely to overeat, or relapse from a diet, in negative emotional states. As well as the early laboratory investigations of fear and eating (Schachter *et al.*, 1968), an association between emotional eating and obesity has also been found in studies in which emotional eating is assessed with one of a number of psychometric instruments; for example, the emotional eating scale of the DEBQ (Van Strien *et al.*, 1986b) or the more recent 'Emotional Eating Scale' (Arnow, 1995).

The idea that emotional cues can lead to overeating is of course fundamental to the psychosomatic theory of obesity (Kaplan & Kaplan, 1957), which suggests links with early childhood experiences in which eating and comfort were linked. The empirical support for this theory is minimal. Schachter *et al.* (1968) found no evidence that eating reduced fear in obese people. Clinical experience indicates that most adults describe only transient comfort from eating, with shame, disgust and frustration being the most common emotions after an episode of binge eating. Furthermore, there is little evidence beyond clinical case histories to support the idea of stronger childhood links between eating and emotions for obese than normal weight adults. However, this area has not been well researched, and the absence of evidence should not be confused with evidence against.

Restraint theory identifies emotional eating to be caused by disinhibition of restraint by emotional arousal (Herman & Mack, 1975). In a more recent formulation, a process of 'escape from self-awareness in response to emotional pain' is similarly hypothesised to disinhibit eating (Heatherton *et al.*, 1993). Investigations of the association between restraint and emotional eating in normal

population samples have found mixed results, with some finding a positive association in at least some sub-groups (Wardle *et al.*, 1992), while others fail to find any effect (Van Strien *et al.*, 1985). A more recent study in obese people also found that emotional eating was not correlated with restraint (Arnow, 1995), although this study may have suffered from range restriction, as few if any clinically obese adults are non-restrained. However, the implication of these results is that emotional eating is not characteristic of all dieters, so although dieting may confer susceptibility to emotional eating, other factors must contribute to its expression.

12.3.3 Food addiction

The concept of addiction is used loosely in the popular nutrition literature to denote a problem of control of eating, which is outside of volition. Behind it lies the medical model of addiction, which proposes that a substance may, by virtue of exposure, modify the central nervous system, so that withdrawal symptoms and craving are experienced when the substance is withheld. Relief of withdrawal also functions as a powerful reinforcer, which amplifies any inherently reinforcing features of the drug. Few addiction specialists would analyse foods in this light, since food consumption is both normal and essential to maintain life. However, there are some features of food intake regulation which have parallels in the addiction field (Orford, 1984) and these include cravings for specific substances and extreme difficulty in self-control. Cravings for foods are widely reported in the normal population, being more common in women than men and reported particularly in connection with pregnancy and the pre-menstrual period (Weingarten & Elston, 1991). The idea that self-control might be especially difficult because of biologically based drives for consumption, is another feature. Hunger is a powerful drive that organises an elaborate repertoire of food seeking and consumption behaviours and consequently, the self-control required to keep energy intake to below the level of energy expenditure may be a psychobiological challenge for people of any weight. Food intake is also rewarding, both in terms of assuaging hunger and the sensory experience of delicious foods. However, at the root of the addiction theory is the idea that some individuals might crave foods because of particular constituents that meet a biological need.

Wurtman & Wurtman (1986) proposed the idea that some people crave, and overeat, carbohydrate because it raises the levels of brain serotonin, which in turn reduces feelings of depression or anxiety. One particular form of depressive illness, seasonal affective disorder (SAD), is characterised by atypical depressive episodes, which tend to occur seasonally. Patients with SAD also commonly report overeating during the depressive episode, particularly on carbohydrate foods. SAD has been hypothesised to be caused by a light-mediated depletion of serotonin, which causes both the depression and the overeating. The strongest support for this theory comes from the efficacy of serotoninergic drugs in the management of SAD, although these drugs are now widely used across the spectrum of depressive disorders. There is experimental evidence that high carbohydrate meals increase the availability of tryptophan (the precursor of serotonin) and, as precursor concentration is the rate-limiting step in serotonin activity, carbohydrate consumption, therefore, increases brain serotonin. However, it has yet to be established that carbohydrate-mediated changes in brain tryptophan have a functional impact. There are a number of experimental studies on carbohydrate and mood, but the results have been inconsistent. The first study (Spring *et al.*, 1982) provided limited support for an antidepressant, or calming, effect of high carbohydrate meals, but the effect varied across time of day, and sex and age of the subjects. Other studies have also failed to produce a definitive result, partly because there are many methodological problems. Not least of these are that carbohydrate cannot be manipulated independently of other macronutrients, without affecting energy content. Adding to these uncertainties is the observation that the foods that SAD patients crave are not solely high carbohydrate, but are sweet, high energy-dense foods, which would not be predicted to increase tryptophan availability to the same extent.

The observation that many obese people report problems controlling their eating and that they crave and binge on sweet foods, led Wurtman (1988) to propose that some obese people were also carbohydrate cravers, because of a neurochemical deficit, and weight gain had resulted from over-consumption of carbohydrate. Again, the specific experimental evidence is limited, or even contradictory. In general, obese people do not eat more carbohydrate that non-obese people. Like SAD patients, obese people usually crave sweet, fatty foods, which are not pure carbohydrate and they rarely crave the pure sugars. Studies of the effects of serotoninergic drugs have also been interpreted as showing a selective reduction of carbohydrate craving among the obese, but this conclusion has been questioned (Fernstrom *et al.*, 1992).

The other food to which the addiction model has been applied is chocolate, resulting in the popular term 'chocaholism'. Chocolate is certainly one of the most craved foods and the craving is specific to real chocolate, and not for other sweets or for white chocolate (Rozin *et al.*, 1991). Chocolate craving is also commonly described among obese patients and particularly among obese binge eaters. The phenomenon of chocolate craving has led to every constituent of chocolate being examined as a possible pharmaco-active substance that could support addiction. Attention has focused on caffeine, theobromine, tyramine and phenylethylamine. However, in an ingenious study in which cravers were given either real chocolate, white chocolate (which lacks any of the putative addictive substances), or white chocolate with these substances added, only the real chocolate satisfied the craving (Michener & Rozin, 1994). This suggests that the craving is for the sensory experience and not any constituent, although longer term studies are required to exclude conditioned effects. Hetherington & Macdiarmid (1993) interviewed 50 self-identified 'chocaholics' and found that while some reported positive effects on mood, the dieters experienced negative effects after eating. In a second study (Macdiarmid & Hetherington, 1995) positive effects of eating chocolate were no more apparent in 'addicts' than controls, while negative effects (e.g. guilt) were more common than in controls. To that extent, the chocolate 'addicts' are not describing the positive reactions that most drug addicts experience following use of their drug.

Overall, the addiction theories have had more success in popular nutrition than in nutritional science, and attract a much larger following than is merited from their empirical base.

12.3.4 Night eating syndrome

Night eating was another of the pathological eating patterns identified by Stunkard (1959). Defined as a syndrome involving nocturnal eating, insomnia and morning anorexia, it was reported by 64% of an emotionally disordered sub-group of obese patients, and 10% of obese patients attending a nutrition clinic. There have been few systematic studies of the syndrome and over the past 36 years, Schenck and Mahowald (1994) identified only nine reports, of which seven were single case studies. They reported data on a series of 38 patients with nocturnal eating, who were seen in their sleep disorder clinic. Most of these patients were women and half were overweight as a result of their night eating. Several notable features were described, including the absence of hunger before the eating episode, the 'automaticity' of the behaviour after waking in the night, and the variable level of consciousness during eating. Most ate fast and carelessly (with 30% having injured themselves), often eating food which was odd or inappropriate. Unlike the patients on whom Stunkard reported, who were seen in a psychiatric context, none of the sleep clinic patients reported any problem with overeating at other times. Most said that they restricted their daytime eating to compensate for the night eating. In a more recent study, 79 overweight women (40 of whom had BED) monitored their nocturnal eating for 8 nights (Greeno *et al.*, 1995). Only six patients, all of whom had BED, reported night eating, but only one episode in most cases. In another survey, Stunkard *et al.* (1996) examined the prevalence of a night eating syndrome, which they operationally defined as comprising: morning anorexia, eating more than 50% of daily intake after 7.00 pm, and sleep disturbance. The prevalence was 8.9% in patients at a weight reduction clinic, 15% in a sample of binge eaters taking part in a trial of medication for BED and 13.7% among women who responded to a television call for women to take part in a trial of medication for BED (among whom only 19.6% met the criteria for BED). Evidently, on present evidence it is not clear whether night eating is properly described as a syndrome, how it is related to binge eating and obesity, or whether it is best understood as a sleep disorder or an eating disorder.

12.3.5 Body image dissatisfaction

No discussion of the psychological aspects of obesity is complete without some discussion of body image. Many, but by no means all, fat people are dissatisfied with the appearance of their body. In some, this reaches the point of intense self-loathing and avoidance of exposure. Obese children may be tormented by their peers and humiliated by teachers, especially in connection with sports activities. Some obese adults try to avoid situations where physical exposure is required, such as sports or close physical contact, thereby compromising their health and happiness still further. Some health professionals regard a negative body image in obese people as normal and they themselves feel disgusted by fat patients (Maddox *et al.*, 1968). Behavioural treatments at one time encouraged body image disparagement as a means of motivating treatment compliance. Now, as part of recent trends towards considering quality of life and not just disease processes, a negative body image is coming to be recognised as part of the problem of obesity and one which might be amenable to treatment. However, there has been virtually no research on body image disparagement among the obese, perhaps reflecting the view that it is normal for someone who is fat to feel self-critical.

Body image dissatisfaction in relation to weight and shape emerges as a consequence of the mismatch between the individual's body image and their concept of their ideal body. Contemporary western ideals for body shape emphasise extreme slenderness, and therefore many people, even those with healthy weights, perceive their own body shape in negative terms. However, the intensity of an individual's reaction to the self-ideal discrepancy varies. Obese binge eaters generally express more body image distress than non-binge eaters, although neither group reaches the level of body image distress of patients with bulimia nervosa (Raymond *et al.*, 1995). Body image distress also varies in relation to social and cultural position. Obese women express more body image distress than men, and white women express more dissatisfaction than black women. Pregnancy seems to be associated with a reduction in body image dissatisfaction (Davies & Wardle, 1994). A number of cognitive-behaviour therapists are beginning to recognise that reducing body image distress among obese adults could make a significant contribution to their well-being (Rosen *et al.*, 1991).

12.3.6 Psychological factors in sport and exercise participation

Low levels of activity are associated with obesity, and participation in sport and organised forms of exercise, provide an important means by which people are able to maintain or step up their energy expenditure. Personality traits have not been strong predictors of physical activity participation either among school children or adults. However, several psychosocial factors are moderately to strongly associated with competitive and recreational sport and attendance at health clubs. Participation in activities that require the demonstration of skill or fitness in public settings is related to perceptions of competence in these activities (Sonstroem, 1997). By late adolescence, physical self-perceptions strongly predict degree and type of involvement in sport and exercise. For those who perceive low competence, this produces a significant mental barrier to future participation in any form of health related activity and hence increases chances of becoming significantly overweight. For instance, the Allied Dunbar National Fitness Survey (HEA/Sports Council, 1992) indicated that 34% and 46% of middle-aged to elderly men and women respectively, reported that they were not active because 'they were not the sporty type'. Similarly, investigations into social physique anxiety, a fear of displaying the body in public settings, have indicated that this presents an additional barrier to attendance at exercise settings (Eklund & Crawford, 1994). These findings are supported by systematic research with middle-aged to elderly populations that show levels of exercise self-efficacy or confidence in ability to perform exercise is associated with low participation rates (McAuley & Courneya, 1993). A meta analysis of 31 studies producing 162 effect sizes (Hausenblas *et al.*, 1997) also indicated that attitudes, beliefs and intentions are related to physical activity participation throughout the life span. Wankel *et al.* (1994) in a national sample of 4000 Canadians, showed that 31% of variance in intentions to be active was explained by a psychosocial profile made up of attitudes, perceptions of confidence and influence of social norms.

Clearly, by adulthood, participation in the more formalised elements of exercise and sport carries a profile of attitudes and beliefs about the behaviour itself, but also self-perception of the ability and ease with which that form of activity could be engaged in. A mental 'set' can be identified that predicts inactivity and the obese score particularly low on such profiles (Fox, 1992; Treasure *et al.*, 1998). It appears that negative profiles are formed early, often during adolescence, as indicated by a high avoidance rate among girls in their early teens. Physical education programmes in schools must address the need to encourage positive attitudes, beliefs and self-perceptions related to activity so that a greater percentage of youngsters emerge from the school years with fewer psychosocial constraints on their activity participation. Similarly, activity programmes for adults, especially those already overweight, need to be carefully tailored to overcome lack of confidence and negative beliefs and attitudes that may have become ingrained over many years.

12.4 Summary

- A number of psychological models have been proposed as possible causes of obesity. These associate obesity with behavioural, cognitive and emotional processes, which themselves can be genetic or environmental in origin.

- In general, it has been difficult to separate cause from effect in the relation between obesity and emotional disorders. A current view is that personality and emotional factors play only a minor role in the aetiology of obesity, but may be important in relation to responses to treatment.

- The externality theory, proposing that obese people are unusually responsive to food cues, has lost favour in recent years, but may have been prematurely discarded.

- The concept of dietary restraint is intimately linked to obesity, but there is controversy regarding cause and effect. In susceptible individuals restraint may precipitate eating disorders and hence may lead to obesity. However, in others restraint is an effective coping strategy in maintaining a healthy body weight.

- Binge eating disorder (BED) has recently been

classified as a specific disorder. Community studies suggest a prevalence as high as 2.5% in the general population and 20–30% among obese patients.

- Emotional eating caused by disinhibition of restraint, resulting from emotional arousal represents a less severe form of binge eating.

- The concept of food addiction (e.g. carbohydrate craving and 'chocaholism') is widely prevalent in lay circles but has little empirical support from the scientific literature.

- Night eating syndrome can be considered as a subset of BED and it is not clear whether it represents a discrete entity and, if so, whether it should be viewed as an eating disorder or a sleep disorder.

- Body image dissatisfaction is highly correlated with obesity. Cognitive behaviour therapies are increasingly recognising that reducing body image distress among obese people can make a significant contribution to well-being and treatment.

- A profile of psychosocial factors is identifiable in adolescents and adults that is closely associated with non-participation in organised sport and exercise. This may predispose individuals to developing obesity.

- Programmes in schools need to be designed to focus on the development of positive attitudes and self-perceptions related to physical activity in all youngsters. Adult activity schemes need to address psychosocial barriers if they are to be successful.

13
Aetiology of Obesity IX: Dietary Factors

13.1 Epidemiological evidence

13.1.1 Secular trends in intake

In the UK, the National Food Survey (NFS) provides the longest running continuous survey of household food consumption in the world (MAFF, 1998). This shows that total energy intake increased from the end of the Second World War to a peak in 1970 and thereafter has declined (Fig. 13.1). One of the drawbacks of the NFS data is that, until 1991, it measured only household food purchases. However, since 1992, information on soft drinks, alcohol and confectionery brought into the home has also been recorded and reported. In addition, since 1994, half of the households have recorded food, alcoholic and soft drinks consumed outside the home. Previously, only the number, and not the content, of meals eaten outside the home was recorded, and this information was taken into account only when nutrient intakes from household food purchases were reported as a proportion of the dietary reference values (Department of Health, 1991). Although the contribution of these additional items (i.e. soft drinks, alcohol and confectionery brought into the home; food and drink consumed outside the home) has progressively increased, they constitute a relatively small proportion of the total energy intake. The downward trend in energy intake recorded by the NFS data is not altered, even when account is taken of these additional items.

The recorded net decrease in energy intake from NFS data is approximately 3 MJ/d (720 kcal), a decrease of about 30% compared to the mean intake in 1970. Although it may be unwise to rely

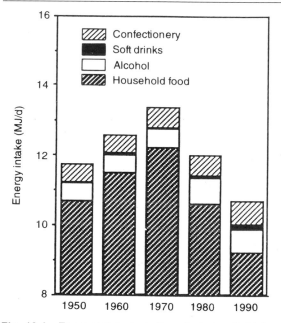

Fig. 13.1 Energy intake including alcohol, soft drinks and confectionery. Data from NFS with additions derived from national supply figures (Prentice & Jebb 1995a).

too heavily on the absolute magnitude of this decrease, given the limitations of the NFS dataset, few would dispute that total energy intakes have declined during the last 10–20 years. Indeed, an analysis of cross-sectional surveys of energy intake in adults in the UK confirms this trend (Prentice & Jebb, 1995b) (Fig. 13.2). Two studies in South Wales have also documented reductions in energy intake over time. In women, between 1966 and 1983, total energy intake decreased by 16%,

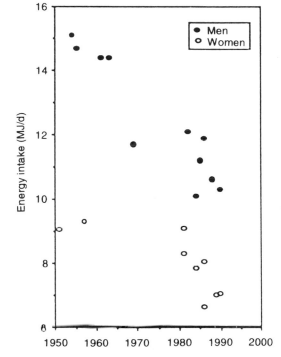

Fig. 13.2 Trends in energy intake from cross-sectional surveys in adults. Each point represents a study. Total sample size 2616 subjects (from Prentice & Jebb (1995b).

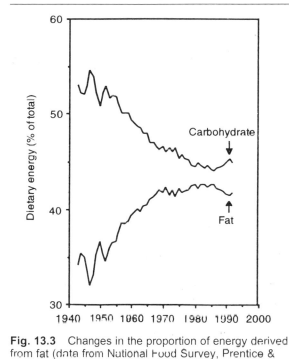

Fig. 13.3 Changes in the proportion of energy derived from fat (data from National Food Survey, Prentice & Jebb 1995a).

(Elwood *et al.*, 1990), while in men, intake declined by 8% between 1980–1983 and 1990 (O'Neill & Fehily, 1991).

The nutritional analysis of the NFS data shows striking changes in the composition of the diet (Fig. 13.3). Although the proportion of energy derived from protein has remained essentially unchanged, there has been a marked increase in the proportion of energy derived from fat, with a reciprocal decrease in the proportion derived from carbohydrate. In the early 1940s, for every kilojoule (kJ) of carbohydrate in the diet, fat provided only 0.6 kJ whereas, in the 1980s, for each kJ of carbohydrate there was 0.95 kJ of fat; an increase of more than 50% (Prentice & Jebb, 1995b).

Data from other affluent nations also show large historical increases in the proportion of energy derived from fat over the past century, with an indication of a slight recent decline in response to healthy eating messages (Willett, 1998). The con-

sumption of high-fat diets is closely related to affluence, as measured by per capita national income. This effect is mediated by greatly increased consumption of animal fats in wealthier nations, while vegetable fat intake shows no gradient with wealth (Drewnowski & Popkin, 1997). A consequence of these relationships, and of increasing income and urbanisation, is that fat intake is also rising sharply in many developing countries (Drewnowski & Popkin, 1997). The 'globalisation' of diets is also modifying the traditionally low-fat diets of countries such as Japan and China, where the formerly low rates of obesity are now rapidly increasing.

There has also been a change in the type of fat consumed. The proportion of saturated fatty acids in the diet has been decreasing for at least the last 25 years, from 19.9% in 1969 to 16.6% in 1990 and 15.7% in 1994. This is because of changes from whole to reduced-fat milks, butter to low-fat spreads and a decrease both in the consumption of carcass meats and their fat content. Mono-unsaturated fatty acid intakes have remained relatively constant at approximately 15% of energy intake.

Polyunsaturated fatty acids have shown a small increase in intake, owing to the increased consumption of polyunsaturates-rich margarine, but this group of fatty acids only contribute approximately 7% of the energy content of the diet. However, since the increase has occurred primarily with respect to n-6 fatty acids, this has led to a marked increase in the ratio of n-6 to n-3 fatty acids in the diets of many affluent nations (e.g. Rizek *et al.*, 1983). Further information on fatty acids can be found in the BNF Task Force Report on *Unsaturated Fatty Acids* (British Nutrition Foundation, 1992).

Overall, it is apparent that, in recent years, there has been a decline in total energy intakes and absolute intakes of each macronutrient. Yet, this has coincided with a rapid increase in the prevalence of obesity in men and women in the UK (Gregory *et al.*, 1990; Bennett *et al.*, 1995). Since positive energy balance is a pre-requisite for weight gain, this implies that obesity has developed as a consequence of a greatly reduced energy requirement and an inability of the physiological mechanisms to down regulate energy intake to a similar extent (Chapter 15).

13.1.2 Cross-sectional trends in intake

i Problems of under-reporting

Studies of diet and health make the tacit assumption that the recorded intake represents the habitual intake of the individual. The difficulties in measuring food intake can be considered in three main categories: precision, random inaccuracy and bias. The precision of dietary assessments can be readily assessed on the basis of repeated measures. The potential for inaccuracy can be overcome by the selection of appropriate sample sizes or within the data analysis. Random inaccuracy will tend to lead to false negative findings, by reducing the strength of true relationships, but will not generate misleading false positive associations. However, bias remains a potentially serious problem, which may generate false conclusions.

Over the last decade, the extent of bias in dietary surveys has become increasingly apparent. Few subjects report consuming food they did not eat, yet many fail to report all the food they do consume. Thus, over-reporting does not counterbalance under-reporting, leading to an overall underestimate of intake of the group. Moreover, the extent of under-reporting may not be consistent across the whole population. There have been particular difficulties in understanding the relationship between diet and obesity, since it appears that the extent of under-reporting in obese subjects is greater than among their lean counterparts (Black *et al.*, 1993).

The problem of under-reporting was recognised by Prentice *et al.* (1986) when it was observed that the habitual energy expenditure of obese subjects greatly exceeded their reported energy intakes. As this situation is incompatible with the long-term maintenance of body weight, it was concluded that dietary intake had been under-reported. Since this time, a similar phenomenon has been observed in many other studies of energy balance (e.g. Lichtman *et al.*, 1992). Under-reporting may occur as a consequence of genuine forgetfulness, underestimation of portion size, a change in dietary habits during the period of recording, or an attempt to conceal true dietary habits in favour of those perceived to be 'better' or 'more healthy'.

In studies that include simultaneous measurements of energy expenditure, it is possible to accurately identify individuals whose reported food intake is inconsistent with their habitual energy needs. In epidemiological surveys, such measurements are impractical but a method has been described to identify datasets in which the reported energy intake can be compared to an estimate of the energy needs of the population. This concept was first suggested by Schoeller (1990) and was subsequently refined to allow the derivation of specific cut-offs to identify under-reporting (Goldberg *et al.*, 1991a). These cut-offs take into consideration the measurement imprecision and individual variability in energy requirements and, therefore, are inevitably conservative in their identification of under-reporting. Nonetheless, application of this method reveals that very many of the major surveys of diet and health are based on erroneous estimates of energy and macronutrient intake (Black *et al.*, 1991).

This procedure to identify under-reporters is based entirely on concepts of energy balance and cannot indicate whether the bias is equal across all foods, or whether some items are selectively under-reported. Measurements of urinary nitrogen excretion have been used to provide an independent biomarker of protein intake (Bingham & Cummings, 1985). However, currently there are no independent biomarkers of dietary fat or carbohydrate intake, and the extent of under-reporting of these nutrients can only be inferred from independent measures of energy or protein intake. There is some evidence that under-reporting of energy intake is approximately 15% greater than under-reporting of protein intake (Heitmann & Lissner, 1995), which has been interpreted as suggesting that snacks may be more likely to be under-reported than main meals. Under-reporting of snacks has also been implied from studies which have found differences in the frequency of meal-eating episodes between high- and low-energy reporters (Summerbell *et al.*, 1996) and also when reported intake has been compared to direct observation (Poppitt *et al.*, 1998).

In recent years, there has been widespread acknowledgement of the phenomenon of under-reporting, but as yet there is no clear resolution of the problem. The exaggerated bias observed in obese subjects causes particular difficulties in the analysis of the relationship between dietary factors and obesity. In consequence, the data concerning differences in food consumption between lean and obese people must be interpreted with caution. The bias that under-reporting contributes into dietary surveys, with respect to total energy intake, macronutrient composition and micronutrient adequacy, clearly has implications for studies of the causation of obesity and also for its successful management. Much more research is required in this area.

ii Changes in intake with age

In adults, average energy intake tends to decline with age (Section 7.6). In a nationally representative sample of over 2000 adults in Britain, Gregory *et al.* (1990) showed that total intake was similar for all ages up to 49 years, but decreased by just under 0.5 MJ/d (119 kcal/d) in the older age group (50–64 years). In a smaller survey in Northern Ireland of around 600 people, men aged less than 40 years consumed approximately 1 MJ/d (239 kcal/d) more than those aged more than 40 years (p <0.05). In

women, the trend was more striking across the whole age range, with a progressive decrease in reported energy intake (p <0.001) from 7.6 MJ/d (1816 kcal/d) in the 16–29 year group to 6.3 MJ/d (1505 kcal/d) in the 50–64 year group (Barker *et al.*, 1989).

Absolute protein intake and the proportion of energy derived from protein increases with age (p <0.05) (Barker *et al.*, 1989; Gregory *et al.*, 1990). There is a modest decline in carbohydrate intake with age. In women, this is related to a decline in the consumption of sugars (p <0.01) whereas in men, there is a decrease in starch intake (p <0.01) (Gregory *et al.*, 1990). There is no significant change in fat intake as a proportion of energy with age (Barker *et al.*, 1989; Gregory *et al.*, 1990). Alcohol consumption appears to increase during young adulthood, into middle age and then to decline. The peak for men occurs at an earlier age than in women (Barker *et al.*, 1989; Gregory *et al.*, 1990; Bennett *et al.*, 1995).

These modest changes in energy and macronutrient intake with age must be set alongside a marked increase in the prevalence of obesity associated with ageing (Barker *et al.*, 1989; Gregory *et al.*, 1990). Together, they imply that the positive energy balance in middle and later life is a consequence of a reduction in energy requirements, which is in excess of the small reductions in energy intake (Section 7.6).

iii Intake and social class

There is a strong social class gradient in the prevalence of obesity, showing that lower social classes are at increased risk of obesity (Bennett *et al.*, 1995). This is particularly evident in women, where there is a fourfold increased risk of becoming obese in social classes IV and V relative to social class I. However, in itself this trend is not well correlated with differences in total energy or macronutrient intake.

Data from the NFS suggest that, in women, the average energy intake decreases slightly in relation to social class from 7.3 MJ/d (1745 kcal/d) in groups I and II to 6.6 MJ/d (1577 kcal/d) in classes IV and V (p < 0.01). In men, there is no significant trend relative to social class. However, men who are working have significantly higher intakes than the unemployed (10.5 versus 8.6 MJ/d [2510 versus

2055 kcal/d]; p < 0.01). Similarly, the Caerphilly Heart Disease Study found significantly higher energy intakes in men with manual occupations, versus those in non-manual occupations (Fehily *et al.*, 1984). Overall, the differences in energy intake relative to social class in Britain and Northern Ireland are small (Cade *et al.*, 1988; Barker *et al.*, 1989; Gregory *et al.*, 1990).

There are marked differences in the types of food consumed in relation to social class; most notably the intake of fresh fruit and vegetables declines in lower social class households. Yet, despite this variation, only modest differences in the intake of macronutrients have been observed (Barker *et al.*, 1989; Gregory *et al.*, 1990). Gregory *et al.* have reported that in social classes I and II, both men and women have higher intakes of protein than in social classes IV and V (men: p <0.05; women: p <0.01). In Britain, the percentage of total energy provided by carbohydrate is lower for men and women in social classes I and II than IV and V (p <0.01) because of significantly lower intakes of both starch and sugar. There were no significant differences in the proportion of energy derived from fat. In the Northern Ireland survey, there were no significant differences in the macronutrient intake as a proportion of total energy. In the Caerphilly Heart Disease study, men in manual occupations consumed significantly more carbohydrate than those in non-manual occupations (Fehily *et al.*, 1984).

Studies of the relationship between social class and total alcohol consumption have shown no clear association in men, but a marked inverse relationship in women. As with the types of food, there are marked differences in the type of alcohol consumed. In both men and women, the intake of beer is higher in low social classes while the consumption of wine and spirits is lower (Bennett *et al.*, 1995).

The lack of a direct association between dietary intake and obesity is because of the multitude of additional covariable lifestyle factors, which confer a relative protection or susceptibility to obesity.

iv Intake and geographical region

National surveys suggest that, in England and Wales, only small regional differences exist in the prevalence of obesity (Gregory *et al.*, 1990) and in total energy intake or the macronutrient composition of the diet. A study by Fehily *et al.* (1990), using 7-day weighed diet records, found only minor differences between energy and nutrient intake in men from South Wales, Northern Ireland, Edinburgh and Bristol. However, there are clear regional differences in the types of food consumed, particularly with respect to the consumption of fresh fruit and vegetables. This may have an impact on the overall energy density of the diet.

13.1.3 Protein and obesity

Protein intake has been implicated in the development of adiposity in young children. Studies of infants weaned onto isoenergetic, low or high protein formulae show that the growth rates of infants on the low protein diet closely resembles that of breast-fed babies, while growth of those on the high protein diet is more rapid (Axelsson *et al.*, 1988). Data, from a French longitudinal study of nutrition and growth, show that the age of 'adiposity rebound' (which is arguably a predictor of subsequent obesity) is significantly younger in children consuming high protein diets (Rolland-Cachera, 1995). Diets containing a high proportion of protein have also been reported in those with established obesity (Rolland-Cachera *et al.*, 1990). However, this finding may be an artefact of selective under-reporting of food intake by obese subjects, relative to their lean counterparts (Section 13.1.2).

Woods *et al.* (1974) have suggested that the growth hormone to insulin ratio may be important in controlling body fatness and it is possible that any effect of a high protein diet on fatness is mediated in this way. High protein intakes are associated with decreases in growth hormone, while insulin is increased, favouring an early adiposity rebound.

13.1.4 Fat, carbohydrate and obesity

As described above, data from the NFS over the last 50 years show that there have been major changes in the principal sources of energy in the diet. There has been a dramatic increase in the proportion of fat in the diet, with a proportionate reduction in carbohydrate. The intakes of protein and alcohol have remained relatively constant and, indeed, these nutrients represent less than one-fifth of the total energy intake and, therefore, make a relatively small contribution to the overall energy budget. This inverse relationship between fat and carbohydrate has also been demonstrated in numerous cross-sectional surveys of nutrient intake in developed countries (Gibney *et al.*, 1995; Hill & Prentice, 1995). Intriguingly, it can also be shown that it is simple sugars in particular, and not complex carbohydrates, which tend to counterbalance the fat energy in the diet. This relationship has been described as the 'fat-sugar see-saw' (Fig. 13.4). The implication of this association is that any sub-group of the population shown to take a high proportion of their energy intake as fat will also tend to derive a low proportion of their energy intake from sugar, and vice versa. In the context of obesity, it may be difficult to separate out the independent effects of fat and carbohydrate (or more specifically sugar) from epidemiological data alone.

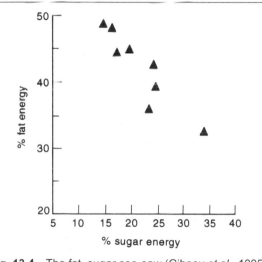

Fig. 13.4 The fat–sugar see-saw (Gibney *et al.*, 1995).

i Ecological studies

Ecological studies have been widely used to investigate the association between dietary composition and obesity, but they are inherently inconclusive because of the plethora of unmeasured factors, which may contribute to the development or maintenance of obesity and which preclude any definitive link to diet alone.

On a world-wide basis, there are very clear differences in the relative contribution of dietary fat and carbohydrate to energy intake. Advances in economic development appear to be associated both with an increase in the proportion of fat in the diet, at the expense of carbohydrate, and with an increase in the prevalence of obesity. However, such associations are inevitably confounded by a multitude of other factors, which track the progress of economic development. Likewise, migration studies, such as the movement of Japanese people to Hawaii, have observed an increase in both the proportion of energy derived from fat and BMI in the migrants, but do not adjust for other confounding lifestyle characteristics (Curb & Marcus, 1991).

Studies in economically similar nations have yielded inconsistent findings. For example, a cross-country analysis of the MONICA surveys in Europe has shown a negative association in women between BMI and the proportion of energy derived from fat, but no significant relationship in men (Lissner & Heitmann, 1995). However, in this case the food intake data were derived from national food disappearance data, which may not equally reflect true food intake across different countries. In the Seven Countries study, which included a dietary survey of the participants, there was no clear evidence of an association between the macronutrient content of the diet and body weight (Keys, 1970).

In countries with robust longitudinal data on both dietary composition and the prevalence of obesity (or mean BMI), there is some evidence of a positive relationship between the proportion of energy consumed as fat and an increase in the prevalence of obesity; for example in Denmark (Lissner & Heitmann, 1995) and in the UK, up until 1970 (Prentice & Jebb, 1995b). However, in recent years, in both the UK and USA, there has been a decline in the proportion of energy consumed as fat, while the prevalence of obesity continues to increase (Heini & Weinsier, 1997). This may reflect the relatively long lag-phase in the development of obesity, such that it may take many years to see a corresponding fall in body weight. However, it reinforces the absence of a direct and immediate link between macronutrient intake and obesity.

ii Cross-sectional studies

Cross-sectional studies have studied individuals, rather than population-based groups, and measured the independent and dependent variables in parallel. These studies are necessarily retro-spective, considering data collected in the recent or distant past, together with an individual's current weight or fatness, which is itself a product of their historical state of energy balance.

Overall, these studies do provide support for the hypothesis that the proportion of dietary fat is positively associated with body weight, while there is a negative association with the proportion of carbohydrate and indeed with simple sugars. The studies have been extensively reviewed elsewhere (Hill & Prentice, 1995; Lissner & Heitmann, 1995). However, in the light of the 'fat-sugar see-saw' described above, these studies can give no indica-tion about whether a high proportion of dietary fat leads to a susceptibility to obesity, or if a high carbohydrate intake confers protection against obesity.

These cross-sectional studies are particularly susceptible to errors caused by under-reporting, especially if the magnitude or nature of under-reporting is, in itself, a function of adiposity. The existence of under-reporting is highlighted by some studies, which fail to find an association between total energy intake and BMI. Some investigators have attempted to correct for this, using a multi-variate nutrient density model, in which the asso-ciation between dietary constituents and BMI is assessed independently of total energy intake. One of the largest datasets is derived from the Scottish arm of the MONICA survey, where the data is analysed with respect to quintiles of intake of fat or extrinsic sugars, as a proportion of dietary energy (Bolton-Smith & Woodward, 1994). This shows a clear positive association between fat consumption and the prevalence of obesity, and an inverse relationship between sugar intake and obesity. When divided into fifths according to the ratio of fat:sugar intake, there is a threefold difference in the prevalence of obesity in men and more than a twofold difference in women (Fig. 13.5).

A remaining caveat to these cross-sectional studies is the possibility that they may reflect a post-hoc event, whereby obese people have assumed a particular type of diet consequent to their obesity. For example, the apparently low sugar intakes of obese people may be generated by increased use of artificial sweeteners in an attempt to reduce their energy intake, in response to their obesity. How-ever, there is also a plausible argument that dietary

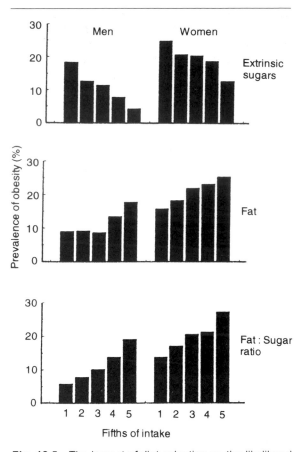

Fig. 13.5 The impact of diet selection on the likelihood of developing obesity. (Data from 11,626 men and women from the Scottish Heart Health and Scottish arm of MONICA studies. Redrawn from Bolton-Smith & Woodward, 1994. Taken from Prentice & Jebb, 1995a) (Quintile 1 = lowest intake.)

habits are notoriously resistant to change, and even cross-sectional dietary surveys are likely to reflect long-standing habits with respect to food prefer-ences and consumption.

In many of these studies, there has been a remarkable absence of an association between BMI and complex carbohydrates, perhaps because of the relatively small inter-individual variability in intake as a proportion of total energy. A notable exception is the Nurses Health Study, which found a negative association between BMI and the intake of crude fibre and alcohol, alongside a positive association with consumption of animal fat (Colditz *et al.*, 1990).

Metabolic studies have implied that the adipogenic potential of high-fat diets is a consequence of the high energy density of such diets. In recent years, there has been an increase in the number of low-fat foods on the market, of which only a proportion have a parallel decrease in energy density e.g. reduced fat milks. Many other low-fat products, particularly in the cake and biscuit sector, which have substituted fat by simple sugars, have a radically different macronutrient composition, but with a similar energy density. It is not yet clear how this will impact upon patterns of consumption with respect both to total energy and macronutrient composition.

iii Prospective studies

The use of prospective studies in the assessment of diet and obesity is complex because of the protracted duration of exposure and the interactive changes that may occur. Individuals gaining weight may make significant changes to their dietary habits in an attempt to reverse the trend and, thus, dietary intake at baseline may not account for the observed weight fluctuation at the end of the observation period. Klesges *et al.* (1992) reported significant positive associations between percentage energy as fat, at the baseline measurement, and subsequent weight gain, in both sexes. However, in men, concurrent increases in fat intake over the course of the study were the strongest predictor. Pudel & Westenhoefer (1992) also reported positive associations between increases in fat intake and intercurrent weight gain, rather than fat intake, at baseline While Colditz *et al.* (1991) suggested that fat intake was positively associated with previous, rather than subsequent, weight increases.

Overall, prospective studies have yielded inconsistent results in relation to fat and carbohydrate intakes and weight gain. For example, Rissanen *et al.* (1991) reported a 70% excess risk of weight gain over 5 years in women in the highest quintile of dietary fat intake, although no association was found in men. Data from the Prospective Study of Women in Gothenburg showed that energy-adjusted fat intake only predicted weight gain over the subsequent 6 years in women who were overweight at the outset and who had at least one obese parent. This suggests that there was an important interaction between genetic predisposition to obesity and the adverse consequences of a high-fat diet (Heitmann *et al.*, 1995). It seems probable that the difficulties of

accurately measuring energy and macronutrient intake, and accounting for other potential cofounders may undermine the likelihood of finding robust associations between macronutrient intake and weight gain in this type of analysis.

In summary, the weight of epidemiological evidence suggests that the fat to carbohydrate ratio is an important aetiological determinant of obesity. However, in isolation it is by no means conclusive. It becomes more persuasive when linked to experimental evidence showing the mechanisms by which fat may disinhibit the control of energy intake (Chapters 9 and 10) and to the results of intervention studies that have successfully reduced dietary fat intake and observed spontaneous weight loss (Chapter 19). Taken together, there is strong evidence that fat is the dominant force in setting the scene for a positive association of obesity with a high dietary fat to carbohydrate ratio, while there is very little indication that carbohydrate confers a specific protective effect.

13.1.5 Alcohol and obesity

Epidemiological studies of the relationship between alcohol intake and obesity are perhaps even more tenuous than other aspects of diet, since the problems of under-reporting are magnified. As with food energy, it is impossible to know whether under-reporting is a uniform effect across all alcohol consumers or whether it is specific to those with particularly high levels of consumption. This confounds the interpretation of any epidemiological associations.

Data from the Health Survey for England shows that, in both men and women, non-drinkers are more likely to be obese than those who consume alcohol (Bennett *et al.*, 1995). However, among alcohol consumers, there is a curious gender difference regarding the effect on body weight. In men, there is a very slight positive relationship between alcohol intake and mean BMI (or the proportion of subjects who are obese). Whereas in women, there is a powerful negative association, such that the highest alcohol consumers are only half as likely to be obese as non-drinkers (Fig. 13.6) are. Epidemiological studies in many other developed countries support the pattern seen in the UK, with a positive association between alcohol consumption and body weight in men and a negative

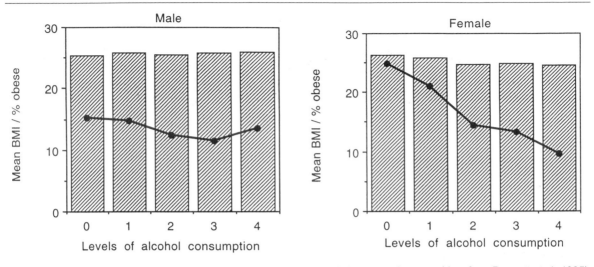

Fig. 13.6   Relationship between alcohol consumption and body weight in men and women (data from Bennett *et al.*, 1995).

association in women (Helderstedt *et al.*, 1990; Colditz *et al.*, 1991).

One possible explanation for this paradox in women, is that alcohol intake suppresses the intake of other foods and, thereby energy. However, self-reported data on food intake does not support this hypothesis (Colditz *et al.*, 1991). Food energy is remarkably constant across the range of alcohol intakes, suggesting that alcohol is supplementing, rather than substituting for, food. Alternatively, high alcohol consumers may have other lifestyle attributes that offset the effect of alcohol, such as higher levels of physical activity. However, a multivariate analysis of the Health Survey for England data concluded that, even after adjustment for age, smoking, social class and physical activity, the inverse relationship between BMI and alcohol intake in women persisted although the magnitude of the effect was greatly reduced (Prentice *et al.*, 1996). This epidemiological evidence is at odds with the experimental evidence relating alcohol to body weight, and the discrepancies between these two investigative approaches have yet to be reconciled (Prentice, 1995a).

13.2 Summary

- There has been a steady decline in energy intake over the last 20 years at a time of continued increases in obesity.

- Since World War II there has been a marked shift in the macronutrient composition of the diet, favouring fat at the expense of carbohydrate.

- There has also been a change in the type of fat consumed, with a decrease in saturated fatty acids and an increase in polyunsaturated fatty acids, especially n-6 fatty acids.

- Studies of the links between dietary habits and obesity are hindered by the under-reporting of food intake, especially among obese subjects.

- There is a modest decrease in energy intake with age, while the prevalence of obesity increases sharply.

- Inter-individual differences in dietary intake between geographical regions or by social class are poorly associated with differences in the prevalence of obesity.

- Epidemiological analyses of nutrient intake and obesity provide modest, but inconclusive, evidence that high-fat/low carbohydrate diets favour the development of obesity.

- Epidemiological evidence, which is suggestive of an inverse association between alcohol consumption and obesity, is in conflict with the metabolic evidence that alcohol consumption may be a risk factor for weight gain.

14
Aetiology of Obesity X: Food Choice, Food Policy and Eating Patterns

14.1 Behavioural responses to food

Biological signals related to satiety and regulation of energy balance are clearly important, but exist among a wide set of factors influencing what are ultimately voluntary decisions of what, when, and how much is eaten (Herman, 1996). Many studies have focused on comparative psychological and behavioural profiles and traits of obese and lean individuals (Chapter 12). However, in relating food intake and obesity, two major cognitive behavioural theories have dominated the eating behaviour research literature over the past 25 years.

i Externality

Formulated in the late 1960s, the 'externality theory' of obesity (Schachter, 1971; Schachter & Rodin, 1974) suggested that, compared with their lean counterparts, both obese rats and humans were more reactive to external cues (time, presence of food, and situational effects) and less sensitive to internal hunger and satiety signals (Fig. 14.1). According to this view, high external responsiveness would, given an environment of an easily accessible, abundant and highly palatable food supply, encourage overeating and hence the development of obesity.

These ideas became widely accepted and generated a large volume of related research in the 1970s. Many of the subsequent studies confirmed the original notion of externality. However, many did not and this view lost favour as it became clear that the relationship between externality and overweight is

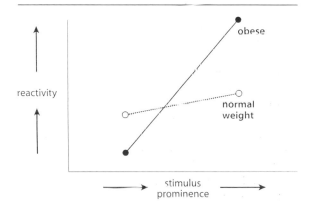

Fig. 14.1 Theoretical curves of the relationship of reactivity to stimulus prominence (from: Schacter, 1971). © 1971 The American Psychological Association. Reprinted with permission.

much more complex than originally proposed (reviewed by Leon & Roth, 1977; Rodin, 1981; Spitzer & Rodin, 1981). Nevertheless, this spawned a number of ideas, which have continued to be the focus of research through to the present. In particular, in experimental studies, better-liked foods are not only consumed in higher quantities than lesser-liked foods, but the magnitude of this palatability effect was reliably found to be exaggerated in obese subjects. However, the relationships among sensory acceptance, actual food choices and intake, and the development and maintenance of obesity have never been fully explored in human research. The possibility that certain traits of externality contribute to, or augment, a pre-

101

disposition to obesity remains a plausible hypothesis.

ii Restraint

The differences in eating behaviour of obese and
non-obese individuals in experimental situations, as
identified by Schachter (1971) and Schachter &
Rodin (1974) (Section 14.1.i), could arguably be a
result of concurrent dieting or a chronic struggle to
restrain their eating against (possibly biologically
based) drives toward an undesirably high body fat
content. However, since dieting and restrained
eating are prevalent among individuals whose
weight is normal or below normal (e.g. Biener &
Heaton, 1995), research has been directed at the
eating behaviour of subjects classified according to
their degree of dietary restraint and dieting, rather
than body weight or fatness alone.

The role of restrained eating in eating behaviour
was initially explored in a series of studies by
Herman and colleagues (Herman, 1978; Herman &
Mack, 1975; Herman *et al.*, 1978) and made use of
their Restraint Scale, assessing concern with dieting
and weight, and short-term weight fluctuation. One
of the crucial, but initially surprising, behavioural
correlates of restraint that they identified is a tendency to exhibit 'disinhibited' eating. In the classic
experiments, intakes of a test meal are found to be
inversely related to the size of a prior pre-load in
subjects scoring low on their Restraint Scale, while
intakes by restrained subjects paradoxically
increase with a greater pre-load (Fig. 14.2). This is a
cognitive effect, as demonstrated by the fact that
restrained subjects also eat more after a pre-load is
identified as 'high calorie', compared to the same
pre-load identified as 'low calorie' (Polivy, 1976).
Many factors, other than food pre-loads, have also
been shown to precipitate overeating in restrained
eaters, such as emotional events, the presence of
other people overeating, the sight and smell of well-
liked foods, and even the anticipation of a forth-
coming high food intake (Herman & Polivy, 1975;
Herman, 1978; Polivy *et al.*, 1979; Baucom & Aiken,
1981; Ruderman *et al.*, 1985; Rogers & Hill, 1989).

This counter-regulatory behaviour apparently
occurs when the perceived intake of energy is sufficient to cause normally restrained eaters to sus-
pend their self-imposed restraint, thereby releasing
an underlying desire to (over) eat (Herman &

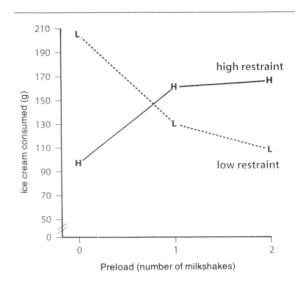

Fig. 14.2 Relationship between restraint and
consumption in an ice cream 'taste' test following
different levels of milkshake preloads (data from Herman
& Mack, 1975).

Mack, 1975; Herman, 1978; Herman & Polivy,
1984). Research in this area has confirmed a major
influence of cognition on short-term food intake
and suggests potential causal links between
restraint and compulsive eating (Wardle, 1987) and,
perhaps, longer-term failure of weight control. The
Restraint Scale of Herman and colleagues (Herman *et al.*, 1978) and more recent eating behaviour
questionnaires (Stunkard & Messick, 1985; Van
Strien *et al.*, 1986b) have been widely used in
behavioural research over the past decade. There
are important theoretical and practical differences
among these scales and the extent to which they
may characterise 'successful' and 'unsuccessful'
aspects of restraint or weight control, and there is
an extensive volume of literature on their behavioural and nutritional correlates (Mela & Rogers,
1998; see also Chapter 12).

In relation to the development or maintenance
of obesity, the role of restrained eating and
related or consequent behaviours, especially the
tendency for disinhibited eating, remains suggestive though unproven. One of the intriguing issues
is whether restrained eating is reflecting an underlying biological predisposition for overeating and
obesity. On the basis of diet records alone, some
authors have concluded that restrained eaters

have lower energy requirements (Laessle *et al.*, 1989; de Castro, 1995). However, self-reported energy intakes of restrained eaters appear to be particularly prone to underestimation (Ortega *et al.*, 1996; Mela & Aaron, 1997; Chapter 13). Studies using more objective measures have generated mixed conclusions regarding the possibility of lower total or obligate energy expenditure amongst restrained eaters (Tuschl *et al.*, 1990; Westerterp-Plantenga *et al.*, 1992; Lawson *et al.*, 1995; Platte *et al.*, 1996). It is also possible that, like obese individuals, restrained eaters may manifest some reduced capacity to raise fat oxidation commensurate with moderate or high fat intakes (Verboeket-van de Venne *et al.*, 1993).

Although dietary restraint of some form is inevitably a component of successful dietary treatments for obesity, certain behaviours that characterise restraint might, in a paradoxical way, contribute to the development and maintenance of obesity in some individuals, or amplify a pre-existing behavioural or biological predisposition. Recent work has continued to refine these concepts and investigate the importance and implications of dietary restraint in an environment where energy-dense foods and opportunities to eat are ubiquitous, while slimness is promoted as the ideal of beauty, self-control and success. One important interpretation of restraint research is that palatable, energy-dense foods may not be of concern solely because of their inherent nutritional composition, and potential for 'passive' over-consumption (Blundell *et al.*, 1993). For many individuals, the consumption, or even the presence, of such foods may present a particularly potent stimulus for the

breakdown of restraint, loss of dietary control, and overeating of these or other foods.

14.2 Sensory and food preferences

i Methodological issues

A wide variety of different tasks may be used to assess, or make, inferences about individual perceptions and acceptance of specific sensory qualities (tastes, smells, textures) or whole foods, in relation to dietary or nutritional criteria (Mela, 1992; MacFie & Thomson, 1994). A discussion of sensory methodology is outside the scope of this review; however, it is important to note and draw a distinction between measures that assess functional aspects of perception and those that consider some aspect of liking or acceptability (Table 14.1). The latter are arguably most likely to show relationships with eating behaviour (Mela, 1992), but can also be assessed in many different ways (Table 14.2). Selection of test items and context are a major issue, and sensory studies vary from the use of highly controlled stimuli consisting of single chemical species (e.g. NaCl or sucrose) in water to more ecologically valid but complex models of real foods. However, many (perhaps most) food preference studies do not actually include tasting of samples, but are based upon questionnaires eliciting ratings of hedonics (liking) or preferred frequency of consumption of specific items. Food acceptability is also inferred from actual dietary intake data, on the (rather dubious) assumption that consumption is a correlate of liking. In fact, purchase and consumption decisions represent an integration of many

Table 14.1 Common assessment methods in sensory perception.

Threshold (detection or recognition)	A measure of absolute sensitivity; the lowest consistently detectable or recognisable concentration of a stimulus in a given medium.
Intensity ratings	A measure of relative strengths of sensations; the relationship between physical concentration and perceived intensity of duration of a stimulus at levels above threshold.
Profiling; multidimensional scaling	Placement or grouping of stimuli (in a multi-dimensional perceptual space) based upon perceptual relationships amongst a range of sensory attributes or liking.
Identification/Recognition	The ability to associate stimuli with their usual or natural sources; used most often for olfaction.
Hedonic (preference)	The absolute or relative liking or acceptability of a stimulus.

Table 14.2 Examples of measurement variables in assessments of sensory and food preferences. (© BBSRC.)

Test items	Simple controlled stimuli Complex real or model foods
Context	Sensory evaluation laboratory test Home trial Actual purchase conditions
Hedonic ratings	Actual tasting Questionnaire
Preferred frequency of consumption ratings	Actual tasting Questionnaire
Behavioural data	Purchase information Diet history or records
Food groupings	Nutritional criteria Sensory characteristics Source or degree of preparation required Typical use/culinary role

different characteristics of a food, in addition to sensory quality (e.g. price, brand, perceived nutritional attributes). This is even true for 'objective' taste test data, which may be considerably influenced by individual attitudes, beliefs, and expectations about the test stimuli (e.g. Aaron *et al.*, 1994). Hence, simple affective measures of liking for specific foods or food groups do not necessarily correspond to actual dietary intake behaviour (Mela, 1992, 1995; Lluch *et al.*, 1995).

ii Sensory preferences in relation to weight status

It is commonly suggested that the preference for selected sensory qualities may be heightened in obesity and that this may be a contributing factor in excessive food intakes. Historically, much of this research has been directed toward sweet taste preferences, although most studies have found that obese and lean individuals do not differ in their general sensitivity to, or perceptions of, intensity of sweetness, or in their liking for sweetness in foods or beverages (Grinker, 1978; Malcolm *et al.*, 1980; Frijters & Rasmussen-Conrad, 1982; Drewnowski *et al.*, 1985; Grinker *et al.*, 1986; Mela, 1996b). No obese–lean differences have been reported for sensitivity to or liking for non-sweet tastes (Malcolm *et al.*, 1980), or a food-related aroma (benzaldehyde) (Thompson *et al.*, 1977). While there appears to be little evidence to associate obesity with specific abnormalities of chemosensory function, many of the pertinent studies may lack eco-

logical validity, as they have used methods or focused on stimuli that may be irrelevant or unrelated to real world perception of normal foods (Mela, 1992).

Much of the recent work on sensory perception and preferences in relation to obesity has focused on fats. Obese and lean subjects have not been found to differ in their intensity ratings for fat content or creaminess of a range of sweetened milk and cream samples (Drewnowski *et al.*, 1985) or model emulsions (Mela *et al.*, 1994). However, Drewnowski *et al.* reported that obese and recently reduced, formerly obese individuals, show enhanced preferences for higher fat levels in a sweetened, milk-based test food system (Drewnowski *et al.*, 1985). Subsequent studies by Drewnowski and colleagues (Drewnowski *et al.*, 1991; Drewnowski & Holden-Wiltse, 1992) have suggested that a greater preference for sweet, high-fat stimuli is particularly associated with a history of weight cycling. Most recently, Karhunen *et al.* (1997) have presented data from obese women, suggesting that relatively lower leptin levels (corrected for fat mass) may be associated with both higher fat intakes and heightened liking for high-fat, low-sugar stimuli (Chapter 6).

Enhanced liking for higher fat levels in foods extends (perhaps more consistently) to savoury, rather than sweet foods and, importantly, appears to characterise non-obese individuals predisposed to obesity. Mela & Sacchetti (1991) found a positive relationship, in subjects of normal weight for height, between per cent body fat and the preferred fat content of a test battery comprising both sweet and savoury foods (Fig. 14.3). Fisher & Birch (1995) assessed fat preferences of young children, using a test battery comprising savoury high fat items and a mix of sweet and savoury low fat items. They found significant positive correlations of fat preferences with measures of both child and parent fatness, and child's fat intake. Kanarek and colleagues found that liking for a higher fat content in a test food (popcorn) was increased by higher salt content among restrained but not among unrestrained women (Kanarek *et al.*, 1995). Measures of restraint did not, however, relate to consistent differences in response to fat content of a sweet–fat combination (Frye *et al.*, 1994). Relationships among fat intakes, sensory preferences, and weight status, would be clarified by improved identification of the sources of variance in fat intakes, and by work linking actual food choices and individual consumer characteristics with subjective (sensory) and objective (nutrient composition) information on specific foods (e.g. Cox *et al.*, 1998), and perhaps also to individual metabolic characteristics. Current views of the acquisition of liking for high fat foods and diets open up the possibility that these preferences could be linked to genetically based/ physiological factors, which predispose to obesity (Mela, 1995; Mela, 1996b; Mela & Rogers, 1998). However, this

is only now beginning to be empirically tested (Chapter 6).

iii Food preferences and intake in relation to weight status

There are few published studies comparing either the expressed food preferences or the actual food or food groups (as opposed to nutrients) consumed by lean and obese individuals. This body of research suffers from problems of interpretation, as specific food categories are usually defined by investigators, and can be based upon subjective similarities in nutrient profile (e.g. high-fat and low energy density), sensory characteristics (e.g. sweet, savoury), source or site of preparation (processed versus home-prepared), role in cuisine ('snacks' versus 'meals'), or various combinations of these. These many different categorisation schemes are clearly incompatible with each other and specific schemes often seem contrived and illogical. Causality is also difficult to establish from these data, since obese individuals may select, or claim to select, or avoid certain foods as a result of their present weight status.

In contrast to data on macronutrient intakes (Chapter 13), dietary intake studies generally reveal few, if any, consistent relationships between measures of weight status and specific food selections (e.g. Coates *et al.*, 1978; Kulesza, 1982; Baeke *et al.*, 1983; Morgan *et al.*, 1983; Pangborn *et al.*, 1985; New & Grubb, 1996; Table 14.3). Food preference studies are more suggestive, but fewer, and also inconclusive. In a summary of their extensive studies of United States armed forces personnel, Meiselman (1977) and Meiselman & Wyant (1981) reported that overweight subjects assigned higher hedonic and preferred frequency ratings to entrées particularly meats. Drewnowski (1985) used a novel, multi-dimensional scaling approach to assess preferences of normal weight and obese subjects for listed foods. Although the range of foods was rather limited, the results suggest greater liking for clusters of foods characterised as 'healthy' (milk, eggs, peanut butter, fruits and vegetables) and as energy-dense 'snacks' (ice-cream, candy, carbonated beverages), by normal weight and obese subjects, respectively. In a later study, Drewnowski *et al.* (1992) reported that while obese males indicated greater preferences for low carbohydrate,

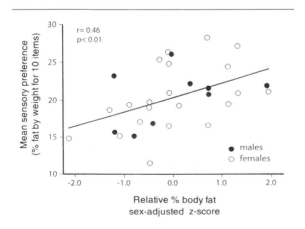

Fig. 14.3 Relationship between relative per cent body fat and mean most preferred fat level in a battery of foods. Sex-adjusted z-scores are used to place males and females on a single scale (from: Mela 1992).

Table 14.3 Examples of results of studies comparing self-reported preferences or intakes of specific foods and food groups of obese and non-obese subjects. Subjects were all adults unless stated otherwise. FFQ = Food Frequency Questionnaire used to assess intakes. (© BBSRC. From Mela & Rogers, 1998.)

Reference and measure	Food groups	Differences, obese relative to non-obese Direction of response and foods		
Meiselman, 1977	8			
Preferred frequency		↑		Entrées
Hedonic		↑		Entrées
Coates *et al.*, 1978	7			
Stored food		↑	(father)	Desserts
		↓	(family)	'Processed' foods
Meiselman & Wyant, 1981	12			
Hedonic		↑		Carbonated beverages
Kulesza, 1982	17	No differences observed		
Baeke *et al.*, 1983	10			
2-day intake (correlation)		↓ (♀)		Fats & oils
		↓ (♀)		Sugars
		↓ (♂)		Fruits & vegetables
Drewnowski, 1985	16			
Hedonic ratings		↑		Energy-dense 'snacks'
		↓		'Healthy' foods
Pangborn *et al.*, 1985	9			
FFQ		↑		Meats
		↓		Avocado, olive
Rolland-Cachera & Bellisle, 1986	17			
FFQ (age 7–12)		↑		Meats
		?		Eggs
Jacobsen & Thelle, 1987	12			
FFQ (correlation)		↑ and ↓		Many low correlations (r <0.1)
		↑		Low fat milk
		↓		Bread
Ortega *et al.*, 1995	13			
Weighed intake (age 15–17)		↑		Fish
		↓		Non-alcoholic beverages
				Miscellaneous foods
Correlations with BMI:		↑		Fish, eggs
		↓		Fruit
Parker *et al.*, 1997				
FFQ	7	None related to 4 year weight change		
Cox *et al.*, 1997				
Hedonic	14	↓		Vegetables
		↓		Fruits

high fat or fat/protein foods (e.g. meats); obese females preferred more fat/carbohydrate combination items and sweet items (e.g. cakes and ice-cream). However, the sex differences reported in that work are not consistently split along these lines and the absence of corresponding responses from normal weight individuals makes it unclear whether these preferences are specific to obese subjects, or characterise the population as a whole. A preliminary report by Lluch *et al.* (1995) also found that an obese subject population assigned high hedonic ratings to high-fat, energy-dense foods, but the work lacks comparative information from normal weight individuals. Cox *et al.* (1997) found no lean–obese differences in overall mean hedonic ratings assigned to a list of common foods, but obese subjects assigned typically lower hedonic ratings overall, and significantly lower ratings to fruits and vegetables. Cox *et al.* (1998) also found no lean–obese differences in mean hedonic ratings assigned to the foods actually eaten over a 4-day period. However, obesity was associated with a higher overall dietary energy density, which was associated with foods having a predominantly salty/savoury taste quality.

iv Sensory characteristics of food, 'palatability' and energy balance

It is commonly assumed that the sensory appeal of foods can exert an effect on energy intake and, consequently, on energy balance. More specifically, it may be believed that presence and ready availability of 'palatable' foods has a causal role in overeating and obesity. This is an intuitively attractive notion and there is little doubt that, at least in the short term, individuals tend to eat greater amounts of a better-liked food and would avoid a truly disliked option. But it is less clear how this influences energy balance over the longer term, in the real world and particularly when food composition is taken into consideration. The fundamental question, of whether the sensory appeal of foods exerts an independent effect on energy balance, or specifically contributes to overeating and obesity, would appear to raise some complex issues (Mela & Rogers, 1998).

There are a variety of ways in which the sensory hedonic value of foods could alter short-term energy intake and expenditure. Positive sensory stimulation can undoubtedly prompt a desire to consume food, even when individuals are not hungry (Cornell *et al.*, 1989) and can enhance the rate and total intake of energy within a meal (Hill & McCutcheon, 1975; Bellisle & Le Magnen, 1981; Bellisle *et al.*, 1984; Hill & McCutcheon, 1984). These findings are in accord with everyday experience, and not necessarily surprising. Sensory stimulation and palatability clearly influence a spectrum of pre- and post-prandial metabolic events, some of which are known to modulate hunger and nutrient utilisation (Feldman & Richardson, 1986; Simon *et al.*, 1986; Teff & Engelman, 1996). However, the effects of the sensory components and hedonic value of foods on post-ingestive appetite ratings are not clear, and studies have found that consumption of a more appealing food may either stimulate (Hill *et al.*, 1984) or suppress (Warwick *et al.*, 1993) later feelings of hunger. A more palatable version of a meal was also found to generate significantly greater post-prandial thermogenesis in one report (le Blanc & Brondel, 1985). A subsequent study, with better control of the food composition, found that sensory acceptability had no appreciable effect on measures of post-prandial resting energy expenditure (Weststrate *et al.*, 1990a). The possible effects of hedonic value or sensory characteristics of foods and meals on post-prandial satiety and metabolism appear to be relatively small, but may warrant further study.

Perhaps most importantly, there is a conceptual problem of distinguishing between effects of hedonic value and effects of food composition. Many well liked foods are also high in energy density. Hence, effects attributed to 'palatability' or specific sensory qualities may actually be fundamental effects of food composition. Furthermore, the link between energy density and sensory appeal is not coincidental, as described below, because the nutritional value of particular foods may be at the root of their hedonic value. Similarly, metabolic responses to sensory stimulation may also be learned, as a result of associations with food composition. As noted elsewhere (Chapters 10 and 13), there is evidence from human studies that diets high in fat or energy density may be associated with overeating and weight gain. However, many short-term and animal experiments have confounded palatability and composition, by comparing (usually) highly liked energy-dense foods or diets to less-liked foods or diets of lower energy density.

Animal studies have been used to try to dissect the differential influences of composition and palatability or flavour variety on intake, but results have led to different conclusions regarding the relative contribution of each factor (Mela & Rogers, 1998). Some of the differences between studies are probably related to the (in)ability of animals to use flavours as a reliable cue to energy density, under conditions where food composition and flavour are independently varied. Thus, variations in sensory quality have the potential to disrupt, or prevent, the development of learned controls of intake. This may, perhaps, contribute to the results of human studies, where volume of food intake remains fairly constant, rather than responding to changes in the (fixed) energy density of varied menus (Mela & Rogers, 1998; see also Chapter 10).

Individual sensory and food preferences are highly adaptable and not distinctly separable from composition (Mela & Catt, 1996). Humans, and other animals, readily learn from the conditions and consequences (metabolic, physiological, and psychological) associated with ingestion of specific foods or sensory qualities (Booth, 1985; Rozin & Schulkin, 1990; Sclafani, 1995). There is abundant evidence for the predominance of these and other learning processes in the formation of sensory likes. Numerous experiments in animals have shown how the physiological consequences of foods, including subtle nutritional and metabolic effects, can markedly alter sensory acceptance, including reversal of 'innate' likes and dislikes. Many examples of human food preferences and aversions can be best explained by such processes, including the apparent liking for the sensory contribution of fats in foods (Mela, 1995; Sclafani, 1995). Flavour preferences in humans have been shown to be influenced by the energy content (as fat or carbohydrate) of test foods (Booth *et al.*, 1982; Birch *et al.*, 1990; Johnson *et al.*, 1991; Kern *et al.*, 1993). These studies provide particularly compelling evidence that these processes are operative in humans. Overall, this area of research convincingly demonstrates that sensory acceptance can be modified by association with differential nutritional properties of foods, and suggests that energy density could be an important contributor to this process.

Repeated exposure to particular foods or sensory qualities (familiarity or 'mere exposure') provides opportunities for the development or continued reinforcement of conditioned preferences, or might possibly represent an additional mechanism for acquisition of particular food likes (Mela & Catt, 1996). Although change in sensory exposure to salt has been shown to reduce preferred salt concentration in foods, the effect of changes in macronutrient (especially fat) intakes on liking or desire to consume particular foods is not clear (Laitinen *et al.*, 1991; Mattes, 1993; Mela *et al.*, 1993; Rolls, 1994). Outside the laboratory, familiarity may also interact with consumer attitudes, beliefs and expectations, rather than directly influencing the hedonic value of foods. This distinction may seem fine, but has potentially important implications for dietary change.

Taken together, this analysis suggests that the sensory quality of foods may have an acute effect, but probably rather more limited, long-term independent contribution to variation in energy balance, when food composition is taken into account. However, this dissection of the issue may have more theoretical, than practical, importance and the sections above also raise the possibility that individuals predisposed to obesity may respond more strongly to the hedonic value of foods and also show a heightened liking for fats. It is conceivable that fat-containing foods might hold greater reinforcing psychobiological effects for such individuals and could, therefore, be more potent stimuli for the acquisition and maintenance of sensory preferences for such items (Mela, 1995; Mela, 1996b). By any mechanism, however, the ready availability of foods having a particular combination of sensory appeal and composition may represent a situation which, combined with a heightened responsiveness to such foods specifically (or to palatability generally) or given a tendency for disinhibited eating, creates fertile nutritional and psychological conditions for excessive intakes and poor weight control.

14.3 Macro-environmental aspects

The food environment is clearly linked to obesity, in so far as the condition is only prevalent among populations that have constant economic and market access to high-fat, energy-dense foods. It is generally agreed that food product availability and cultural norms are the primary factors determining the range and frequency of items likely to be consumed by a given population. However, this level of analysis is very broad, laden with social and historical antecedents and does not necessarily map onto nutrient or energy intakes. Beyond this, linking specific characteristics of the production, distribution, and marketing of foods, to the development of overeating and obesity, becomes much more speculative. The fundamental question seems to be, are there practices within the industrial food chain that specifically facilitate or promote lifestyles or diets implicated in the development or prevention of obesity?

Many interrelated variables are known to influence an individual's food purchasing behaviour. The food industry clearly has an impact on what is eaten, although the extent of this effect is difficult to tease out. Food availability is another of the many factors that are clearly linked to food choice. Reviews by Shepherd (1989, 1990) of descriptive models of food preference and choice, highlight common characteristics of personal, product and environmental factors influencing food purchasing decisions. Ritson & Hutchins (1995) place buying decisions in an economic context.

A relevant background to macro-environmental aspects is that during the post-war period, in spite of the price-raising effects of agricultural policies, the prices of agricultural raw materials have declined relative to prices of other products. This, together with the growth in personal incomes, means that, according to National Food Survey data, the proportion of income spent on food in the UK has declined from over 30% in the mid-1950s (immediately after the period when it was controlled by rationing) to 18% in 1995. The proportion of income spent on food is much higher for lower-income groups than for high-income groups, but the capacity of the vast majority of people in this country to choose a nutritious diet, not constrained by income, has increased significantly.

Obesity is generally prevalent only among populations or population groups that have economic and market access to more than sufficient energy intakes, and to high-fat energy-dense foods. However, there is no evidence from which to conclude cause and effect, i.e. that obesity results from positive economic circumstances and a wide availability of food. The fundamental question to be addressed is: to what degree do macro-environmental factors associated with the industrial food-chain distort eating patterns compared to the pattern that would be expected in a resource-constrained supply system responding to freely expressed consumer demand? The principal ways in which such influences might occur are highlighted below.

i Food industry and marketing policies

Aspects of food industry marketing policy have been criticised for encouraging the consumption of 'unhealthy' foods, i.e. of undesirable nutritional value (e.g. Fine *et al.*, 1996; Lang *et al.*, 1989). However, reviews of the influence of marketing on eating behaviour indicate a paucity of information, which is perhaps unsurprising in such a complex subject area (Schutz & Diaz-Knauf, 1989). Marketing policies typically involve a combination of product promotion, distribution and pricing strategies to supply a pre-identified target market with a product that meets its needs. Food manufacturers, operating in a highly competitive environment, aim to innovate and keep abreast of competition by satisfying demands linked to changing consumer tastes, preferences (Buisson, 1995) and requirements. Although, for example, 'value-added' products have been claimed to offer poor nutritional value (Lang *et al.*, 1989), it is important to emphasise that food manufacturers provide consumers with food products, not 'diets'.

Aspects of consumer lifestyles that contribute to eating patterns such as 'grazing' and factors such as the desire for convenience foods are also relevant to discussions on obesity. Lang *et al.* (1995) argue that, in particular, time constraints and a loss of cooking expertise induce a 'snacking' and convenience food culture. The 'industrialisation of food', typified by the availability of convenience products, is believed by some commentators to have been developed to meet the needs of producers in search of a competitive advantage, rather than the needs of consumers. Gussow (1987), reporting on research examining promotional strategies of US food manufacturers, suggested that although the food industry responded to consumer demands for product innovation, the industry fostered negative public attitudes towards food preparation, thus paving the way for further innovations and reliance on convenience foods.

The strongest allegations of potential for distortion of eating patterns have been levied at the promotional strategies, in particular advertising, used by the food industry. The highly competitive global marketplace necessitates huge expenditure to assist brand survival. Ennew *et al.* (1995) state that approximately 80% of the 100 largest advertising expenditures are made by food companies each with an advertising spend of over £1 million. However, are energy-dense, high-fat foods selectively promoted? A recent National Food Alliance survey (Dibb & Castell, 1995) reported that foods high in fat and sugar, which are recommended to comprise no more than 7% of an individual's diet, were the most heavily advertised, accounting for 44–76% of all food advertisements (depending on the time period) and were, therefore, 'grossly out of proportion to recommended consumption level'. The study concluded that 'the cumulative effect of food advertising undermines progress towards a healthy diet' (Dibb & Castell, 1995).

Although advertising seeks to inform, and thereby challenge knowledge, beliefs and hence attitudes, this does not necessarily result in changes in purchasing behaviour. The inability of the mass media to bring about long-term improvements in eating habits has been used to highlight this (Schutz & Diaz-Knauf, 1989). For example, although the majority of UK adults are aware that fresh fruit and vegetables are essential for a healthy diet, this has not translated into a substantial increase in consumption (Leatherhead Food Research Association, 1996). This does not necessarily mean that consumer behaviour is not responding to the healthy eating message; it may reflect the fact that some other factor (for example, the desire for convenience) is overriding consumers' desire to act on their knowledge.

The success of advertising in influencing product choice varies according to the product being promoted, the individual receiving the message and other external circumstances (Lannon, 1986). Whether or not advertising consciously or subconsciously changes beliefs and attitudes, adults do not have a passive role in the process of communication, and may be able to rationalise and understand the context of advertisements. On the other hand, children are seen as impressionable and vulnerable to media messages. Here the question raised is what action results as a consequence of the media message on children? Young *et al.* (1995) argued that advertising was not a principal influence on children's eating behaviour; rather, the factors were more complex and should be considered in the context of a child's physiological, psychological and socio-cultural domains. Thus, the influence of advertising on changing food choice and eating behaviour remains inconclusive.

The price of food products and its ability to impact on food choice and eating behaviour is highly complex. Price is exclusionary in terms of a consumer being able and willing to pay for a product. However, the price of an individual product is complicated by consumer perceptions of price as an indicator of quality, which may lead to greater desirability of higher priced food products (Monroe & Petroshius, 1981). One aspect of price, twinned with the distribution of food products, is the price of the theoretical 'healthy basket' of groceries compared to the 'unhealthy basket', and the price differentials of each according to the retail outlets of purchase. These are discussed below.

ii The structure of food retailing

Major changes in the modern UK distribution chain, and food retailing, in particular, have been well-documented (e.g. Dawson, 1995). Five companies now account for approximately 65% of retail food sales. Store size of the multiple retailers has increased and stores have been relocated to edge-of-town or out-of-town positions on major transport routes, thus favouring the car-owner. This leads to the questions: to what degree is consumer food choice influenced by the food products on offer at such multiple retail outlets, and to what degree are the diets of some low-income consumers adversely affected by the location of stores and product prices? The latter is complicated by retail pricing policy. Some food products are offered for sale as 'loss leaders', e.g. bread, on which the retailer does not make a unit profit. Retailers are also known to use various polices such as 'averaging' and 'levelling' on some seasonal products in an effort to standardise the price of products throughout the year, on the assumption that consumers prefer stable prices (Digby, 1989). Furthermore, there is conflicting evidence as to which type of retail outlet, discount or non-discount, presents the best 'value for money'. In a recent survey comparing the costs of 'healthy' and 'unhealthy' baskets of food of equal energy content, it was found that while discount supermarkets offered lower prices for the 'unhealthy' basket, the 'healthy' basket was more expensive than in other non-discount supermarkets (Zeffler & Adamson, 1995). Moving supermarkets to edge-of-town locations has been criticised for the creation of 'shopping deserts', risking the diets of low-income consumers to be adversely affected as a result (Lang, 1995). However, White *et al.* (1996) found that, in a socio-economic study of the spatial distribution of retail outlets, proximity to supermarkets did not have a significant effect on food choice.

iii Government policies and food prices

Government policies can have both direct and indirect effects on food purchasing behaviour. For example, fiscal and social welfare policies have an indirect effect on a household's disposable income and, hence, purchasing power. Inequalities in health between high- and low-income groups have increased over the past two decades. However, a combination of factors that cause deprivation have been shown to be more illuminating than low income alone, when trying to explain such inequalities (Dowler & Calvert, 1995).

One publicly visible reflection of government policies concerns decisions that fall under the aegis of the Common Agricultural Policy (CAP). These have been criticised from a nutritional viewpoint because of the release of cheap butter and beef to old age pensioners and the periodical destruction of fruit and vegetables. In fact, these are only minor issues; butter subsidies only affect other CAP policies which discourage its consumption, and most fruit and vegetables destroyed would never reach consumers (Ritson, 1997a). Although only a relatively small number of studies have looked specifically at the impact of the CAP on the UK diet (e.g. Colman, 1987; Ritson, 1983, 1992, 1997a; Henson, 1992; Swinbank, 1992; Cawley *et al.*, 1994), all broadly came to the same conclusion. The main impact has been on food prices. By a mixture of minimum import prices, intervention and export subsidies, the CAP has sustained the prices of most food products above the level that would otherwise apply, but does so in an uneven way. Although it is possible that the CAP may have a negative impact on some aspects of nutrition for low-income consumers, its main impact has concerned the balance of food consumption throughout the nation, and has been broadly positive from a nutritional point of view.

It is, of course, extremely difficult to estimate the extent to which the prices of individual foods have been raised by the CAP, and thus to what extent and in which ways, patterns of food consumption have been influenced. Table 14.4 ranks major agricultural products according to the degree to which the CAP has increased prices, and thus discouraged consumption. It would be possible to

Table 14.4 Agricultural products ranked according to the price raising effect of the CAP[1].

Products	EU price as a % of world market prices (Average 1968–1993)
Milk and dairy products[2]	300
Sugar[3]	172
Lamb	222
Beef	177
Pork	131
Poultry	128
Bread and cereal products[4]	125
Most fruit and vegetables[5]	110
Vegetable oils[6]	105
Potatoes[7]	100

[1] Most of these figures are derived from estimates by the European Commission and OECD, listed in Tables 1.1 and 1.2 in Ritson (1997b). For much of the history of the CAP, prices in individual member states may have differed significantly from these because of monetary compensatory amounts (see Ritson & Swinbank, 1997).
[2] Estimates for milk and dairy products are based on butter and skim milk powder 1968–1980; and whole milk equivalent 1980–1993.
[3] This is at the production level. Under the CAP, export subsidies for sugar are financed by a sugar tax, which has a substantial additional price raising effect.
[4] Based on estimated cereal content of products.
[5] Crude estimate on the basis of limited periods when cheap imports are restricted; plus impact of import tariffs.
[6] Impact of small import tariffs.
[7] No CAP policy.

dispute the order in which some items appear, but not that the CAP had a substantial effect on the price of those commodities at the top of the list and a broadly neutral effect on those at the bottom.

Thus, by virtue of its reliance on price support, the CAP tends to **discourage** the consumption of those products for which it gives the greatest stimulus to production. These are also products that consumers have been recommended to eat less of. Such findings are compatible with research in other EC countries, for example, Georgakopoulos (1990) has analysed the implications of the CAP in the Greek market. Recent changes to the CAP are, if anything, strengthening this effect. For example, the MacSharry reform of the CAP and the changes necessitated by the GATT Agreement, have resulted in a fall in the price of cereal products and grain-fed livestock, but milk and dairy product prices are largely unaffected.

iv Changes in food composition

In the UK and other western nations, most consumers have economic and market access to a diet of virtually any composition. However, cultural and culinary 'rules' largely dictate that certain individual foods and food combinations are deemed appropriate and are, therefore, more widely and frequently accessible and consumed. Therefore, changing dietary habits, implies either changing people (attitudes, preferences and choices) within the same food environment, or changing the composition of traditional foods.

In the early 1980s, a number of reports were published by expert committees advocating substantial changes in the UK diet (National Advisory Committee on Nutrition Education, 1983; Royal College of Physicians, 1983; Department of Health and Social Security, 1984). Since this time, there has been tremendous growth in the development and marketing of foods intended to aid compliance with public health nutrition guidance, including new or reformulated products reduced in fat, sugars or energy. In particular, there has been considerable expansion in the availability, marketing and sales of low and reduced-fat dairy products, ready meals with controlled fat and energy contents, and low and reduced-fat desserts and ready-to-eat 'snack' foods. The fat content of many cuts of meat has also declined significantly (Paul & Southgate, 1978; Chan *et al.*, 1995, 1996).

It is not clear how such apparently beneficial changes in the market relate to actual nutrient intakes, or to the concurrent rise in prevalence of overweight and obesity. Although the major macronutrient composition of the diet changed relatively little between 1970 and 1995 (Ministry of Agriculture, Fisheries and Food, 1995, 1996), there has been a substantial decline in reported energy intakes and evidence of a modest decline in the proportion of energy coming from total fat and from saturated fatty acids between 1983 and 1995. Given that many changes in the composition or marketing of manufactured foods have been prompted by, or largely directed at, concerns about weight status, it seems appropriate to consider the implications for the development of obesity of foods with a modified composition.

Studies have assessed the potential influences of sugar and fat replacement on appetite and energy intake. Most of this literature comprises short-term experiments, based in the laboratory and/or using covert manipulations of pre-loads or foods in order to investigate the biological regulation of hunger, satiety, and eating (reviewed by Rolls, 1991a,b; Bellisle & Perez, 1994; Blundell & Rogers, 1994; Mela, 1996a, 1997a,b). As a very gross generalisation, this research suggests that, under most conditions, normal weight individuals with access to a mixed diet tend to compensate for moderate reductions in energy density, associated with casual use of sugar and fat substitutes in place of traditional ingredients. With few exceptions, these studies also indicate that energy compensation would be through eating a mixed diet of normal composition, i.e., the composition is not macronutrient specific.

Most of these types of experiments, however, have not been designed to characterise the actual dietary behaviour of consumers in natural situations, although often they are interpreted in that way, and are potentially sensitive to many details of experimental design. These short-term studies also allow limited opportunity for involvement of regulatory processes, which may become meaningful in studies of longer duration. Furthermore, most of the studies have used covert experimental manipulation and, therefore, knowledge or beliefs about the test foods and their energy or macronutrient content has not been a major focus of interest. Nevertheless, the general findings are confirmed by longer-term studies of free-living subjects under normal food purchase and consumption conditions (Gatenby *et al.*, 1995, 1997; Westerterp *et al.*, 1996; de Graaf *et al.*, 1997; Lawton & Blundell, 1998). Unfortunately, though, there are presently few studies which have exploited large dietary intake databases to assess the dietary or anthropometric profiles that characterise macronutrient substitute use or users.

Although the general trend is for good energy compensation, if use of macronutrient-substituted foods is extensive enough to yield significant changes in macronutrient composition of the diet, this may have implications for the development of obesity. However, this could depend upon whether it is fat or carbohydrate (sugars) that is being removed from the food, what is used in place of these macronutrients, and the energy density of the resulting products. Given that there is little evidence for a direct causal role of sugar intakes in obesity (Mela & Rogers, 1998; Section 13.1), the specific removal of, or substitution for, sugar should not necessarily be expected to prevent or treat the condition. Correspondingly, despite the widespread use of non-nutritive sweeteners, there is a lack of evidence that this reduces the risk of becoming overweight, or even impacts upon total sugars intake (Anderson & Leiter, 1996). Indeed, one concern is that energy from sugars might be replaced by a mixture of macronutrients, including fat, leading to an overall increase in the fat and energy density of the diet (Beaton *et al.*, 1992; Mela, 1997a). However, despite inverse relationships between fat and sugar intakes (Chapter 13), there is no support for a direct link between fat intake (or measures of fatness) and use of intense sweeteners. The limited experimental data (e.g. Chen & Parham, 1991) suggest that, in practice, foods containing intense sweeteners may be largely additional to the diet, rather than actually substituting for other sugar-containing foods. Since the major dietary sources of intense sweeteners are non-caloric ('diet' beverages, tabletop sweeteners), the overall nutritional impact of such products could be negligible if used in this manner (Mela, 1997b).

Given the experimental and epidemiological evidence linking high fat intakes with an increased risk of obesity (Chapters 9, 10 and 13), replacement of fat in foods by non-fat ingredients appears to be a potentially helpful industrial and public health approach to the problem. However, fat replacement may only be helpful in weight control if it contributes toward meaningful overall reductions in the fat content and also the energy density of diets (Mela & Rogers, 1998; see also Chapter 10). The actual consumer response to casual or extensive use of modified foods, in terms of nutrient and energy intakes or food selection patterns, is not well established (Mela, 1996c, 1997a,b). Predictive analyses of the impact of macronutrient-substituted foods (e.g. Beaton *et al.*, 1992; Lyle *et al.*, 1991) largely assume that these products would be used in place of the traditional items, not in addition to them, while market and research data suggest that this is not necessarily true. Furthermore, a focus on modified foods alone may undermine efforts to promote a wider range of desirable dietary and nutritional goals. Nevertheless, use of reduced-fat

products may afford opportunities for altering intakes within the existing traditional diet and seems likely to be a useful and acceptable adjunct to a broader strategy for achieving desired changes in the types and composition of foods consumed (Kristal *et al.*, 1992; Mela, 1997a). An effective contribution of such products to the prevention or treatment of obesity may, however, require that they are reduced in energy density as well as fat content, and incorporated into a programme of other lifestyle behaviours (Lawton & Blundell, 1998).

14.4 Eating frequency and circadian distribution

Interest in 'meal patterns' was largely stimulated by a combination of animal research and epidemiological studies in the early 1960s. These studies suggested that consumption of larger, less frequent 'meals' was associated with a greater fat deposition and risk of obesity, compared to a more frequent pattern of eating (Leveille, 1970; Fábry & Tepperman, 1970). Human research in this area has been plagued by problems with definition of eating occasions and lack of data on eating frequency *per se*. Non-standardised, colloquial terms such as 'meals' and 'snacks' are common even in the scientific literature, but are often poorly quantified and conflate aspects of timing, frequency, amount and type of food consumed. Furthermore, overweight or dieting subjects may choose to alter eating frequency as part of their personal strategy for restraining intake in the hope of achieving weight reduction, or may have different criteria for what constitutes a 'meal'. This would point to reduced eating frequency as a result of overweight or obesity, rather than as a cause (Kant *et al.*, 1995a), as inferred from some epidemiological analyses. This also suggests that additional behavioural characterisation of subject populations would aid the interpretation of such data. It is also likely that individuals with higher levels of physical activity eat more frequently (e.g. Durrant *et al.*, 1982; Butterworth *et al.*, 1994) and this could generate results suggesting higher energy intakes (but lower fatness) in association with more frequent eating.

Although a number of epidemiological studies have supported an inverse relationship between measures of eating frequency and body weight status (Fábry & Teppermann, 1970; Ries, 1973; Kaufman *et al.*, 1975; Metzner *et al.*, 1977; Kulesza, 1982; Kant *et al.*, 1995a), many recent investigations have not found this relationship (Morgan *et al.*, 1983; Dreon *et al.* 1988; Summerbell, 1989; Edelstein *et al.*, 1992; Basdevant *et al.*, 1993; Anderson *et al.*, 1995; Ruxton *et al.*, 1996). However, limitations in the methods used to quantify eating patterns make it difficult to draw definitive conclusions from these data. Some epidemiological investigations of the circadian distribution of energy intake, have suggested that the obese consume a greater proportion of energy intake in the latter half of the day compared to lean individuals (Beaudoin & Mayer, 1953; Baeke *et al.*, 1983; Bellisle *et al.*, 1988; Fricker *et al.*, 1990). Other studies have failed to find such a relationship (Maxfield & Konishi, 1966; Durrant *et al.*, 1982; Anderson *et al.*, 1995; Kant *et al.*, 1995b). Overall, the current consensus is that evidence for a causal link between the patterns and circadian distribution of energy intake and obesity is weak, especially when possible influences on diet composition are taken into account (Bellisle *et al.*, 1997; Mela & Rogers, 1998).

Increased meal frequency may have beneficial metabolic effects (e.g. on glucose handling and lipoprotein metabolism), but prospective studies of regimens of varied meal size and frequencies have not documented substantial effects on energy intake and fat deposition. Although Fábry *et al.* (1966) reported greater fat deposition among adolescents eating 3 meals per day (versus 5 or 7) over a year, other prospective studies have generally found little effect of meal frequency on normal energy balance (Dallosso *et al.*, 1982; Verboeket-van de Venne *et al.*, 1993; Bellisle *et al.*, 1997). Some investigators have suggested that high eating frequency in the form of 'snacking' is common in the obese (Björvell *et al.*, 1985; Basdevant *et al.*, 1993) and possibly causally related to obesity (Booth, 1988); however, empirical support for this is lacking. The question of whether certain eating patterns favour excessive energy intakes may be resolved with better understanding of the regulation of meal-to-meal energy intake (Westerterp-Plantenga *et al.*, 1994). In particular, there is a need for experimental work to determine the effects of changes in eating frequency, and particularly the timing of insertion of extra eating events ('snacks'), and their composition, on long-term energy balance.

14.5 Summary

- Obesity and dietary restraint can be associated with a heightened responsiveness to specific food and other environmental stimuli and emotions and this may manifest in a loss of dietary control or excessive eating in general or isolated bouts. Palatable, high-fat, energy-dense foods may, therefore, provoke behavioural problems of weight control.

- Obesity has not been clearly linked to preferences for, or intakes of, any specific foods or food group, or to altered taste or smell function, or (despite extensive research) to an enhanced sweet taste preference. However, the predisposition to obesity has been consistently linked to a sensory preference for fat-containing stimuli.

- Sensory stimulation or food 'palatability' influences short-term energy intake and possibly also expenditure, but appears to be secondary to food composition over the longer term. However, sensory variety may disrupt learning of diet-sensory associations, and undermine its role in appetite control. Sensory and food preferences are also not independent of food composition, which may be a major determinant of the acquisition and maintenance of these preferences.

- There is no strong evidence to suggest that the marketing policies of the food industry directly impact an individual's predisposition to obesity. The argument remains inconclusive for two principal reasons:
  (i) a number of factors influence an individual's selection of foods (including, for example, advertising)
  (ii) the food industry makes available individual foodstuffs rather than 'diets'.

- The main impact of the EU's Common Agricultural Policy on the UK diet has been via altering the relative price of major food product groups and has been broadly positive from a nutritional point of view.

- Based on the role of fats and sugars in the diet, and existing research, there is a lack of evidence supporting the efficacy of non-nutritive sweeteners in weight control, whereas fat replacement/

reduction in foods appears to offer greater potential benefits. In either case, use of modified foods presumably can only be helpful in weight control if it contributes toward meaningful overall reductions in the energy density of the diet, or comprises one part of a broader and wilful effort. This approach may offer certain benefits to consumers, but the actual dietary response to casual or extensive use of modified foods is not well established.

• The distribution and frequency of eating has not been found to have a consistent independent relationship with weight status or long-term control of energy balance, and appears to be secondary to food composition and other factors.

15
Aetiology of Obesity XI: Physical Inactivity

15.1 Physical activity

The human body has evolved to accommodate vigorous physical activity and inactivity can be regarded as the abnormal, rather than normal, state. It should, therefore, not be surprising that inactivity is associated with ill health. Similarly to high energy intake, chronic low energy expenditure has the potential to produce a long-term positive energy balance and consequent weight gain. Energy expenditure is a function of basal metabolic rate (BMR), dietary induced thermogenesis (DIT), adaptive thermogenesis (shivering and non-shivering heat production) and physical activity. Of these, physical activity offers the greatest scope for an individual to increase energy expenditure. Evidence of this is provided by contrasting a triathlete in training, who may be expending as much as four times his/her BMR throughout a 24-hour period, with a sedentary person, whose physical activity may be lower than 0.5 × BMR. In effect, physical activity for the triathlete represents 70–80% of total energy expenditure compared to 30% or less for the sedentary person.

15.1.1 The nature of physical activity

Definitions of physical activity have varied considerably and this has produced difficulties and confusion in the literature. Recently, the terminology has been clarified by Caspersen *et al.* (1985) and these definitions have now been widely accepted.

- **Physical activity** is an umbrella term describing any bodily movement produced by the skeletal muscles, which results in energy expenditure.

- **Exercise** is a subset of physical activity, which is volitional, planned, structured, repetitive and aimed at improvement or maintenance of an aspect of fitness or health.

- **Sport** is physical activity that involves structured competitive situations, governed by rules. In Europe, sport is often used in the wider context to include all exercise and leisure time physical activity.

- **Physical fitness** is a state or product. It is a multi-dimensional indicator of several functional capacities such as cardiovascular endurance, muscular strength or mobility, which in varying degrees are a result of genetics and stage in the life span, as well as physical activity levels.

- **MET** or **metabolic equivalent** is the energy requirement of an activity expressed as a multiple of energy requirement at rest or resting metabolic rate. Work at 5 METs requires 5 × the energy expended at rest.

Physical activity can be a feature of a complex range of behaviours, from very minor movements such as fidgeting and restlessness to levels of high intensity exercise involving large muscle groups such as running or lifting heavy weights. Within this range are light intensity activities such as household work, gardening or walking, and more moderate intensity activities such as brisk walking, cycling, or swimming. Activity can be generated, therefore, within the context of daily routines, occupational settings, or leisure time (Table 15.1).

In the past, greater emphasis has been placed on

Table 15.1 Examples of light, moderate and vigorous physical activity (adapted from: Pate *et al.*, 1995).

Light	Moderate	Hard/Vigorous
<3.0 METs* or <17 kJ (4 kcal) min^{-1}	3.0–6.0 METs* 17–29kJ (4–7 kcal) min^{-1}	>6.0 METs* >29 kJ (7 kcal) min^{-1}
Walking slowly or strolling 1–2 mph	Walking briskly 3–4 mph	Walking briskly uphill or with load or jogging
Cycling, stationary <50 W	Cycling, steadily for pleasure or transport 5–10 mph or up slopes	Cycling faster than 10 mph or up hills
Swimming slowly	Swimming with moderate exertion	Swimming fast or treading water
Easy stretching or conditioning exercises	Specific conditioning exercises such as sit-ups	Conditioning exercise with stair ergometer or ski machine
Home care such as hoovering	Home care such as heavier cleaning	Moving furniture
Garden work such as weeding	Mowing the lawn with a power mower, sweeping and raking	Mowing the lawn with a hand mower, digging

(*Note:* *MET or metabolic equivalent is the energy requirement of an activity expressed as a multiple of energy requirement at rest or basal metabolic rate.)

moderate to vigorous physical activity. Activity of this type is particularly relevant when considering coronary heart disease, where higher training loads produce greatest improvement in the cardio-respiratory system. However, energy expenditure as a result of movement, is also of great importance when addressing weight gain and obesity. The amount of time spent in sedentary pursuits, such as television and video viewing, is also significant when considering weight gain, as it constrains the opportunity to be active and, therefore, reduces overall energy expenditure.

15.1.2 Assessment of physical activity

The range of components of physical activity and the variety of contexts in which it can take place has caused great difficulties in its measurement. Where energy balance is the consideration, then it is important to measure all movement, including incidental activity, involved in household tasks, transport, work and in planned recreation. It may also be useful to assess the amount of activity undertaken at different levels, such as light, moderate and high intensities, to view the effect on different health parameters. No singular field or laboratory method exists to provide this information simultaneously. Calorimetry and doubly labelled water techniques provide accurate estimates of total energy expenditure as a result of movement, but no indication of patterns or intensities of activity (Murgatroyd *et al.*, 1993a). Heart-rate monitors appear more useful in the assessment of moderate to high intensity exercise than low intensity exercise. Motion sensors can now detect and record minute-by-minute movement in three planes, providing estimates of patterns and amounts of activity, but this technique has yet to be fully validated. In some studies (e.g. Blair *et al.*, 1989), aerobic fitness, assessed by a timed treadmill walk, has been used as a substitute measure for exercise participation, as the two are moderately related. Other studies have used observational systems to code activity. However, in the large population-based epidemiological studies that are required to examine trends in activity, there remains no alternative but to rely on self-reported activity levels through questionnaire or interview.

As with dietary intake, self-report of physical activity is fraught with problems. Structured and more intense activity is easier to recall. Minor movements that are habitual, but frequent, are often neglected yet may significantly add to energy expenditure over a 24-hour or weekly time span. The period of recall (such as the last seven days, a typical week, or the last month) influences results because subjects, particularly children, have limited recall beyond 24-hours. Seasonal variation is also difficult to quantify without losing precision. Daily movement patterns are a result of such a wide variety of behaviours that it is very difficult to include them all in a questionnaire that is still manageable to the participant. The Allied Dunbar National Fitness Survey (Health Education Authority & Sports Council, 1992) demonstrated the fallibility of questions, which are not carefully anchored by specific activity reference points. For example, 56% of men believed they were sufficiently active for health, whereas only 36% are even moderately active when judged by objective criteria. Equivalent figures for women are 52% and 24%.

For these reasons, many surveys are limited to the measurement of leisure time physical activity or sustained periods of moderate or vigorous exercise of 20–30 min length, that are easier to recall. This will provide a limited view of total energy expended through movement and will attenuate any activity/energy balance relationship. Similarly, in a cultural climate that influences the public value attached to activity, self-report may reflect intentions or socially desirable responding and this may confound evidence for trends found in longitudinal studies.

15.2 Epidemiological evidence

15.2.1 Trends in inactivity

i Adults

Two studies in England, the Allied Dunbar National Fitness Survey and the Health Education Authority National Survey of Activity and Health were recently combined (Fentem & Walker, 1995) to provide data on 6583 adults aged 16–74 years. Using a criterion of less than one 30-min period of moderate activity per week, 29% of men and 28% of women were classed as sedentary. A further 35% of men and 48% of women engage in only irregular bouts of moderate activity (Fig. 15.1). Only 16% of men and 5% of women participate in regular vigorous intensity activity. Inactivity increases with age (Figs 15.2, 15.3) and is lower in ethnic minority groups. Social class differences are not strong because occupational activity is balanced with leisure-time activity.

Similar patterns of low activity are found in the USA, with 60% not regularly active and 25% reporting no significant activity at all (US Department of Health and Human Services, 1996). Similar

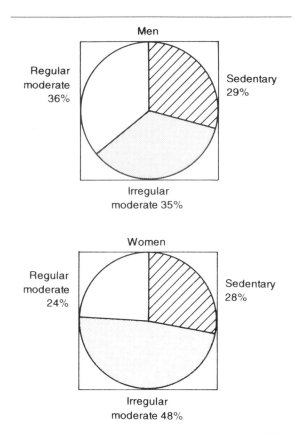

Fig. 15.1 Physical activity levels among adults aged 16–74: England 1990–91 (data from: Fentem & Walker, 1995).

levels of activity are reported in Australia and Canada.

Unfortunately, there are no comprehensive data sets available to establish trends in activity. Almost all longitudinal data are restricted to leisure time activity and sport participation. Using the Health in Wales surveys to compare activity between 1985 and 1993 (Moore, 1994), the proportion of respondents reporting three or more periods of moderate to vigorous activity each week rose significantly in all groups except those aged 55–64 years.

Evidence is provided by the Health and Lifestyle Survey (Cox, 1993) indicating increases in participation rates in leisure-time activity from 1984/5–1991/2, with the greatest differences shown in non-manual males (from 43–52%) living in the south. The Health Education Authority (1995), using data

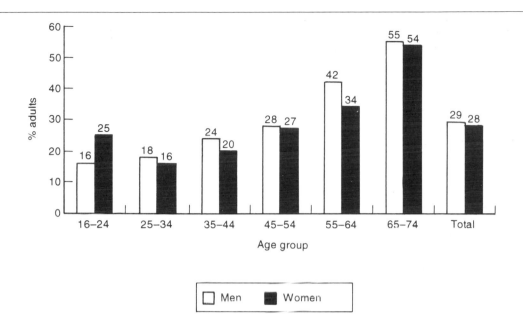

Fig. 15.2   Adults with sedentary lifestyle by sex and age group: England 1990–91 (data from Fentem & Walker, 1995).

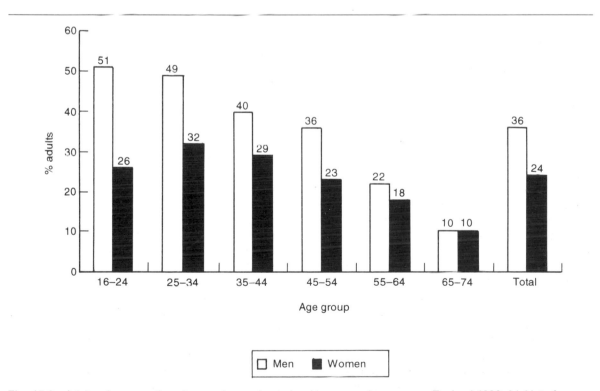

Fig. 15.3   Adults who are active at a regular moderate level by sex and age group: England 1990–91 (data from Fentem & Walker, 1995).

from the General Household Surveys of 1987, 1990 and 1993, found comparable results. Small increases were shown in participation in swimming, keep fit activities, yoga and cycling, suggesting a gradually increasing awareness of the health benefits of exercise, at least in some sectors of the population.

Similar small increases in leisure-time activity have been reported in the USA by Caspersen & Merritt (1994), using the Behavioural Risk Factor Surveillance System (BRFSS). Between 1986 and 1990, inactivity (as measured by no reported active leisure during the previous month) reduced in all sectors except for non-whites and those with fewer than 12 years education. Jacobs *et al.* (1991) used the Minnesota Leisure-Time Physical Activity Survey to investigate change between 1957–1960 and 1985–1987. Higher levels of activity were recorded from the 1970s in men, with the greatest population increases seen in the white-collar groups. Greater activity was seen in women from the 1980s but only in the blue-collar group.

Estimates of leisure time physical activity provide only a limited description of energy expended during discrete and relatively infrequent sessions. Energy expenditure through all movement, regardless of intensity, is likely to be more salient in the activity–weight management relationship. Unfortunately, this information is much more difficult to gather. However, there are several indirect indicators that suggest that many aspects of our lifestyles are becoming less active, thereby contributing to lower daily energy expenditure. Fewer than 20% of males and 10% of females have active occupations. Modern technology and increased disposable income have together brought greater availability of labour-saving devices and motorised transport. There has been a boom in electronic home entertainment and the average time spent watching television has doubled to 27 hours per week in the last 30 years (Office of Population Censuses and Surveys, 1994). It is clear that in many people's lifestyles it is now possible to restrict physical activity to very low levels. This would need matching with a low energy intake if energy balance is to be maintained and weight gain avoided.

In summary, participation in moderate or vigorous activity, at a level that is likely to optimise health benefit, is low and becomes lower with increasing age, a time when there is likely to be greatest benefit. Furthermore, there has been a critical reduction in incidental lifestyle-related activity, resulting in reduced energy expenditure among the population in the last 30 years. This has resulted from fewer active jobs, increased technology and affluence, which together have led to greater reliance on motorised transport, sedentary home entertainment, and labour-saving devices at home, at work and in the shopping environment. Several surveys show small increases in the type of moderate to vigorous activity associated with leisure time activity and sport. Increased activity of this nature is more readily seen in some socio-demographic groups than in others, with those in lower educational attainment, ethnic minority and older age groups being less responsive. However, evidence presented later suggests that any increase in active leisure has been unable to compensate for the reductions in general expenditure caused by gradual elimination of physical work from the daily routine.

ii Children

Of particular interest to the prevention of obesity are the levels and patterns of activity among children, particularly as there is now evidence that children are steadily increasing in fatness (Hughes *et al.*, 1997). As with adults, little is known about the total energy expenditure that occurs as a result of physical activity among children and adolescents. It involves a broad range of behaviours such as walking or cycling to and from school, informal play, organised exercise and sport at school, and a wide variety of formal and informal activities at evenings and weekends.

Using heart-rate telemetry to monitor the activity of 11- to 16-year-old British children, Armstrong *et al.* (1990) found that almost 50% of girls and 38% of boys did not achieve one 10-minute period equivalent to sustained brisk walking in a period of 3 school days. Weekends were even less active. Similar results were found with a survey of over 3000 11- to 18-year-old children in Northern Ireland (Riddoch *et al.*, 1991). The most striking feature of these data is the sharp decline in this type of activity for girls beyond the age 13 or 14 years. Unfortunately, there are no equivalent reliable data to establish that there has been a significant decline in recent years.

International comparisons of participation in

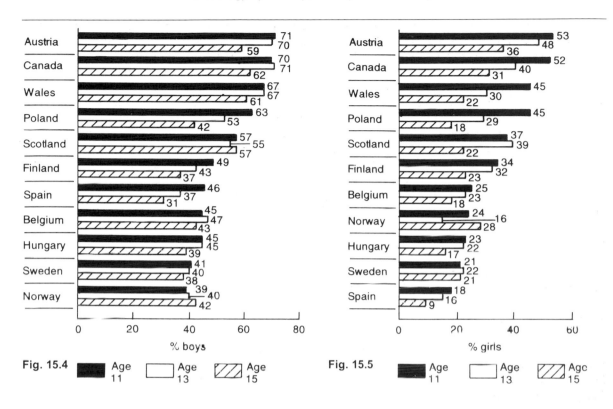

Fig. 15.4 ■ Age 11　□ Age 13　▨ Age 15

Fig. 15.5 ■ Age 11　□ Age 13　▨ Age 15

International comparisons of boys (Fig. 15.4) and girls (15.5) who exercise vigorously at least 4 times a week out of school: 1990 (from: King & Coles, 1992, © Health Education Authority).

moderate to vigorous physical activity show considerable variations across countries, ranging from 12% in Austrian 11-year-old boys to 73% of Spanish 15-year-old girls reporting no vigorous activity. International comparisons of vigorous activity among boys and girls are shown in Figures 15.4 and 15.5.

Compared with adult levels of activity, surveys of children's exercise and sport participation provide a more optimistic picture. The Health and Lifestyle Survey (Health Education Authority, 1991), conducted in 1989 with 10 000 9- to 15-year-olds, indicated that children were on average involved in 4.7 hours of exercise each week. Children from lower socio-economic groups, and some minority ethnic groups reported lower levels of activity. Using the World Health Organisation's Health Behaviour in School-Aged Children Study (King & Coles, 1992), it is possible to extract trends for some countries between 1983–1984 and 1989–1990. There is a trend towards increased vigorous activity over this period

for some countries. However, the time allocated to physical education in schools is declining. In Britain, less than 90 minutes a week, on average, is dedicated to physical education, making Britain among the lowest in Europe at both primary and secondary level.

Hillman (1993) has shown indirect evidence of a decline in the levels of lifestyle activity in British children. In a report based on schools surveyed in 1971 and again in 1990, he found that the percentage of children being driven to school had risen nearly four times to 36%. Other aspects of their freedom, and hence their independence for physical activity, had also been affected. In 1971, half of the children were permitted to travel unaccompanied by bus, whereas by 1990 this had fallen to just one in seven. By 1990, over 90% of children owned a bike, but only a quarter of them were allowed to cycle on the roads and fewer than 5% biked to school, compared with over 60% in some other European countries. There were also increased restrictions on children's outdoor play and a decrease in weekend activities. These constraints were being imposed on the grounds of safety, with parents worried about traffic accidents and abduction.

Hillman (1993) suggested that remaining inside the home, for a variety of reasons, has become a more appealing and convenient environment for children to spend their leisure time. The majority of children now own computer games units, many have televisions in their bedrooms and the volume of programming for children has increased, particularly during holiday time. This is reflected in increased time spent playing with home computers (Balding, 1997) and children, on average, watch 2–3 hours of television per day. Most adults would agree that the lives of children involve less activity than their own did when they were children.

In summary, children seem to be influenced by the same pressures to be inactive as their parents, with an additional barrier presented by the safety concerns of parents. The extent to which this reduces their total energy expenditure is not fully known. Studies using heart-rate monitoring suggest that many children participate in little or no sustained moderate to vigorous activity, and this is particularly the case for adolescent girls. As with data for adults, surveys focusing on exercise and sport tend to be more optimistic, perhaps in part reflecting socially desirable responses to the trend in greater interest in fitness and active leisure that has taken place in some sectors. However, there is a tendency in studies with children and adults to focus on mean outcomes. The key to the activity/weight gain relationship is more likely to be found in the identification of children who are inactive across the range of social settings, including travel to school and opportunities to play in informal and formalised games. Of particular significance for the development of obesity, is the extent to which children spend their spare time on inactive leisure pursuits such as watching television and playing computer games.

The available literature on the activity of young people was reviewed as the basis of a consensus conference held by the Health Education Authority (Health Education Authority, 1997b). The rationale underpinning the ensuing recommendations for children's activity was based on the need to reverse the trend in increasing fatness in children. These recommendations can be found in Table 15.2.

15.2.2 Inactivity and weight gain

Several studies have shown that physically active people have lower body fat levels than inactive people. For example, using the doubly labelled water method, Schulz and Schoeller (1994) found a correlation between per cent body fat and non-basal energy expenditure of:

$$r = -0.83 \text{ in females and}$$
$$r = -0.55 \text{ in males}$$

Similar data are available from the Allied Dunbar National Fitness Survey (Health Education Authority and Sports Council, 1992). However, this data provides no indication as to whether inactivity is a determinant or result of overweight and obesity.

Prentice & Jebb, (1995) have graphically documented two indicators of inactivity (hours per week of television viewing and cars per household) against the current secular trend in obesity in Britain (Fig. 15.6). A strong relationship exists. At

---

Table 15.2 Recommendations for health-related physical activity in young people. From Health Education Authority (1997b). *Young and Active: A Policy Framework*. London: Health Education Authority.

Primary recommendation:

All young people should participate in physical activity of at least moderate intensity for an average of at least half an hour and preferably one hour per day.

Secondary recommendation:

At least twice a week, some of these activities should help enhance and maintain muscular strength, flexibility, and bone health.

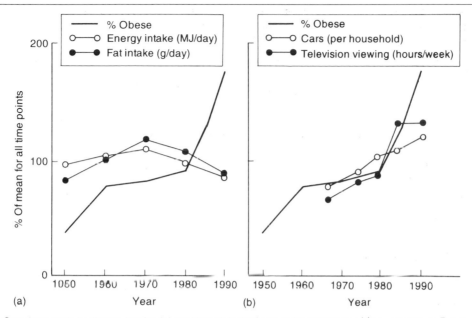

Fig. 15.6 Secular trends in dietary intake (a) and inactivity indicators (b) in relationship to obesity in Britain. The values show percentage for each time point based on an average of 100% timespan (from: Prentice & Jebb, 1995a).

the same time, similar data for total energy consumption and fat intake show downward trends. This points convincingly towards reduced energy expenditure, as a result of increased availability of labour-saving technology, as a major contributor to obesity.

In this paper, the authors also plotted the obesity and activity levels of women across social class categories. They found a matching gradient from classes I and II to classes IV and V, which was paralleled by an increase in the hours of television watching per week (Fig. 15.7).

The Behaviour Risk Factor Surveillance System (BRFSS) study (DiPietro *et al.*, 1993) provides data on over 6000 men and 12 500 women, who reported trying to lose weight (Fig. 15.8). The prevalence of obesity (BMI >30) decreased significantly with increasing level of activity. The weights of those who reported taking part in specific activities, including walking, running, cycling, aerobics and golf, were plotted by age against the weights of those reporting no activity. Patterns showed lower weights in the active subjects, with differences increasing with age and the intensity of the activity. Walking produced significant differences after age

40 years. All differences were independent of height, race, education, smoking and energy intake restriction.

French *et al.* (1994) studied behavioural predictors of body weight in 1629 males and 1913 females, over a 2-year period, in a work-site intervention study for smoking cessation and weight control. Prospectively, dietary variables, such as increased consumption of high-energy foods, independently predicted increases in body weight in women. An increase of one walking session per week predicted a decrease in body weight of 0.8 kg, and the addition of one high intensity activity session per week predicted a 0.6 kg weight loss over 2 years. Equivalent figures for males were 0.4 kg and 1.6 kg. Participation in sports or an active job did not significantly predict weight loss.

A similar prospective study was conducted with a large Finnish population (Rissanen *et al.*, 1991). Subjects were assessed between 1966 and 1972, and again between 1973 and 1976. Significant weight gain (>5 kg/5 years) was found in 17.5% of men and 15.1% of women. Using categories of baseline leisure-time physical activity (frequent, occasional, or rare), a dose-response relationship was seen in

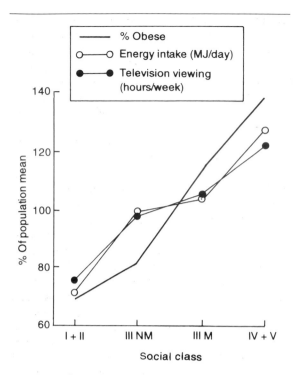

Fig. 15.7 Social class trends in inactivity and obesity, 1990 (from: Prentice & Jebb, 1995a).

relative risk of weight gain of 1.0, 1.5, and 1.9 in men, and of 1.0, 1.5, and 1.6 in women.

A more recent longitudinal study conducted in Finland (Haapanen *et al.*, 1997), compared leisure-time physical activity and weight change over a 10-year period in over 5000 working adults. Odds ratios (OR) were calculated for the chance of a weight gain of greater than 5 kg over the period. For both males and females, those who self-reported no physically active leisure on both occasions, or a reduced activity level by the second occasion, had significantly higher risk of gain (OR 1.62–2.49) than those who reported at least two sessions of vigorous activity per week on both occasions.

Williamson *et al.* (1993) used data on over 9000 subjects from the National Health and Nutrition Examination Survey (NHANES) telephone survey in the USA to compare activity and body weight over a 10-year period (1971/75–1982/84). Recreational physical activity was assessed by a single question to categorise respondents as low, moderate or high in activity. Relative risk results are presented in Tables 15.3 and 15.4. Men who reported low activity at both points were 3.9 times more likely to gain 8–13 kg over the 10-year period than men who reported high activity on both

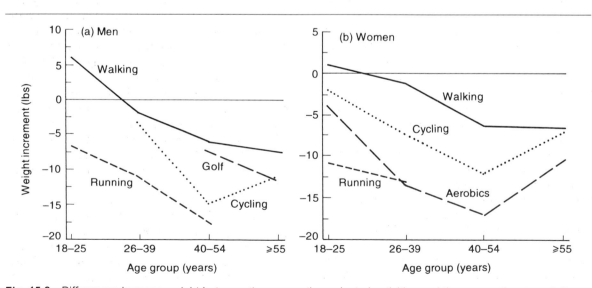

Fig. 15.8 Differences in mean weight between those reporting selected activities and those reporting no activity (baseline) by age for males (a) and females (b). Data is cross-sectional from the Behavioural risk factor surveillance system, 1989, and based on multiple linear regression adjusting for race, height, smoking and caloric restriction (from: DiPietro *et al.*, 1993).

Table 15.3 Estimated relative odds of weight gain categories by recreational physical activity levels: men (from: Williamson *et al.*, 1993).

Base-Follow	Weight gain category (kg)		
	3–8	8–13	>13
Hi–Hi	1.0	1.0	1.0
Mod–Mod	1.0	2.0	1.6
Lo–Lo	1.2	3.9	2.3
Increased	1.0	2.4	1.3
Decreased	1.1	3.3	2.3

Table 15.4 Estimated relative odds of weight gain categories by recreational physical activity levels: women (from: Williamson *et al.*, 1993).

Base-Follow	Weight gain category (kg)		
	3–8	8–13	>13
Hi–Hi	1.0	1.0	1.0
Mod–Mod	1.7	1.0	3.4
Lo–Lo	2.1	1.5	7.1
Increased	1.7	0.9	3.4
Decreased	2.4	1.3	6.2

occasions. The risk for moderate activity on both occasions was 2.0 and those who decreased their activity had a threefold increase in risk. The risk of very high weight gain (>13 kg) for women was high for those who reported low activity on both occasions, although confidence intervals are wide (RR = 7.1 [2.2–23.3]). Relative risk of serious weight gain for women who decreased their activity was 6.2. An increase in activity level was also associated with an increased chance of weight gain. This may be explained by a sector increasing their activity **because** their weight had increased, in an attempt to reduce it again.

The NHANES survey relies on self-report and is, therefore, rather weak but DiPietro *et al.* (1998) have recently replicated the findings in a more rigorous study with 4599 men and 724 women. Here, cardio-respiratory fitness levels were measured by maximal time achieved on a treadmill-walking test, accompanied by self-reported activity measures. Changes in fitness were assessed between three visits, with the first and last visits on average 7.6 years apart. In 14% of men and 9% of women, each one-minute increase in treadmill time was associated with a reduction in risk of weight gain of 5 kg or more. There was also a reduction in risk of a weight

gain of 10 kg or more in 21% of men and 21% of women. Analysis of an interim measure of fitness change at 2 years indicated that increased fitness preceded weight gain. As with the study by Williamson *et al.* (1993), decreases in physical activity were associated with risk of weight gain. In further support, a recent 2-year longitudinal study (Ching *et al.*, 1996) showed that increased physical activity and reduced television/video watching time over the period, was associated with attenuated weight gain.

It has been difficult to show anything more than a weak relationship between inactivity and fatness increase in children. The relationship is heavily confounded through the pubertal years, as body composition changes with stage of sexual maturation. To date, stronger relationships have been detected between patterns of sedentary living (such as the amount of time spent watching television) and obesity, than with physically active pursuits (Dietz & Strasburger, 1991). Recently, Gortmaker *et al.* (1996) examined longitudinal data, on the number of hours spent watching television, throughout the period between 1986 and 1990, and the prevalence of obesity, using a nationally representative sample of 746 children. The odds of being overweight were 4.6 (2.2–9.6) times greater when television viewing exceeded 5 hours per day, compared with 0–2 hours per day. Additionally, the odds of developing or recovering from obesity were linked to time spent watching television, with estimates of risk attributable to obesity, linked to degree of television watching, as high as 60%. The conclusion of the authors is that reductions in television time may be effective in preventing some of the incidence of obesity. This is supported by intervention studies concerned with the treatment of obesity. Epstein *et al.* (1995) demonstrated more success for weight loss by reducing sedentary pursuits than through introducing more physical activity sessions.

To summarise, long-term activity habits, whether recorded as leisure or recreation time activity, non-basal energy expenditure, or changes in aerobic fitness, appear to be associated with weight change patterns. This represents a robust finding. Those who remain active or increase their physical activity or reduce their time in sedentary pursuits do best in sustaining healthy weight levels throughout the period in which they practice one or more of these options.

15.3 Control mechanisms and physical activity

15.3.1 Appetite and physical activity

Although exercise will implicitly produce health benefits, any concurrent stimulatory effect on appetite could prove counterproductive to weight reduction and management. In addition, there is a public perception that 'exercise makes you eat more' and this is often used as an excuse not to exercise. It is, therefore, important to assess accurately the long-term effect of increased physical activity on appetite, macronutrient intake, energy intake and, subsequently, on energy balance, and to convey these findings to the general public.

i Does exercise affect energy intake?

Many exercisers report that exercise is followed by an acute suppression of hunger. Although at least 5 well-designed experimental studies with lean subjects have documented this effect, it is apparently short lived and more likely to occur after higher intensity exercise. It does not result in reduction in later energy intake when compared to a similar period following no exercise. Some studies that have induced exercise of long duration, such as 75 minutes of swimming or 120 minutes of activity, and compared it with rest, have documented increased energy intake after exercise (Verger *et al.*, 1994). However, most studies have not calculated relative energy intake (i.e. any extra intake minus the extra amount expended through exercise). When this has been done, there is usually a net deficit in energy balance, suggesting that exercise does have immediate potential for weight reduction.

Cross-sectional studies indicate that active individuals have higher energy intakes than sedentary individuals. In males, there is some support for a general linear increase in energy intake with increasing habitual physical activity (Tremblay *et al.*, 1983) or fitness level (Broeder *et al.*, 1992). This relationship is only evident when intake and activity are measured over several days. This linear trend is less clear in females. It has been suggested that the relationship may be confounded by a greater tendency of females to be practising dietary restraint. Additionally, although selection bias

might operate, it cannot be denied that few people who are highly active, either through recreational exercise or through their work, are obese or overweight. It appears that in conditions of high energy expenditure, people are able to eat more yet remain in energy balance.

There have been several experimental studies manipulating the amount of exercise taken by obese and non-obese subjects over periods of several weeks or months. At least eight of these studies indicate that there is no increase in energy intake during phases of exercise training. However, in those studies that have detected an increase in energy intake, the subjects still tended to remain in relative energy deficit because the compensatory intake did not match the additional expenditure that occurred as a result of exercise (Woo *et al.*, 1982a,b). When the results of a number of studies are considered, it appears that obese subjects are less likely than lean subjects to increase their intake during the exercise phase. This is supported by a direct comparison of lean and obese subjects in a study by Durrant *et al.* (1982). These data suggested that either there was a difference between obese and non-obese subjects in the regulatory capacity of energy intake, or that the obese already had intakes that exceeded the increased energy requirement of the exercise.

In a recent review, King *et al.* (1997) report that very few studies have indicated a strong coupling effect between energy expenditure changes and energy intake. If anything, there is a tendency for exercise to normalise the appetite response. Mayer *et al.* (1954) reported that, when the opportunities for physical activity were restricted in mice, body weight became poorly regulated. It may be possible that one effect of exercise is to help 'tune up' the regulatory system to stimulate a more appropriate feeding response for the level of energy expenditure.

Recent research has suggested that endocrinological links may be possible but this has yet to be substantiated. It has also been proposed that exercise can help in regulating energy balance because of an asymmetry in appetite control, in which the hunger drive operates more powerfully and precisely than the satiety drive. Thus, active people, whose energy needs generally exceed the societal norm for food intake, will regulate by means of a more efficient physiological mechanism (hunger) than sedentary people, who have to regulate by means of satiety and restraint (Blundell & King, 1998).

There are great individual differences in response to an increased exercise level, suggesting that any physiological links between exercise and energy intake may be overridden by environmental or psychological factors. It may be, for example, that some individuals use exercise as a means of weight control, allow themselves more dietary indulgence and place themselves in positive energy balance. One study has supported this notion in females (Westerterp *et al.*, 1992), perhaps explaining why females tend to be less successful than males in reducing body fat through exercise.

Overall, the short- and long-term experiments and cross-sectional comparisons of groups provide little evidence to suggest that exercise causes an increase beyond compensation for the amount expended through the extra exercise. Furthermore, there is some evidence that there is usually a net energy deficit. This may be even more apparent in obese people, who appear less appetite responsive to exercise.

ii Does exercise affect macronutrient intake?

Interest has also focused on the impact of exercise on selection of macronutrients, particularly fat and carbohydrate, in the diet. It is assumed that the mix of fuels expended through exercise should at some point be redressed in subsequent food intake. Fuel utilisation and, thus, respiratory quotient (RQ) are partially dependent on intensity and duration of exercise, with greater dependence on fat oxidation in low to moderate intensity endurance exercise and greater carbohydrate use in higher intensity exercise. It is possible, therefore, that differential use of fat or carbohydrate as fuel sources will influence food choice, as the body attempts to maintain macronutrient balance.

Few studies have addressed the impact of exercise on macronutrient intake. Tremblay & Buemann (1995) and Almeras *et al.* (1995) found that individuals showing reduced RQ during exercise (suggesting greater fat oxidation) had lower subsequent energy intakes. The suggestion is that there is a greater drive to restore glycogen levels than there is for fat because of limited stores, and that

those exercisers who rely less on carbohydrate during exercise eat less after exercise. If this is the case, exercise of low to moderate intensity and long duration, such as walking for distance, is likely to be more beneficial than higher intensity exercise for long-term energy balance. However, King *et al.* (1997) maintain that the physical stress associated with high intensity might confound the issue. A recent study (King *et al.*, 1994) indicated that, whereas glycogen depletion had occurred when exercising at high intensity, this did not result in an increased energy intake on completion of the exercise. The suggestion was that intense exercise might suppress subsequent food intake through neurochemical mechanisms, such as corticotropin release.

Some studies have manipulated diet after exercise. When exercisers are provided with a low-fat diet, over a 2-day period, they remained in negative energy balance. The opposite occurred with a high-fat diet. Suggestions to explain this have been that exercisers in the high-fat situation eat more in an attempt to take in carbohydrate and replenish glycogen stores. Alternatively, they may simply be victim to 'passive over-consumption' (King *et al.*, 1997) as a result of high-fat foods being higher in energy density. In either case, it seems prudent that low to moderate intensity exercise, which utilises a higher level of fat as a source of energy, should be accompanied by a low-fat diet to encourage weight loss (Tremblay & Buemann, 1995).

15.3.2 Exercise and substrate utilisation

It has been suggested that the only way to establish the mechanisms involved in exercise and weight management is to study the source of fuel used and the subsequent demand and supply of macronutrients for replenishment (Tremblay & Buemann, 1995). Protein metabolism largely remains in balance under a wide range of conditions of supply, and any shortage or excess is unlikely to affect energy balance. Similarly, carbohydrate intake is stored in only small amounts and stores are usually adjusted post exercise to match demand. The key to understanding the link between exercise and weight loss is therefore found in the way that exercise can cause a lipid deficit and the demand of exercise on stored lipids.

i The effect of exercise intensity on substrate utilisation

How hard we exercise determines the amount of each fuel used. Low intensity exercise, such as easy walking, which achieves no more than 40–50% of maximum aerobic capacity, relies primarily on energy from the oxidation of free fatty acids found in the plasma. As the demand of exercise increases, the extra energy is derived from carbohydrate stored as muscle glycogen and from intramuscular triacylglycerol. During very heavy workloads, such as sprinting or lifting heavy weights, energy is supplied almost exclusively by glycogen. This has led many exercise practitioners to recommend low to medium intensity exercise for long periods ('long and slow'), where weight loss or weight maintenance is the major goal, as it utilises more fat as the energy source. This strategy is also supported by the previous discussion on appetite, which suggests that the link between usage and demand is tentative for fat, probably because of the availability of ample stores, in contrast to carbohydrate.

This has to be taken in the context of the overall energy expenditure of the exercise bout. Intense exercise will cause a greater energy deficit, overall, if sustained for the same period as low intensity exercise. It will also utilise greater absolute amounts of fat, even though the proportion of fat usage may not be as high. However, there are other important and, perhaps, overriding practical considerations. The muscular and cardio-respiratory endurance of overweight individuals is usually low, they are burdened with a heavier load, and they also carry risk factors for coronary heart disease. It will, therefore, be both motivationally counter-productive and unsafe to advise higher intensity exercise, at least in the early stages of an exercise programme.

ii The effect of exercise duration on substrate utilisation

The contribution of lipids to the fuel mix increases as the period of exercise is extended (Fig. 5.9). One study with untrained men indicated an increase from 37% at 40 minutes to 62% after 240 minutes of bicycling (Ahlborg *et al.*, 1974). In addition, after long periods of exercise, there is evidence of compensatory lipid oxidation; to re-synthesise depleted

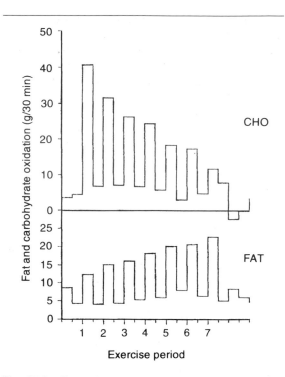

Fig. 15.9 Fat and carbohydrate metabolism over time during a single exercise bout (from: Murgatroyd *et al.*, 1993b).

glycogen stores during the following 24 hours. This process increases with the duration of the exercise. Unfortunately, beta-blockers, which may be prescribed for many overweight people, appear to inhibit this effect. Also, the duration of exercise indicated here is unlikely to be a regular feature of the exercise programmes of overweight and obese individuals, although long weekend walks may be feasible. It remains unclear whether frequent bouts of low level activity, interspersed with rest, as might be achieved through a busy job routine or household work, can have a similar effect to aerobic exercise sustained without a break for extended periods.

iii The effect of exercise training on fat oxidation

As individuals improve their endurance fitness, they increase their capacity to use fats as a source of fuel, both during the range of exercise intensities and at rest. The rate of mobilisation from adipose tissue is improved, and the storage and use of intramuscular triacylglycerols is increased. Consequently, the proportion of energy derived from fatty acid oxidation is greater in the trained individual (reviewed by Martin, 1996). This increase in fat burning capacity may have an impact on long-term energy balance, particularly if it exists during light activity and rest. However, results from studies that have attempted to clarify a difference in RQ at rest, between trained and untrained subjects, remain equivocal. The degree of training required for these effects to be experienced also remains unclear.

15.3.3 Impact on thermogenesis and EPOC

It is obvious that during physical activity the muscles do extra work and hence energy expenditure increases. The effect of heavy manual work on total energy expenditure was studied by Garry *et al.* (1955), who compared workers underground in the coal fields of Fife with sedentary clerks on the surface. The Fife coal fields were chosen because the seams of coal were only 1.5 m thick and the miners had to hew the coal with pickaxes in a crouching or kneeling position, this was deemed to be an extremely strenuous occupation. However, the researchers showed that it was not possible for these workers to maintain an average energy output of more than 21 kJ (5 kcal) per minute throughout an 8-hour working shift. On average they expended 15.4 MJ (3660 kcal) per day, while the control clerks expended 11.8 MJ (2800 kcal) per day. Elite athletes can maintain an output of about 84 kJ (20 kcal) per minute for 2 hours, so during the race they expend about 10.5 MJ (2500 kcal).

People who take regular exercise tend to remain thin, despite an apparently high energy intake, so this has stimulated research to show that physical activity has a greater influence on energy expenditure than can be accounted for by the extra work done during exercise. Possible explanations are as follows.

- Athletes have a higher resting metabolic rate than non-athletes with similar body composition.
- Exercise potentiates the thermogenesis induced by food.
- After exercise there is only a slow decrease in metabolic rate, so the excess post-exercise oxygen consumption (EPOC) makes a significant

extra contribution to the energy cost of the exercise.

The evidence for each of these explanations will be reviewed in turn.

In each case there are conflicting results in the literature, with some researchers finding an effect, while others using a similar protocol do not. The reasons for these conflicts are related to the difficulty of designing a satisfactory experimental protocol. First, athletes and sedentary subjects have different body compositions, so differences in metabolic rates are to be expected. Second, it is not clear what dietary regimen should be used. Suppose two groups of subjects are to be compared who both, at rest, are in energy balance with an intake of 8.4 MJ (2000 kcal) per day. One group now undertakes exercise to increase energy expenditure by 2.1 MJ (500 kcal) per day. Should the diet for both groups be 8.4 MJ (2000 kcal) per day, or should the exercising group have 10.5 MJ (2500 kcal) to restore energy balance? If the latter design is used, and a higher energy expenditure is observed, is this attributable to the exercise or to the additional energy intake of the exercising group? Taking these factors into account, there is no evidence that either short- or long-term exercise training has any significant effect on resting metabolic rate in either lean or obese subjects (Tremblay *et al.*, 1983; Segal & Pi-Sunyer, 1989).

Several workers have investigated the influence of exercise on diet-induced thermogenesis but no consistent effect has been shown. Schutz *et al.* (1987) measured energy expenditure for five hours after a meal providing about 3.8 MJ (900 kcal), which was preceded by different workloads on a bicycle ergometer. The absolute increase in energy expenditure in obese subjects after the meal was 339 kJ (81 kcal), or 402 kJ (96 kcal) in the exercising or resting condition. After weight loss their thermic response to food was highest in the obese subjects, lowest in the lean subjects and intermediate in the obese subjects after weight loss. In every case, the thermic effect was less after exercise than in the control condition. However, the results of Segal *et al.*, 1992 are very different; the thermic effect is greater in the lean subjects than in obese ones and, after a period of exercise training, the thermic effect increased in the obese subjects but not in the lean ones. It is fair to conclude that if there is an effect of exercise on the thermic response to food it is a small and inconsistent effect, and cannot contribute much to the maintenance of lean body weight in exercising subjects.

An effect of high-intensity exercise on EPOC was convincingly shown by Maehlum *et al.* (1986). They exercised eight very fit young men and women at 70% of their maximum VO_2 (workload 152.5 watts) for an average of 80 minutes and measured their energy expenditure for the next 12-hour period under resting conditions. After the exercise, their energy expenditure was 14% higher than during 12 hours after a control run without exercise. During the bout of exercise, these subjects consumed 170 l of oxygen and, post-exercise, an extra 26 l of oxygen. Therefore, the EPOC increased the apparent cost of the exercise by 15%. Elite athletes are able to perform work greater than that supported by oxidative reactions because they will also (for a time) use anaerobic pathways. However, this 'oxygen debt' has to be repaid after the exercise, so that the lactic acid can be converted to pyruvate. Several subsequent studies have shown that, in subjects undertaking less intense and prolonged exercise, there is no significant EPOC. For example, Freeman-Akabas *et al.* (1995) exercised subjects at their aerobic threshold for 20 minutes, and Pacy *et al.* (1985) used 30% of VO_2 max (21 kJ or 5 kcal/min) for four periods of 20 minutes. Weststrate *et al.* (1990b) used a load of 100 W or 175 W on a bicycle ergometer for 90 minutes, but do not report the oxygen consumption during exercise. Goldberg *et al.* (1990) used four periods of 30 minutes each, in a chamber calorimeter with peak energy expenditure of 29 kJ (7 kcal) per minute. Although exercise at the highest intensities are followed by a slight increase in resting metabolic rate, none of these later studies show EPOC near the proportion of original work load reported by Maehlum *et al.* (1986). We may therefore conclude that significant EPOC is a phenomenon that can be demonstrated only among elite athletes who are trained to achieve a considerable oxygen debt during exercise.

15.3.4 Psychosocial effects

Several studies have indicated that exercise is associated with successful long-term weight loss

(Section 20.2). This has led some researchers and practitioners to believe that exercise carries psychological as well as physiological effects that enhance sustained weight loss (Wilfley & Brownell, 1994). Exercise can have both acute and long-term effects on aspects of psychological well-being. For example, it has been shown to be effective in reducing mild depression and anxiety (Martinson & Morgan, 1997) and in improving self-esteem (Sonstroem, 1997b). It can also improve aspects of physical self-perception such as body image, physical self-worth and self-confidence in the presentational and functional aspects of the body (Fox, 1997). Some of these properties have been shown to have emotional adjustment benefits in their own right, and higher self-esteem is associated with better health behaviours (Sonstroem & Potts, 1996).

It may be possible, therefore, that success with exercise produces a more positive psychological profile that helps people manage their diet and helps them avoid relapse (Grilo *et al.*, 1989). Although there is sufficient evidence to establish that exercise can improve the mental well-being of overweight people, the degree to which this causes better weight loss, or weight loss maintenance, has yet to be fully addressed in controlled studies. Furthermore, the problem still remains as to how to produce adherence to exercise programmes among overweight people, for the psychological benefits to occur. Systematic study of exercise adherence is in its early days, although several promising lines of research using the stages of behaviour change model (Prochaska & Marcus, 1994) and a range of clinical and community interventions (King, 1994) are emerging. Clearly, the impact of exercise and the psychological mechanisms involved in long-term weight management, provide important targets for future research.

15.3.5 Interactions with genotypes

Research into the effects of incidental physical activity levels and formal exercise training on the prevention and treatment of overweight and obesity is relatively new and sparse, in contrast to the volumes addressing dietary issues. Consequently, little is known about the interaction of exercise with different genotypes. There is evidence to show that, among child and adult populations given a fixed exercise training stimulus, a range of cardiovascular improvements are found, but the mechanisms for this effect are not yet known, although muscle fibre typing may be implicated. There may be a similar sensitivity in response to exercise for weight loss. For example, throughout the literature, there is weak but consistent evidence that males are more responsive to exercise for weight loss than females. Reasons may be psychological, in that men may be more motivated. However, there may be several genetically determined variables that interact with exercise, such as central versus peripheral fat deposition, and fast versus slow-twitch muscle fibre typing. This is clearly an area for future research.

15.4 Summary

- Clearly, the link between exercise and subsequent energy and macronutrient intake is an area that requires further investigation. More work is particularly needed on the effect of different modes, intensities and duration of exercise, in order that exercise prescription for weight loss and prevention of weight gain can be more precisely determined.

- Overall, the available research indicates that there is only a very weak coupling between energy expenditure and subsequent food intake or patterns of eating. There appears to be no evidence to suggest that exercise results in eating more food than would be expected in order to compensate for the extra expenditure.

- In contrast, the evidence is stronger that exercise may work to improve feeding regulation to better match energy expenditure. For a more extensive summary of this area of research, including full tables of studies, see King *et al.* (1997).

- This presents an optimistic view of the potential of exercise for long-term weight management. Where exercise produces disappointing results for weight loss, this is probably a result of inappropriate food choices following exercise, over-compensatory eating to reward for exercise, unrealistic views of the capacity of exercise to expend energy, or failure to comply with the exercise programme.

- The evidence suggests that exercise is likely to be most effective for weight loss if it:
  (a) is undertaken at low to moderate intensities;
  (b) lasts for extended periods beyond 40 minutes;
  (c) results in an endurance training effect.

16
Significance of Within Person Weight Variation

16.1 How normal is weight stability?

Research on energy balance is considerably helped because pure-bred laboratory rodents, under constant conditions, follow a predictable weight trajectory during life. Some distinguished researchers assume that a similar constancy characterises normal people. Bray (1976) observed that in the Ten State Nutrition Survey the weight of white males 'remained within 2 kg of weight at age 30 until after age 60'. More recently, Liebel and colleagues wrote,

> Body weight in adults is remarkably stable for long periods of time. In the Framingham study the body weight of the average adult increased by only 10% over a 20-year period. Such a fine balance is evidence of the presence of regulatory systems for body weight. (Liebel *et al.*, 1995)

In fact, it is not true that the average adult in Framingham regulated weight within 10% (around 8 kg) over 20 years, the average weight of adults was remarkably constant, which is not the same as the weight of the average adult. Figure 16.1 shows the fluctuations in body weight (maximum minus minimum) during the 10 two-yearly examinations in the first 18 years of the Framingham study (Gordon & Kannel, 1973). Only about 30% had changes of less than 8 kg, but the mean weight in the population remained fairly constant because gainers and losers largely cancelled each other out.

It is true that some individuals (especially workers in the field of energy balance) report remarkably stable body weight over their adult lifetime. For example, the doyen of nutritional physiologists, Professor R. Passmore, had recounted how a tail-coat obtained when he was an undergraduate still fitted him some 40 years later (Passmore, 1973). That is indeed remarkable, but why is his control of energy balance so much more precise than that of most inhabitants of Framingham? It might be that his tail-coat provided feedback about his weight change, so if it did not fit him he made appropriate adjustments to his energy balance.

Information about weight variability in older women comes from the analysis by French *et al.* (1995) of data collected for the Iowa Women's Health Study (IWHS). Participants were asked by mailed questionnaire about their weight status at the ages of 18, 30, 40 and 50 years. They were also asked how often they had intentionally lost 2.3–4.0 kg, 4.5–8.5 kg, 9.0–22.0 kg or 22.5 kg or more, and how often they had unintentionally lost 9 kg or more. Of the 29 015 respondents, only 1.9% reported no weight change of as much as 5% of body weight, while 21.3% reported cycles of change of 5–10% of body weight, and 19.5% reported cycles of >10% of body weight.

Investigators who estimate weight stability from two measurements about five years apart find many more people with stable weight. For example, among 7735 middle-aged men, Wannamethee & Shaper (1990) found 55.1% who had changed weight by <4% in 5 years, and Rissanen *et al.* (1991) found that 71.1% of 6165 women, and 72.0% of 6504 men changed weight by less than 5 kg over 5

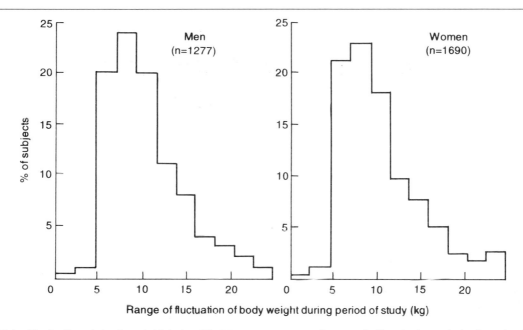

Fig. 16.1   Fluctuations in body weight during 18 years among men and women in Framingham study. Age at entry 30–59 years (data of Gordon & Kannel, 1973 from Garrow, 1988).

years. However, this must overestimate weight stability, because if all the subjects were in fact cycling in weight, it must happen by chance that two surveys 5 years apart will find some of the subjects at the same phase of the cycle on each occasion, and they appear to have a constant weight.

Obesity is a condition in which the mechanism that should regulate energy balance has failed to work effectively. It is, therefore, important that we should understand the mechanism that has failed. The correct therapeutic approach will differ if the mechanism is primarily physiological, or primarily cognitive. It is also important that, in an attempt to help obese people to achieve a normal weight, we do not inadvertently harm them by causing weight cycling. The evidence concerning whether weight cycling is harmful is considered in Section 16.2.

The conclusion by Liebel *et al.* (1995) that there is evidence of 'the presence of regulatory systems for body weight' is, of course, correct. Homeostatic systems are well known that maintain the constancy of many physiological parameters, such as pH, plasma calcium concentration and blood pressure. It is impossible that these should be regulated by cognitive mechanisms, as we are normally unaware

of changes in pH, calcium or blood pressure. Other important parameters, such as body temperature and respiration rate, are under dual control. In most conditions, the physiological controls work without conscious effort, but in extreme conditions of heat or cold we take measures (change of clothing or use of heating or cooling devices) to extend the efficacy of physiological controls.

Regulation of body fat stores requires a different type of control system to that needed for temperature or pH. Human metabolism is designed to operate at a pH of 7.4 and a temperature of 37°C. There is clearly an optimum state, which does not vary with circumstances. However, it was to the advantage of our primitive ancestors that they should overeat when food was plentiful, in order that they had an energy store to tide them over when food was scarce. It appears, however, that the physiological regulation works more effectively to prevent under-nutrition than over-nutrition, presumably because abundant food was seldom available to our ancestors.

Consequently, it is not surprising that there are physiological systems that tend to reduce or increase food intake, or reduce or increase energy expenditure, in order to restore energy balance. These are reviewed in later chapters of this book. It is also clear that there are cognitive mechanisms that regulate body weight. In the IWHS, 47.2% of women reported having lost >9 kg: 16.6% reported that this was intentional, 19.2% that it was unintentional and 11.4% that it was a combination of intentional and unintentional loss. The question, which is addressed here, concerns the component of the regulatory system, physiological or cognitive, which is most likely to cause obesity in man.

16.1.1 Distribution of weight changes with time in prospective studies of populations

There is very little published information about the time-course of weight changes of individuals in a representative population sample. Most information is anecdotal and derived from studies on atypical individuals who had a professional interest in energy balance and body composition. Figure 16.2 was published to illustrate that while fat-free mass (here labelled LBM) decreased gradually over an adult lifetime, body weight (i.e. fat) fluctuated in an unpredictable manner (Forbes & Reina, 1970). It is evident that subject AB (a pioneer in the measurement of body density) increased in weight by about 15 kg between the ages of 36 and 52, and again between the ages of 53 and 60 years. Thanks to four periods of rapid weight reduction at age 65, he weighed 90 kg, which was the same as his weight

30 years previously. Subject EA (a pioneer in the measurement of total body potassium) weighed 67 kg at age 36 and at age 48; with excursions to a maximum of 72 kg at age 42 and a minimum of 60 kg at age 45.

Figure 16.3 provides more detailed information over a shorter period for another nutrition scientist, who was trying to find out if fat cell number altered in an adult who experimentally altered fat mass (the experiment was a failure in this respect). The changes in weight, between days 100 and 160, were induced by maximal tolerable overfeeding and, between days 365 and 415, by underfeeding in order to restore weight to the baseline condition (Garrow & Stalley, 1975). At all other times, weight regulation was left entirely to physiological control. A sequel to this study, extending the measurements up to 1000 days, is shown in Fig. 16.4 (Garrow & Stalley, 1977). In this case, weight was experimentally reduced, by underfeeding, from the baseline of 76 kg, to 69 kg and then allowed to self-regulate, in the hope of finding a 'set-point' (Chapter 10). No such physiological set point was found, but at 1000 days the experiment was no longer 'blind', because the fit of clothing informed the subject that his

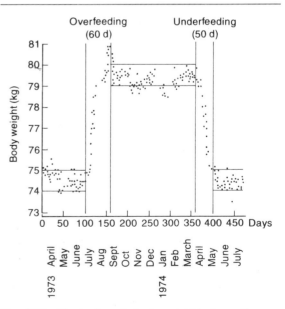

Fig. 16.3 Fluctuations in body weight in the author, induced by deliberate overfeeding and underfeeding (from: Garrow & Stalley, 1975).

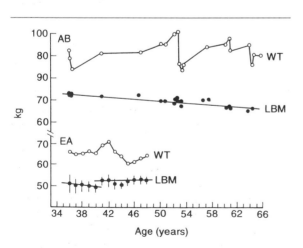

Fig. 16.2 Longitudinal study of body weight and lean body mass of 2 subjects (from: Forbes & Reina, 1970).

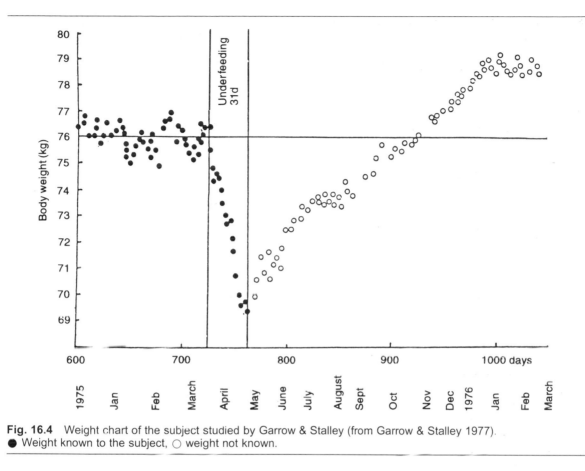

Fig. 16.4 Weight chart of the subject studied by Garrow & Stalley (from Garrow & Stalley 1977). ● Weight known to the subject, ○ weight not known.

weight was at an upper tolerable limit. Over the subsequent 21 years, his weight has remained about 79 kg, probably mostly by cognitive regulation (J.S. Garrow, personal communication, 1998).

Data on weight fluctuation in randomly selected populations does not provide detailed time-course information, but does show that the weight fluctuations discussed above do not occur only in nutrition researchers, or particularly in lean or obese individuals. Figure 16.5 shows a plot of weights of 411 women in the Rhondda Fach region of Wales, who were participating in a study of hypertension. Miall (personal communication, 1973) made measurements of body weight, in 1960 and 1964, on women who were apparently healthy. On average, the weight of the population did not change much, but some people who weighed 90 kg in 1960 weighed 60 kg in 1964, and vice versa.

16.1.2 Characteristics of weight-stable and weight-labile individuals

Rissanen *et al.,* (1991) studied 6165 adult Finnish women and 6504 men, who were examined on two occasions with a median interval of 5.7 years. Over this period, the mean weight change among both men and women was <0.6 kg, but there were 15.1% of women and 17.5% of men who gained more than 5 kg in 5 years and 13.8% of women and 10.5% of men who lost this amount of weight. The weight change was greatest for those men and women with low levels of education (p <0.001), chronic diseases (p <0.01), little physical activity (p <0.001) or heavy alcohol consumption (p <0.05 for women, p <0.001 for men). Weight change was greater for those who became married or quitted smoking between the examinations (p <0.001 for both men and women). In gen-

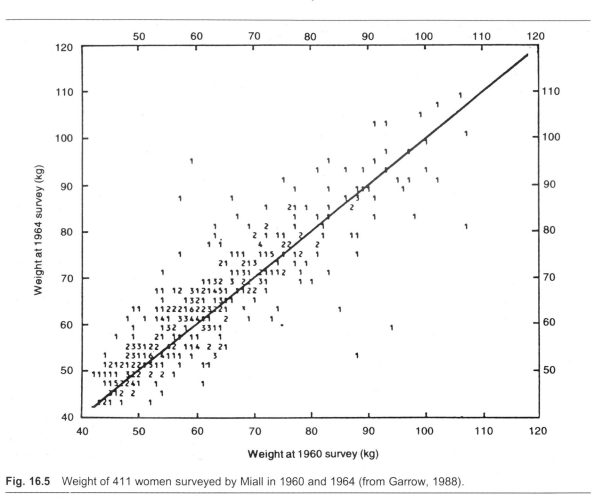

Fig. 16.5 Weight of 411 women surveyed by Miall in 1960 and 1964 (from Garrow, 1988).

eral, the mean weight gain and risk of rapid weight gain increased with the number of children born between the two surveys, but was not related to the number of children at the baseline survey. The adjusted relative risk of obesity with the number of children born (relative to no children = 1.0) for one child was 1.3, for 2–4 children was 1.3, and for 5 or more children was 2.1. However, there was an interesting interaction between level of education and parity in the risk of rapid weight gain. Among highly educated women, the relative risk for one child was 0.8 (CI 0.3–2.1) and for two or more children 0.6 (CI 0.2–5.0). Among the women with lower educational levels the corresponding risks were for one child 1.6 (CI 1.0–2.8) and for two or more children 3.3 (CI 1.6–7.1).

In the IWHS, the variability of weight was not associated with age or use of current hormone replacement therapy, but was related to other baseline characteristics (French *et al.*, 1997). The quartile with the highest weight variability (compared with the least variable quartile) had a higher percentage of women with BMI >28 (56 versus 17) and more with a waist-hip ratio >0.8 (74 versus 53). More women smoked (37 versus 31), fewer currently drank alcohol (36 versus 49), more were physically inactive (52 versus 44) and there were more that did not complete high school education (24 versus 16). Fewer were currently married (74 versus 80), more were diabetic (12 versus 1.7) and more were hypertensive (46 versus 27).

16.2 Associations between weight cycling, mortality and morbidity

Lissner *et al.* (1989) analysed the relationship between body weight variability and mortality in the Gothenburg prospective studies of men and women. A cohort of people from Gothenburg (855 men born in 1913 and 1462 women born in 1908, 1914, 1918, 1922 and 1930) underwent a series of medical examinations some 50 years later, at which body weight was measured. Among the women, the variability of three weights was calculated; a recalled weight relating to 1963–1964 and measured weights taken in 1968–1969, and in 1974–1975. Among the men, measured weights taken in 1963, 1967 and 1973 were used for the calculation of weight variation. The mean (s.d.) of change in BMI among the women was +0.94 (2.47), and among the men was +0.65 (1.74). At a height of 1.73 m, a change in BMI of 1 is equivalent to a change of 3 kg. Therefore, the average weight increase of the women over 11 years was about 2.8 kg and among the men over 10 years it was about 2 kg. The larger change among the women may be attributable to error in the recalled weight relating to 1963–1964. The standard deviation of weights, about the mean weight, for each individual was about 7.4 kg for women and 5.3 kg for men. Among both men and women, mortality rates (between 1976–1988 for the women and 1975–1985 for the men) were significantly associated with the variability of weight (p <0.03 for women, p <0.003 for men). Reported adherence to weight reduction diets did not correlate with mortality.

Other longitudinal sets of weight data have been examined. Some studies depended on reported weights, and some (e.g. the Framingham Heart Study, the Baltimore Longitudinal Study on Ageing (BLSA), the Multiple Risk Factor Intervention Trial (MRFIT), the Charleston Heart Study and the Zutphen Study) provided measured weight at regular intervals. This literature has been reviewed by Lissner & Brownell (1992), who note that a positive association has consistently been observed between body weight fluctuation and all-cause mortality, and usually (but not in BLSA and Zutphen) with coronary mortality, in particular. This finding is very robust, further confirmation is found in the British Regional Heart Study (Wannamethee & Shaper, 1990), in the Seven Nations Study (Peters *et al.*, 1995) and in the Iowa Women's Health Study (French *et al.*, 1997). It is clear from all these data that a constant weight, even at moderate degrees of overweight, is associated with a better health outcome that a weight which varies.

The reasons for this robust association remain unclear. We do not know if changes in weight in otherwise healthy individuals cause ill health, or if people with chronic ill health tend to have a variable weight as a result of relapses and remissions in their disease. These observations present a challenge to those of us who advocate weight loss for people who are overweight. If weight is lost and then regained, is the subject worse off than if weight had not been lost in the first place?

16.3 Confounding factors in the study of weight variation and health

It is obvious that people with a chronic relapsing disease, such as irritable bowel syndrome or infections such as tuberculosis, are likely to fluctuate in weight and also have poor health outcomes. People with heart disease (or a family history of heart disease) will probably be advised to lose weight and will achieve this intermittently. So, they too are likely to show variable weight and a poor health outcome. It is also possible that people with a certain impulsive personality will adopt extreme methods to achieve weight loss and will rebound when the rapid reduction in weight has been achieved. Thus, it is possible to suggest mechanisms by which disease causes the weight variability, but it is equally possible to suggest mechanisms by which the weight fluctuation causes disease. Both starvation and overfeeding reduce glucose tolerance; therefore, weight variation might predispose to diabetes. This possibility has been investigated in a retrospective study of diabetics by Podar *et al.* (1996). They failed to find any evidence that glucose tolerance deteriorated to any greater extent among patients who cycled in weight, than among those whose weight was stable. Muls *et al.* (1995) reviewed the literature and failed to find evidence that weight cycling *per se* was detrimental to health.

16.4 Summary

- Variable weight is associated with poor health and increased mortality, but we do not know if it is the socio-demographic and disease profiles of the subjects which cause weight variability, or if weight variability causes disease. Probably both factors act, but we do not know in what proportion.

- It will be very difficult to obtain a definitive answer, because a randomised controlled trial of the long-term health effects of weight variation versus constant weight would be very difficult (and probably unethical) to set up.

- Those who seek to help obese people lose weight must remember that weight lost and then regained does the patient no good, and may do harm. It is, therefore, essential that any programme seeking to achieve weight loss is linked to a plan to ensure that the weight loss is maintained.

17
Prevention of Obesity

17.1 Introduction

It is very easy to list behaviours that should prevent the occurrence of obesity in the population. Bouchard (1996) writes, 'The tools available to reverse this unhealthy trend' (of increasing obesity) 'are remarkably simple in appearance.'

Despite the apparent simplicity of the solution, all writers on the subject agree that there is sparse evidence of efficacy of health education programmes to promote these behaviours. As discussed in Chapter 4, the prevalence of obesity in the UK has increased markedly despite such attempts to reverse the trend. Some writers have a quite pessimistic outlook: 'We have not been able to prevent obesity in the past, and we do not have the tools to do it better in the future' (Stunkard, 1995). Of course, with sufficiently draconian measures, obesity can be prevented. Scrignan (1980) describes the virtual elimination of obesity in a police force where being overweight was considered a disciplinary offence, punishable by loss of leave, money and promotion prospects. The weight was regained when the law courts ruled that this edict was an infringement of the policemen's constitutional rights.

If the public health burden of obesity is to be reduced, somehow, we must find a means whereby potentially obese people who have obesity-promoting habits are persuaded to change these habits, without applying pressure, which is unacceptable in a democratic society. This will probably involve changing the public perception of obesity and removing the barriers to change (James, 1995; Egger & Swinburn, 1997).

A major problem is to identify the 'potentially obese people' in this group. Why should an individual change his habits if he sees people who have had apparently similar habits for many years, but who have not become obese? If individuals who are at particularly high risk for obesity can be identified, it is more likely that they would heed advice about prevention and, if the target population can be more accurately focused, that advice should be more effectively delivered.

17.2 Identification of groups at high risk for adult obesity

17.2.1 Obese children, or children with obese parents

Children of obese parents are more likely to be obese than children of lean parents (see Chapter 6). Probably the most positive evidence of effective prevention of adult obesity comes from Epstein *et al.* (1994). They recruited children aged 6–12 years and treated them by a family-based behavioural programme. The children and their parents were randomised to three groups, and all the subjects received the same advice on diet and exercise. However, in one group, parent and child were rewarded for behavioural change, in another, only the child was rewarded and in the third group, the control group, the families were rewarded for attendance only. At 5 and 10 years follow-up, the average percentage by which people were overweight in the first group reduced by 11.2% and 7.5% respectively. In contrast, in the control group the average percentage by which people were overweight increased by 7.9% and 14.3% respectively.

Flodmark *et al.* (1993) recruited overweight children aged 10–11 years. Of these, 25 were treated for 14–18 months with diet, exercise and family therapy; 19 were given conventional treatment; and 50 acted as an untreated control group. The first group showed a smaller increase in BMI than the controls after 1 year (5.1% versus 12.0%, p = 0.02).

17.2.2 Rapid weight gainers

When populations are studied several times, with intervals of a few years between measurements, it is common to find individuals who change weight by more than 5 kg between one examination and the next one (Section 16.1). Rissanen *et al.* (1991) found that individuals who gained more than 5 kg in 5 years were more likely than the general population to have a low level of education, chronic disease, little physical activity and high alcohol consumption. These are also characteristics that are associated with an increased risk of obesity. It is likely, therefore, that rapid weight gainers are an identifiable high-risk group who might be targeted in an attempt to prevent obesity, but it seems that this strategy has not been investigated, nor do we know if rapid gainers do in fact become obese, or merely show large fluctuations in weight.

17.2.3 Post-obese

It is a common experience in hospital obesity clinics that obese patients, who attended several years previously and lost a substantial amount of weight, are likely to return having regained this weight. This has given rise to the view that almost all individuals who lose 10% of body weight in weight-loss programmes, regain this weight within 5 years (NIH, 1993). This interpretation may be too pessimistic, as those who maintain their weight loss have no need to return to the hospital clinic, whereas those who do not maintain their weight loss do have an incentive to return. Even so, it is likely that the most powerful predictor of becoming obese is to have been obese in the past. In practice, preventing obesity in post-obese individuals is exactly the same as achieving weight maintenance after treatment of obesity, which is discussed further in Section 18.4.

17.2.4 Pregnancy

Weight gain in pregnancy, and postpartum weight retention, are discussed in Section 7.5.1. There is a strong relation between gestational weight gain and postpartum weight retention. Among women with gestational weight gain less than 12 kg, there is very little mean weight retention. However, a gestational weight gain of more than 20 kg is likely to result in a postpartum gain of about 7 kg.

The susceptibility to weight gain after pregnancy is greatest in women with the highest pre-pregnancy weight and with later pregnancies, this is shown in Fig.17.1. Therefore, overweight women with third or later pregnancies are particularly at risk of excessive postpartum weight retention (Beazley & Swinhoe, 1979). The amount of weight gain that is advisable in pregnancy is discussed in Section 7.5.1. However, pregnancy is not an appropriate time at which to try to achieve weight loss, because this may impair fetal growth. In overweight pregnant women, the best compromise is to attempt to achieve modest weight gain during pregnancy (for example a 6 kg increase in weight, rather than a 12 kg increase in weight). On this

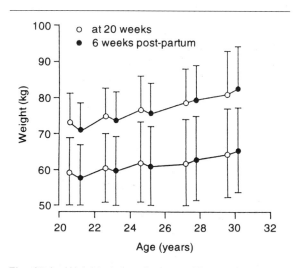

Fig. 17.1 Weight change between 20 weeks gestation and 6 weeks postpartum in 50 women followed through five successive pregnancies. The lower line shown is the Mean ± SEM weight for the whole series, and the upper line is for the heaviest quartile of mothers. The tendency for postpartum weight to be less than weight at 20 weeks gestation disappears after the third pregnancy. (Data of Beazley & Swinhoe, 1979). (From Garrow, 1988).

basis, after delivery, the woman's weight will be less than pre-pregnancy, and the obstetric outcome is likely to be favourable (Naeye, 1979).

17.2.5 Smoking quitters

People who stop smoking cigarettes, frequently gain 5 kg in weight (Rissanen *et al.,* 1991). The health benefits of stopping smoking are much greater than the health risks of this modest weight gain. It is, therefore, inappropriate to highlight the risk of weight gain, because this may discourage the smoker from stopping smoking. Behavioural therapy does not seem effective in preventing this weight gain and may reduce success in smoking cessation, but regular use of nicotine gum is often helpful (Klesges, 1995)

17.2.6 Physically inactive

Individuals who are habitually active are much less likely to become obese than those who are sedentary (Chapter 15). However, successful approaches to persuade habitually inactive people to become more active have yet to be fully established.

17.2.7 Ethnic groups

There is no evidence that obesity prevention programmes specifically targeting ethnic minority groups are generally effective. In some circumstances, they may cause resentment because they may be interpreted as racial discrimination, but in other circumstances, they may be successful.

17.2.8 Genetic markers of susceptibility

Future research may identify genetic markers that are associated with susceptibility to obesity or leanness, either by acting through food intake or through physical activity. No such markers have been identified at present.

17.3 Strategies for prevention applied to the whole population

17.3.1 Education about the diet, exercise, and the risks of obesity

The conventional response to public health problems is to seek to inform the public about the risks

and how they can be avoided, e.g. 'hand washing' and safe sex. One of the *Health of the Nation* targets (Department of Health, 1992) was to reduce the prevalence of obesity to the level of 1980. To help with this target, prevention orientated messages were transmitted through the usual media channels. This met with a resounding lack of success. The public received and understood the message, but the prevalence of obesity continued to increase.

Formal evidence of a similar lack of efficacy of conventional public health approaches comes from two expensive and well-controlled studies in the USA. The Minnesota Heart Health Programme (MHHP) was a 13-year research and demonstration project, designed to reduce cardiovascular risk. The project compared three pairs of matched communities. All six communities were observed for a period of five years (baseline observation). Then, one community in each pair received seven years of community intervention activities. These included risk factor screening, mass media education, adult education classes, work-site interventions, home correspondence programmes, school-based programmes, restaurant programmes and point-of-purchase education in supermarkets. Weight gain prevention was emphasised for all adults and weight loss was encouraged for those who were obese. About 3500 men and women were followed in the three intervention cities and a similar number in the three control cities. The mean baseline BMIs in the intervention and control communities were 25.6 and 25.8, respectively. During the five years of baseline observations, BMI increased in both the intervention and the control communities, and during the seven years of intervention, the average BMIs of both groups of communities continued to increase at the same rate. As a result, they both finished with a mean adjusted BMI of 26.8 (Jeffery *et al.,* 1995). The authors offer four possible explanations for the fact there was no detectable effect on BMI, despite so large an input of effort. First, that the health message was overwhelmed in a media environment in which opposing messages were also widespread. Second, that the MHHP message was presented in an environment already saturated with such programmes. Third, that messages about obesity were in conflict with other MHHP messages, such as smoking cessation. A final possible reason is that the fundamental idea behind this and similar intervention approaches is flawed. A guiding principle of such programmes is that increasing the level of **knowledge** in the population about obesity risk, dietary choices, and exercise behaviour will enable people to lose weight or prevent weight gain. Thus, education *per se* may have limited success.

The other large intervention study was the Stanford Five City Project, which was presented in a somewhat more upbeat manner (Taylor *et al.*, 1991). However, the outcome in terms of BMI was the same; there was no significant effect of intervention on BMI and all groups gained weight.

17.3.2 Individual incentives

In view of the dismal results achieved by general population programmes to reduce obesity (Section 17.3.1, above), several suggestions have been made about methods by which overweight or obese individuals might be motivated to reduce weight. To some extent, this happens already in the case of life insurance companies who impose 'added years' (in effect higher premiums) on customers, who are severely overweight, because their life expectancy is decreased. However, such financial incentives are only applicable for relatively affluent people. Financial sanctions may be effective in reducing obesity, but may be socially (and sometimes legally) unacceptable (Section 16.1). Essentially the problem is one of seeking to change the behaviour of people, in a manner that they do not see as particularly beneficial to themselves.

17.4 Secondary prevention

17.4.1 Motivate doctors to take overweight seriously

Job satisfaction in primary care is derived mainly from making correct diagnoses and then dealing with the problem using the facilities available within the practice or, if necessary, referring the patient for specialist care. The management of overweight or obesity does not sit easily in this scheme. There is no intellectual challenge in making a diagnosis if the problem, when identified, requires a disproportionate amount of the doctor's time to deal with adequately. It is not surprising that, with some notable exceptions, general practitioners are not inclined, or trained, to take on the management of

weight disorders in their patients. However, because the problem is so prevalent, and the health risk is so serious, it is vital that primary healthcare professionals should contribute to the solution.

The Scottish Intercollegiate Guidelines Network has devised a weight management scheme for primary healthcare which is shown in Fig. 17.2 (SIGN, 1996). If generally implemented, this would go a long way towards providing the early detection and management of overweight. However, the report recognised that implementation of these guidelines will require co-operation between many organisations and individuals, as well as a resource to develop these services both in general practice and community groups. Also specialist services would be necessary, to which patients could be referred as appropriate.

17.4.2 Non-profit weight control courses, or endorsement of appropriate commercial clubs

A major resource implication of the scheme shown in Fig. 17.2 is operating the facility that will provide the 3-month weight loss programme; including diet, exercise, behavioural advice and social support. One solution is to set up locally non-profit-making but self-financing slimming clubs on the model described by Bush *et al.* (1988). The model comprises groups of 15–25 people (usually women, men do better in unisex groups) who meet weekly from 19.30–21.30 for 10 weeks, in local authority school clinic premises. A state registered dietitian, who has access to suitable audio-visual teaching material, leads the group. The cost is covered by the fee paid in advance by individuals registering for the course, but is lower than the fee for a commercial weight loss group because the premises are made available without cost and no profit is made. Typically, those enrolling for such clubs are women aged 30–60 years, with a BMI of 25–35, who lose on average 4.4 kg in 10 weeks. The demand for such services in one Health District is indicated by the enrolment of over 1,000 people on 50 courses over 10 years, all at no cost to the National Health Service.

In some circumstances, it may not be possible to set up weight control groups on this model, either because staff with the necessary qualities to lead the group are not available or because local commercial groups provide a very good service. In these

Note: This scheme is for guidance only but provides a logical management process to be evaluated and modified in each centre. See text for graded recommendations and supporting evidence for each stage of the scheme.

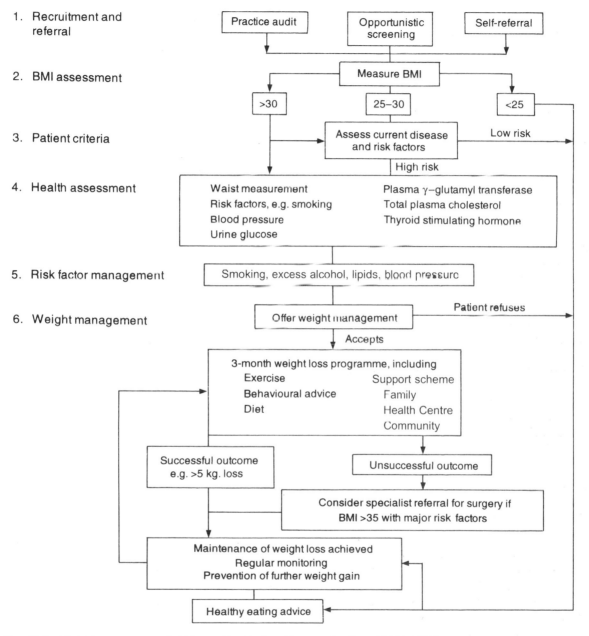

1. Recruitment and referral

Practice audit · Opportunistic screening · Self-referral

2. BMI assessment

Measure BMI

>30 · 25–30 · <25

3. Patient criteria

Assess current disease and risk factors · Low risk

High risk

4. Health assessment

Waist measurement
Risk factors, e.g. smoking
Blood pressure
Urine glucose
Plasma γ–glutamyl transferase
Total plasma cholesterol
Thyroid stimulating hormone

5. Risk factor management

Smoking, excess alcohol, lipids, blood pressure

6. Weight management

Offer weight management · Patient refuses

Accepts

3-month weight loss programme, including
Exercise   Support scheme
Behavioural advice Family
Diet   Health Centre
          Community

Successful outcome e.g. >5 kg. loss · Unsuccessful outcome

Consider specialist referral for surgery if BMI >35 with major risk factors

Maintenance of weight loss achieved
Regular monitoring
Prevention of further weight gain

Healthy eating advice

Fig. 17.2 Weight management in Primary Health Care/Community (from SIGN, 1996).

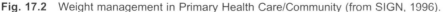

circumstances, endorsement of well-run commercial groups may be the best option.

17.5 Summary

- A successful and acceptable procedure for preventing obesity in the population has not yet been found, although many individuals develop their own strategies. Conventional population-wide health education programmes are ineffective.

- Individuals at high risk of developing obesity can be identified, but there is no evidence that focused health education with these groups is effective; probably, education *per se* is not enough.

- The only trial concerning obese children that has shown good results, aimed to limit the development of obesity in overweight pre-pubertal children with the co-operation of their families.

- The alternatives are: some form of legal coercion of behaviour, which would have to be acceptable to the majority of the population (as is legislation about motorcyclists wearing crash helmets), or a broadly based 'ecological' approach, which has proven effective in public health problems ranging from infectious disease to industrial accidents. The latter seeks to modify not only the 'host' (in this case the individual) by education and behaviour change, but also the environment (economic, physical and socio-cultural) to promote lower energy intake and greater physical activity, and also the 'vehicle' (in this case food and drink) towards the same objectives.

- Primary healthcare professionals, working in a properly integrated manner, must support collectively effective obesity prevention. SIGN (1996) has proposed a scheme by which this may be achieved. It remains to be seen if there is a political and economic will to implement these strategies.

- At present, opinion-formers in the media see obesity as mainly a social and cosmetic problem, not a serious public health hazard (Appendix 1). Progress on prevention will not be made until obese people are seen to have a physical disability, for which they need help both from health-carers and from society in general.

18
Treatment of Obesity I: Introduction

18.1 To treat or not to treat

Any treatment programmes for obesity should address not only the problem of weight reduction but should also include measures to help with the maintenance of lowered weight. The primary aim for a programme is a reduction in body fat, with the assumption that this will reduce risk of conditions associated with the obesity. Nevertheless, a successful programme should also lead to improvements in the quality of life, self esteem, social functioning, anxiety and depression. Obesity is a condition that may not respond to conventional methods of treatment; its management may require an approach that is tailored to an individual's need. The ability of a treatment to maintain a long-term weight reduction is as important as its ability to cause the initial weight loss.

18.1.1 Children

Childhood is an important stage at which to prevent obesity (Section 17.2.1) but it may also be a very difficult stage at which to treat established obesity. A child needs to grow physically and to become psychologically secure. To achieve these objectives, the child needs adequate nutrition and the reliable support and encouragement of his or her family. These constraints are in conflict with the requirements for the successful treatment of obesity, i.e. an energy intake that is less than that required to maintain body weight, and a change of lifestyle.

For a specialist in a hospital obesity clinic there is no more discouraging sight than that of a thin, anxious mother, dragging into the consulting room her fat, sulking adolescent. All three parties to the consultation feel justifiable resentment. The mother is resentful because despite her best endeavours to provide all the right 'diet' foods, her adolescent is becoming increasingly fat and ungrateful. The adolescent is resentful because his or her parents alternate between accusations of 'cheating' on the awful diet they provide, and visits to yet another 'useless' specialist in the hope that he or she will be found to have some hitherto-undescribed metabolic cause of obesity. The specialist is resentful because he or she knows that little progress will be made in the diagnosis and management of the obesity. The best that can be hoped for, is not to make the situation worse.

The age and degree of obesity of the patient determine possible damage-limitation strategies. It is always useful to have a short conversation with the child in the absence of the parent to determine what outcome, if any, the child would consider satisfactory. This can usually be achieved during a brief physical examination of the child in an adjacent room. If the child is between the ages of 5 and 10 years, then a policy of limiting weight gain, rather than attempting weight loss, is ideal as the height–growth spurt is still to come. Post-pubertal children who are brought up by a parent are the most difficult group; this is the group in which mutual resentment is likely to be so strong that co-operation between child and parent is unlikely. It is almost always fair to say that the cause of obesity in a teenager is the failure of his or her parents to prevent the development of obesity at the stage when they were in a position to do so. The debate about who is to blame is unrewarding, and a constant source of resentment on both sides. Teenagers, who come to the clinic unaccompanied, have thereby shown that they are taking personal responsibility for the situation, and the parent will not immediately claim credit for any progress. This is a hopeful situation if sensitively handled.

18.1.2 Pregnancy

The effect of pregnancy on the subsequent risk of obesity is reviewed in Section 7.5.1. The evidence indicates that there is no great difference between the weight at menopause, of women who have had many or few children, when other social factors have been adjusted for, but parity increases the rate of weight gain in young women (Newcombe, 1982). A point, on which there is little evidence, concerns the correct management of an obese woman who is already pregnant. In pregnant women of normal weight, a gain of about 12 kg during gestation is associated with the best pregnancy outcome (Hytten, 1991). However, this rule does not apply to women who start pregnancy with a BMI >28, in whom the lowest perinatal mortality is associated with a weight gain of only 4 kg (Naeye, 1979). It is reasonable, therefore, to try to achieve a total weight gain of 4 kg in obese women; this should provide the best situation for the baby, and should ensure that, following the postpartum weight loss, the mother is less obese than she was when the pregnancy started.

In practice, this objective is hard to achieve for several reasons. During pregnancy, there is a quite powerful physiological drive to increase fat stores as an energy reserve to support lactation. Furthermore, obstetricians have an entrenched belief that faltering of weight gain in pregnancy is an ominous sign (as it is in normal-weight women). It is, therefore, almost inevitable that the obese mother who succeeds in limiting her weight gain to one-third of the normal rate will be discouraged from this policy by health-care professionals in the antenatal clinic. Certainly, pregnancy and lactation are two states in which rapid weight loss is not appropriate. It is understandable that obstetricians, who have delivered a normal child from an obese woman, may think that their job has been well done and that pre-existing obesity in the mother is not their problem. However, if several pregnancies occur between the age of 20 and 30 years, and the woman is obese at age 30, it is hard to see who, other than obstetric health-care professionals, could have intervened to prevent this obesity.

18.1.3 Other groups

It has been stated elsewhere that the objectives in obesity treatment are to:

- achieve weight loss to a point at which the health risks to the patient are reduced as far as possible
- maintain that weight loss indefinitely, and
- restore, if necessary, the self-esteem of the patient.

Sometimes, obese patients present for treatment with other problems (mental or physical diseases, or social circumstances) which are so devastating that the risks associated with the obesity become relatively trivial by comparison. In such situations, it is unethical to treat the obesity without carefully considering if the trouble involved in achieving weight loss will really produce commensurate benefit in such a patient.

18.2 Cost benefits of weight loss

In Section 18.1, the obvious point was made that the treatment of obesity should not be attempted unless it is likely that the benefit to the obese patient of weight loss will be greater than the cost of achieving this weight loss. The benefit of even modest weight loss, in terms of reduced complications of obesity and related diseases, is discussed in Section 18.3. However, evaluating the cost involved with any useful accuracy is very difficult, since the cost is borne by the patient, not the therapist, and the two may differ markedly in their assessment of the difficulty of following a given treatment strategy.

The costs we are concerned with are mainly psychosocial, not financial. Of course, it is possible for treatments to be very expensive if, for example, the patient selects a diet consisting of prime cuts of lean steak along with fresh pre-prepared salads and fruits, and takes exercise in a fashionable fitness club. However, effective treatments for obesity need not be more expensive than the previous lifestyle. For example, selecting lean minced meat and adding lots of vegetables, which are in season, will help to ensure food costs are not excessive. Also, diets such as the milk diet (Section 19.1.3) can hardly be more expensive than the diet that was previously being followed. Increasing energy expenditure by walking or jogging, rather than taking public or private transport, must reduce total financial expenditure and will eliminate the need to join an expensive health club.

It is very disheartening for an obese patient to be confronted by thin doctors or dietitians (or, worse still, fat doctors or dietitians) who seem to think that keeping to a diet for months on end is a very simple matter, but who have no experience of doing so themselves. The qualification to be a group leader in a commercial slimming club is most often that the group leader should have personal experience of substantial weight loss, which is maintained over time (Garrow, 1995). Such people can speak with authority about the cost, as well as the benefit, of weight loss. The psychosocial costs of weight reduction were well described by a patient in 1885, who addressed his physician as follows:

> Sir, I have followed your prescription as if my life depended on it, and I have ascertained that during this month I have lost three pounds or a little more. But in order to reach this result I have been obliged to do such violence to all my tastes and all my habits – in a word I have suffered so much – that while giving you my best thanks for your kind directions, I renounce entirely any advantages from them and throw myself for the future entirely into the hands of Providence.
>
> (Astwood, 1962)

The treatment of obesity is euphemistically described as advocating a change in lifestyle, but this change can, for some patients, represent a 'violence to all their tastes and habits', and the cost of this should not be underestimated. It is clearly set out in the chapters on the aetiology of obesity, in this book, that the lifestyle of the obese person involves a larger intake from food and drink, and/or a smaller energy output from physical activity, than that of the non-obese person. It is of no use for the non-obese therapist to think that their non-obese lifestyle is 'normal', and that it should, therefore, be easy for the non-obese person to follow it, because this is not the case. If it had been the case, the obese person would not now be seeking help to lose weight.

The psychosocial cost of dietary restriction does not merely relate to a change in diet, it also involves 'violence' to all the social, as well as nutritive,

aspects of eating. Obese people often have low self-esteem, their family and friends are familiar with their cycle of dieting, failing to lose weight and relapsing again, with an even lower self-esteem. It takes courage to attempt a diet, and risk failure once again. The motivation to persist with a given regimen is not constant over time. Eyton (1987) observes that the main factor that motivates obese people to keep to a regimen is the observed weight loss, if the weight loss falters, so does the motivation, just at the stage when it is most required. The friends and family of an obese person may regard attempts at weight loss as a suitable subject for ridicule, or may be jealous that the patient seems likely to succeed in an enterprise at which they have failed (Garrow, 1991b). It is part of the job of the therapist to be aware of these costs to the patient and to seek to decrease them as much as possible; this will alter the cost/benefit ratio in favour of weight loss. More information on this subject is given in Chapter 24.

18.3 Effect of modest weight loss on complications of obesity and associated disease

Patients or primary health-care professionals do not always appreciate the benefits of weight reduction in the management of associated diseases such as diabetes, hypertension and hyperlipidaemia. Short-term weight loss corrects, or eradicates, many of the metabolic abnormalities associated with overweight, including insulin resistance, diabetes mellitus, hypertension, dyslipidaemia and blood coagulation abnormalities as well as obesity-related physical impairments (Chapter 2). Moreover, weight loss by obese individuals consistently improves negative emotions such as depression and anxiety. It also improves psychosocial functioning, mood and quality of life; but these beneficial effects may be transitory and sometimes are offset by the adverse psychological and psychosocial consequences of subsequent weight regain (Stunkard & Wadden, 1992; Rand & MacGregor, 1991). Data on the long-term consequences of weight loss on health are presently scanty. A review of the evidence for reduced mortality rates in people who have lost weight is inconclusive, because of methodological problems. However, the initial findings from the Swedish

Obese Subjects (SOS) study confirm that a substantial weight loss, of approximately 30 kg is, after 2 years, associated with a 60% reduction in plasma triglycerol insulin, a 25% decrease in glucose and a 10% reduction in blood pressure. Furthermore, this degree of weight loss resulted in a 14-fold reduction in risk of developing diabetes and a three- to fourfold risk reduction of developing hypertension, hypertriglyceridaemia and low HDL cholesterol levels (Sjöström *et al.*, 1995).

18.4 Long-term strategies including weight maintenance

Obesity and overweight are chronic conditions. Short-term programmes are likely to be ineffective, with rapid weight regain once treatment is stopped. Treatment programmes must be for the longer term and include measures to prevent relapse. A better understanding of the characteristics of those who are particularly at risk from obesity is needed to ensure appropriate use of resources. Those at risk will include subjects who are moderately over-weight, with a BMI 27–30, who have central obesity. Weight gain in infancy, adolescence and pregnancy are important aspects that have already been discussed in this book (Chapter 7). A family history of obesity or associated diseases, body fat distribution, and risk factors for coronary heart disease are individually important factors which influence the choice of treatment.

18.5 Assessing the individual

It is now suggested that the initial contact with the obese individual should be primarily an assessment interview. The physician and/or dietitian should seek information on the following.

- medical history, risk factors and complications,
- weight history,
- history of previous treatments for obesity,
- BMI and waist/hip ratio,
- family history of related diseases and risk factors, i.e. diabetes mellitus, hypertension, premature CHD, and gallstones,
- eating behaviour pattern,
- diet history,
- activity and lifestyle,
- relevant social history, finance and culture.

Basic medical investigations may be necessary, e.g. assessment of thyroid function and cholesterol levels. Although most health professionals do not have access to facilities to measure energy expenditure, approximate calculations can be made using formulae, e.g. the Schofield equation to estimate energy expenditure (Schofield, 1985). The history of previous treatments will include the range of dietary, behaviour and drug treatments tried, and the involvement of health professionals (if any).

It is known that individuals, especially obese individuals, under-report what they eat and over-report their activity levels (Prentice *et al.*, 1986; Southgate, 1986; Lightman *et al.*, 1992; Heitmann & Lissner, 1995). However, taking a diet history is still invaluable in giving an insight into eating patterns, beliefs and social and economic factors. A large discrepancy between the outcome of the diet history and estimated energy expenditure does suggest that the individual does not accept responsibility for tracking their weight problem, and long-term success is questionable. Individuals who believe that their eating habits are instrumental in their obesity, have been shown to be more likely to lose weight (Rodin *et al.*, 1977).

It is important at this stage that the health-care professional does not offer advice, but gathers and gives information in an objective and non-judgemental manner. Offering advice may increase resistance to change, as the individual may look at the personal implications rather than future benefits (Rollnick *et al.*, 1993). Rollnick suggests that health professionals should be flexible in their approach, allowing counselling skills (if they have them) to guide the negotiations of behaviour change. There is a move towards using the 'stages of change' model by Prochaska & DiClemente (1986) to assess 'readiness of change', i.e. the motivational state of the patient (Fig. 18.1).

The 'stages of change' model is a dynamic model, describing the behaviour changes that individuals may undergo. Pre-contemplation refers to the stage when individuals are not interested in changing their 'risky' lifestyle. Contemplation is the stage when the individual is 'thinking about change'. Preparing to change refers to the stage when the individual is gathering the knowledge or skills needed to facilitate the changes. Action is the period during which the individual makes changes in his or her lifestyle, and maintenance is the period

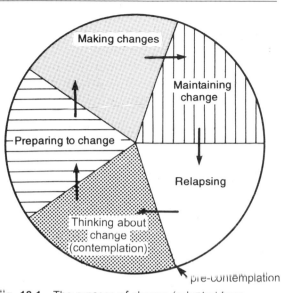

Fig. 18.1   The process of change (adapted from Prochaska & DiClemente, 1986. From Helping People Change © Health Education Authority, 1994)

during which those changes become more established, resulting in a 'more stable, safer lifestyle'. Relapse occurs when the individual finds it difficult to maintain the changes; this may result in a return to the contemplation stage before further action is taken (Prochaska, 1991).

18.5.1 Motivation

The conventional approach to the management of obesity has been to tell an obese person to 'go on a diet'. Giving advice to an individual who is not already making lifestyle changes, may increase their resistance to change (Prochaska & DiClemente, 1986; Rollnick *et al.*, 1992) and result in the breakdown of the relationship between the patient and the doctor (Garrow, 1992).

Some researchers have found subjects to be more responsive to health promotion programmes when they have already passed the initial stages of pre-contemplation and contemplation. For instance, among smokers, intervention aimed at their giving up cigarettes, has been shown to be most effective in those who were 'in action' or 'ready for action' (Ockene *et al.*, 1992). The rates of smoking cessation in pre-contemplation, contemplation and

action groups, were 22%, 44% and 80%, respectively. It is, therefore, important to identify which stage of change the individual is at. Rollnick *et al.* (1992) describe a process which enables the interviewer to select a strategy which matches the patient's readiness for change. Rollnick (1996) also suggests that the use of negotiating strategies encourage the patient to become an active decision-maker. He discusses four examples of negotiation based strategies:

- setting the agenda,
- quick assessment of motivation and confidence,
- making decisions and setting targets,
- exchanging information.

If faced with an individual who is not motivated to lose weight, it is suggested that the health professional may encourage the individual to explore the benefits and costs of making changes and of not making changes (Rollnick *et al.*, 1992; Rollnick, 1996). A brief form of motivational interviewing is described, which may facilitate this process (Rollnick *et al.*, 1992). Although it may not result in the patient deciding to make changes, it may help avoid confrontation between the health professional and the patient, enabling the patient to seek help in the future.

Patients who are motivated but lacking in confidence may need help with their confidence skills. Rollnick (1996) states that asking individuals open questions about what would help increase their confidence will aid identification of areas of need. The Health Education Authority (1997) has adopted an approach based on the 'stages of change' model. This approach, along with motivational interviewing, needs to have further exploration.

18.6 Realistic goals

18.6.1 Weight

The success or failure of any treatment programme may be judged by an arbitrarily chosen target weight or percentage weight loss. A true measure of success will depend on the type of patient, the initial degree of obesity, the prevalence of associated risk factors or complications, and previous attempts at weight control. The use of ideal weight tables to set target weights for obese patients may result in unrealistic and unachievable weight goals. A weight loss of between 5–10% of the initial body weight is associated with clinically useful improvements in terms of blood pressure, plasma cholesterol, triacylglycerols and HDL cholesterol, and a significant improvement in diabetic control (Goldstein, 1992; Stamler *et al.*, 1980; Kanalay *et al.*, 1993; Wood *et al.*, 1988). It is suggested that an initial loss of 10% is an appropriate goal for significantly obese individuals as it is achievable, results in improvements in health indices and can be maintained (Wadden & Steen, 1996; Wadden *et al.*, 1996). However, there is a need to agree the goal weight, as cessation of treatment before the individual has achieved his or her target weight may leave the individual with the feeling of failure, which may result in relapse (Wolfe, 1992). Goals for older patients will be different from those who are young. Data suggests that a population becomes heavier with age, whereas the risk from obesity does not increase proportionally. In some older patients, prevention of further weight gain may be more appropriate. It is suggested that setting small weight goals, followed by a focus on developing weight maintenance skills, will improve long-term results (Fairburn & Cooper, 1996). Setting targets to increase activity has been demonstrated to be of benefit; however, more research is needed in this area of obesity treatment.

18.6.2 Rate of weight loss.

The weight history of the individual usually illustrates that there has been weight gain at significant life stages or that it has happened over a period of years. Although, often obese patients claim to have gained several kilograms in a short space of time, rarely can this be demonstrated by verified weights. An acceptable rate of weight loss for obese individuals is 0.25–1 kg per week, resulting in 13–52 kg (2–8 stone) per year (Garrow, 1981). Many individuals are dismissive of this rate, claiming it to be too 'slow', although this rate is usually significantly greater than the rate at which they gained the excess body weight.

18.6.3 Other goals

It is important that goals, other than target weight and rate of weight loss, are focused upon. These goals may be medical in nature, e.g. an improvement in plasma lipids, blood pressure or diabetic control, which may not only reflect weight loss but also alteration in the composition of the diet. The obese person may also be persuaded to increase their activity or participate in an exercise programme.

18.7 Summary

- The objectives in obesity treatment are to:
  - achieve weight loss to a point at which the health risks to the patient are reduced as far as possible
  - maintain that weight loss indefinitely, and
  - restore, if necessary, the self-esteem of the patient.

- Successful treatment requires intelligent co-operation by both patient and therapist. Failed treatment is probably worse than no treatment, therefore, goals and methods must be agreed and realistic. Treatment of a severely obese patient involves a major long-term commitment by both parties.

- Even a modest weight loss (5–10 kg) will result in an improvement of health indices in an obese person.

- In some obese people, the disability arising from obesity is overwhelmed by other social or health problems. In such cases, it may be unethical to treat the obesity, as the benefits from any weight loss will be trivial compared with the other problems.

19
Treatment of Obesity II: Dietary Treatment of Obesity

For successful dietary treatment, changes are not just for the short-term alone. Long-term changes in food choices, eating behaviour and lifestyle are needed, rather than a temporary restriction of specific foods. Support should be available to the individual, who may pass back and forwards along the 'stages of change' model, and mechanisms for dealing with relapse need to be incorporated. In addition, the maintenance of weight loss should be an important feature of any weight loss programme.

The modern dietary treatment of obesity, which is the foundation of any management programme, must be a healthy diet in terms of prevention of hypertension and coronary heart disease, and must be in line with the general recommendations for the population as a whole. The reports from COMA on *Dietary Reference Values for Food Energy and Nutrients for the United Kingdom* (Department of Health, 1991) and on *Nutritional Aspects of Cardiovascular Disease* (Department of Health, 1994) and *Nutritional Aspects of the Development of Cancer* (Department of Health, 1995) recommend an increase in wholegrain cereals, fruit, potatoes and vegetables, and a decrease in sugar, fat and sodium intakes (Table 19.1).

19.1 Types of dietary treatment

There are a variety of dietary treatments available in both clinical and commercial settings. The following factors should be considered.

- The diet should provide the essential nutrients to minimise loss of lean body mass and maintain health, while providing a negative energy balance.
- The diet should be adapted to the patient's dietary preferences, financial circumstances and lifestyle. However, a diet should be encouraged that meets the COMA guidelines.
- The patient should realise that long-term changes in diet, activity and lifestyle are necessary not only to lose weight, but maintain the degree of weight loss.

The treatment programme should contain both weight loss and weight management elements. Diets can be divided into three main classes:

- low calorie diets
- very low calorie diets
- milk diets.

These are each described in more detail in the following sections.

19.1.1 Low calorie diets

Low calorie diets are energy-restricted diets and usually provide in the range of 3.4–6.3 MJ (800–1500 kcal) per day. They should contain a balanced ratio of protein, carbohydrate and fat, but in reduced quantities. They may be tailor-made for the individual, using food exchanges or a selection of meals. Usually, the diets within this category follow the same basic principles, recommending an increase in wholegrain cereals, vegetables and fruit, and a decrease in fat. The following types of diets fall into this category.

Table 19.1 Dietary Reference Values for fat and carbohydrate as a percentage of daily food intake and Reference Nutrient Intake for sodium (mmol/day), and non-starch polysaccharides (g/day), for adults (adapted from COMA, Department of Health, 1991).

	% Food Energy
Fat	
Total Fat	35
of which	
Saturated fatty acids	11
CIS monounsaturated fatty acids	13
CIS polyunsaturated fatty acids	6.5
Trans fatty acids	2
Carbohydrate	
Total Carbohydrate	50
of which	
Non milk extrinsic sugars	11
Intrinsic and milk sugars and starch	39
Non-starch Polysaccharides (g/day)	18 (Individual minimum 12 g and individual maximum 24 g/day)
Sodium (mmol/day)	70 (equivalent to 4 g salt)

Note: Many individuals will derive some energy from alcohol, however the food energy values exclude a contribution from alcohol (Department of Health, 1991).

(a) High fibre diets

High fibre diets reduce calorie density by increasing the consumption of low energy density foods. Duration of eating is longer, because foods are bulkier and other high-energy foods are displaced. Such diets are used in clinical settings and by many reputable slimming organisations, encouraging long-term changes in diet that are in line with the general recommendations for the population as a whole.

(b) Calorie counting diets

These diets rely on the individual counting the calories provided by all the foods that they eat and drink, keeping to a daily allowance. This approach allows flexibility in the food items chosen. However, it is dependent on the individual knowing the calorific value of a large number of foods, as well as being able to estimate portion sizes accurately. The individual will also need some knowledge, or will need to receive some guidance, on the 'healthier' food choices, otherwise there may be no move towards a high carbohydrate, low fat diet. While some individuals respond very well to calorie counted diets, with others it may result in an increase in dietary restraint. Fairburn (1993) suggests that, in the treatment of obese binge eaters, restricting the calories to below 6.3 MJ (1500 kcal) may result in an increase in binge eating.

(c) Fat units

Foods are given a fat unit score, based on the amount of fat per portion. A fat unit allowance is then assigned in the same way as a calorie allowance. It is a means of restricting fat intake, and hence energy, without counting calories. It was devised by *Slimming Magazine* and does require that the user has a comprehensive list of foods with assigned fat units.

(d) Energy prescribed diets

Energy requirements of the individual are estimated and a diet devised to provide an energy intake of 2.1–4.2 MJ (500–1000 kcal) below energy expenditure. As a result, the prescribed diet will often be in excess of 3.4–6.3 MJ (800–1500 kcal) per day. Dietitians and reputable slimming clubs may use this approach, in conjunction with a high fibre, low fat diet. It avoids the huge differences between energy intake and expenditure that may result from the prescription of a standard 4.2–5.0 MJ (1000–1200 kcal) diet. It may be used in combination with calorie counting or fat units.

(e) Formula diets

The recent definition of formula diets is 'Foods for use in energy-restricted diets for weight reduction are specially formulated foods which, when used as instructed by the manufacturer, replace the whole or part of the total daily diet.' (Commission Directive, 1997)

The Commission Directive (1997) defined two categories of formula diets:

- products presented as a replacement for the whole of the daily diet
- products presented as a replacement for one or more meals of the daily diet.

If the product is the replacement for the whole of the daily diet, it must provide between 3.4–5.0 MJ (800–1200 kcal) per day. If it is a meal replacement, it must provide between 0.8–1.7 MJ (200–400 kcal) per meal (Commission Directive, 1996).

Some formula diets may be in liquid form, having a novelty value, while others may be ready-prepared meals. Liquid formula diets, while resulting in weight loss, do not help educate the patient about improving their eating pattern. The prepared meals may aid compliance through ease of use. However, they may be expensive compared with meals cooked and prepared in the home. The individual may still need to make additional alterations in their diet to meet the recommendations of COMA (Department of Health, 1991).

(f) Low carbohydrate diets

The carbohydrate content of this type of diet is low, resulting in a restricted intake of cereals, bread, rice, pasta and potatoes. The individual is often allowed to include protein foods such as meat and cheese more freely. Weight loss may be fast initially, as a consequence of a decrease in glycogen stores and resulting fluid loss, however, it is often quickly regained once the individual includes carbohydrate foods again. Although many individuals may lose weight with this diet, the individual would need to increase the contribution of carbohydrate during weight maintenance, to meet the recommendations of COMA (Department of Health, 1991).

Low energy diets may be used in isolation, but are often combined with health counselling, behavioural therapy and/or physical activity. Many researchers have shown that, although weight may be lost in the short term, it is often regained over a period of time. Bennett (1987) reviewed interventions between 1977–1985, which were primarily aimed at energy restriction. The maximum average weight loss was 8.5% of the starting weight; however, over a period of five years the weight loss was zero. Hakala (1994b) reviewed conventional weight reduction programmes between 1981–1993, which used various combinations of dietary counselling, health counselling, behavioural therapy and physical activity. Some programmes offered contact post-treatment. Again, the studies show short-term weight loss, which may be maintained at the one-year follow-up. However, those studies, which follow their subjects for a period of five years, show that many regain the weight that they lost.

The role of maintenance programmes

Some researchers have tried to improve the long-term results by offering post-treatment programmes. Perri *et al.* (1984) offered three treatment conditions (dietary advice with non-behavioural therapy, behavioural therapy, or behavioural therapy plus relapse prevention training), combined with either no contact post-treatment or post-treatment contact by telephone and mail. The groups that received no behaviour therapy, or behaviour therapy plus relapse prevention training with post-treatment contact, maintained their lower weight significantly better than those who had no contact post-treatment. Post-treatment contact made no impact on weight maintenance for those obese subjects who had behavioural therapy only. Those who had behavioural therapy and relapse prevention training without post-treatment contact were unable to maintain their weight, suggesting that post-treatment contact is necessary to enable individuals to implement the strategies that they have learnt. The most successful were those subjects who had behaviour therapy plus relapse prevention training and post-treatment contact. They maintained their weight loss and did not suffer significant relapse at one year of follow-up (Table 19.2).

Perri *et al.* (1988) examined the effects of four post-treatment maintenance programmes and compared the results with those of behaviour therapy without post-treatment contact. An average of 82.7% of the mean post-treatment weight loss was maintained at the 18-month follow-up in the four maintenance programmes, compared with 33.3% in the group who had behaviour therapy only. These studies suggest that post-treatment programmes may facilitate the maintenance of weight loss (Perri *et al.*, 1984, 1988).

Perri *et al.* (1989) examined the effect of the length of treatment on weight loss. Obese subjects were assigned to either 20 or 40 weekly sessions. After 20 weeks, both groups had comparable weight losses (8.9 kg for the 20-week group, 10.1 kg for the 40-week group). At week 40, the 20-week group had gained a non-significant amount of weight (2.5 kg) while the 40-week group had lost an additional amount of weight (3.6 kg, p <0.5), making their average weight loss 13.6 kg, compared with 6.4 kg in the 20-week group. At week 72, both

Table 19.2 Maintenance strategies for weight loss (data from Perri *et al.*, 1984).

Programme content	Mean and standard deviation for kg lost at the end of treatment and at one year				Percentage of subjects achieving a net weight loss of 9.1 kg or more at the end of treatment and at one year	
	End of treatment		1 year		End of treatment	1 year
	M	SD	M	SD	M	M
DC+PA (N = 15)	8.2	3.8	3.2	4.8	33.3	13.3
DC+PA+C (n = 16)	8.5	4.4	6.3	5.0	37.5	31.3
DC+PA+BT (n = 21)	7.5	3.8	6.3	6.1	19.0	23.8
DC+PA+BT+C (n = 15)	8.7	3.6	5.8	4.2	46.7	26.7
DC+PA+BT+R (n = 15)	8.5	7.3	3.0	3.6	40.0	0
DC+PA+BT+R+C (n = 17)	9.6	7.2	10.3	11.4	41.2	41.2

DC = Dietary counselling   PA = Physical activity   BT = Behaviour therapy
R = Relapse prevention   C = Contact post-treatment

groups had gained some weight. However, the mean overall weight loss in the 40-week group was statistically significantly greater than the mean loss of the 20-week group (9.9 kg versus 4.6 kg, p < 0.05). The authors suggest that extending the treatment time and providing maintenance programmes may improve long-term results. Wolfe (1992) suggests that the success may be partially related to the fact that subjects in the 40-week group had reached 'personally meaningful weight loss goals', which they had greater motivation to maintain.

In the study by Björvell & Rössner (1985), patients participated in either a 6-week in-patient programme or a jaw-wiring programme. In the 6-week programme, subjects were provided with 2.5 MJ (600 kcal) and behavioural therapy, with relapse prevention training. This was followed by 4 years of maintenance support, which included an opportunity for a 2-week in-patient admission to prevent relapse. In the jaw-wiring group, patients had their jaws wired until their weight plateaued. Following this, they had a 2-week in-patient programme plus the opportunity for maintenance support. At 4 years, among those who had the initial 6-week programme, there was a significant mean weight loss of 12.6 kg for the men and women. In the jaw-wiring group, there was a mean weight loss of 8.7 kg. However, half the jaw-wiring group was lost to follow-up and their weight loss is, therefore, unknown. In those participating in the initial 6-week programme, a positive correlation was seen between the change in weight at the 4-year follow-up and the number of booster sessions. At the 10–12 year follow-up, significant weight losses were still maintained (Björvell & Rössner, 1992).

The effect of high carbohydrate diets

Many researchers have looked at the effect of manipulating the composition of the diet. It is suggested that protein and carbohydrate, unlike fat, will reduce subsequent energy intake (Stubbs *et al.*, 1995b; see also Chapter 10). Lawton *et al.* (1993) have shown that when obese individuals are hungry, they are more likely to overeat when provided with high fat foods than high carbohydrate foods, as dietary fat has a weak effect on satiety. Shah *et al.* (1994) compared the effects on weight loss of a low fat, *ad libitum*, complex carbohydrate diet, with a calorie restricted diet, and found that although the former resulted in comparable weight losses it was associated with improved palatability and quality of life. A study by Jeffery *et al.* (1995) compared a diet containing 20 g fat/day with an energy-restricted diet (4.2–5.0 MJ [1000–1200 kcal] per day). Both diets resulted in modest weight losses in the first 6 months. However, these losses were not maintained, and by 18 months the average weights had returned to base-line levels. However, it was reported that participants on the fat reduced diet were more compliant, rated their diets as more palatable and had decreased binge-eating scores. It is likely that both groups under-reported their intake at follow-up. The fat reduced group reported an intake of about 5.0 MJ (1199 kcal), 26% fat, and the energy restricted an intake of about 5.0 MJ

(1181 kcal), 33% fat, at 18 months. Yet both groups had returned to their base-line weight. The effects of energy restriction (4.2–6.3 MJ (1000–1500 kcal) per day, and <30% fat) versus energy and fat restrictions (4.2–6.3 MJ (1000–1500 kcal) per day, and 20% fat) were compared in obese individuals with NIDDM or a family history of diabetes (Pascale *et al.,* 1995). Both groups took part in a behavioural weight loss programme, where behavioural and self-management strategies were used to modify eating and exercise habits. Individuals with NIDDM lost significantly more weight with a combined energy and fat restriction, than with calorie restriction alone. At one-year follow-up, a significant amount of weight loss was maintained in the energy and fat restricted group, whereas almost all of the weight was regained in the calorie-restricted group. In those individuals with a family history of diabetes, there was no significant difference on weight loss or weight maintenance with the two diets. It is suggested that, as the diabetic subjects were older, and had more health problems, they had had more attempts at energy restriction in the past, and so found the combined energy and fat restriction more novel. Neither the group with energy restriction alone, nor the group with combined energy and fat restriction, managed to achieve the level of fat restriction in their food intake diaries. This suggests that subjects found it difficult to achieve the degree of restriction required.

Ad libitum, high carbohydrate diets may have a greater role in weight maintenance than in weight loss. Siggaard *et al.* (1996) studied the effects on weight loss of a 12-week *ad libitum* carbohydrate rich diet in overweight and normal weight subjects. The intervention group lost 4.2 ± 0.4 kg (5% initial weight), compared with 0.8 ± 0.5 kg (0.9% of initial weight) in the control group. In the intervention group, the overweight subjects lost significantly more weight (5.2 ± 0.4 kg, 6.1 ± 0.2% of initial weight) than the normal weight subjects (2.5 ± 0.4 kg, 3.7 ± 0.3% of initial weight). At 52 weeks follow-up, 50% of the normal weight group had lost 0–2.5 kg, while 50% had gained weight. In contrast, 28% of the overweight group had lost more than 5.0 kg, 41% lost 2.5–5.0 kg, and 31% 0–2.5 kg. This suggests that a low fat, high carbohydrate diet may aid the maintenance of weight loss. Toubro & Astrup (1997) assigned obese patients, who had

undergone weight reduction programmes resulting in a mean weight loss of 13 kg, to a year-long weight maintenance programme of either an *ad libitum*, low fat, high carbohydrate diet or a fixed energy diet (7.8 MJ (1864 kcal) per day). The mean weight loss after following the weight reduction diet for 2 years was greater in the *ad libitum* group (8.0 kg) compared with the fixed energy group (2.5 kg). In terms of weight maintenance, 65% of the *ad libitum* group, compared with 40% of the fixed energy group, maintained at least 5 kg or greater of the original weight loss.

Wing *et al.* (1996) have demonstrated that compliance with dietary advice may be improved by providing specific meal plans and grocery lists. Subjects who had help with menu planning, lost a significantly greater amount of weight compared with those subjects who had healthy eating advice combined with an energy restricted diet, with 20% of the calories from fat. At one year follow-up, a significantly greater weight loss was maintained in the group who received the specific meal plans and grocery lists. It is suggested that the provision of menu plans and grocery lists, re-introduced at high-risk times, may help improve long-term results.

Group versus individual therapy

Little is known about the effectiveness of group versus individual therapy. Jeffery *et al.* (1983) recruited overweight men to participate in a weight reduction programme that combined energy restriction, increased physical activity and behavioural techniques. The men were assigned to either individual contract groups or groups with group contract conditions. The contract involved making an initial monetary deposit. In the individual contract group, the men received individual refunds based on individual weight loss. The men in the group contract conditions received refunds based on the average weight loss of the group. Individuals in the group contract conditions initially lost more weight than those in the individual contracts group, however, at the one-year follow-up there was no significant difference.

In obese patients with NIDDM, Heller *et al.* (1988) found that those allocated to group education by the diabetes specialist nurses and dietitians had lost more weight and had better diabetic control, six months after diagnosis, than those seen individually in the clinic setting. However, at one year, the difference in weight loss was less and diabetic control was similar. Re-examination of the data in this study by Lean & Anderson (1988) suggests that the rate of weight loss is 44% poorer in those patients receiving group education, when the patient's time spent in education is considered.

Hakala *et al.* (1993) compared the effects of two weight reduction programmes which both began with 2 weeks of inpatient treatment, followed by either individual or group counselling over a 2-year period. It was found at the 5-year follow-up, that individual counselling resulted in a greater weight loss than group counselling and that men, in particular, were more likely to benefit from individual counselling.

In another study (Hakala, 1994a) obese subjects were allocated to either a 3-week in-patient weight reduction programme or a 10-week outpatient weight reduction programme, followed in both cases by individual counselling by the patient's general practitioner for up to 24 months. Although both programmes resulted in weight reduction, at the end of two years the weight loss achieved was better maintained in the group that had the initial in-patient period. At the 5-year follow-up, only the men who participated in the initial in-patient period maintained a significant weight loss. Many general practitioners in this study considered that they were not the appropriate people to offer follow-up support and this may have affected the results.

Hayaki & Brownell (1996), in their review of group interventions, call for further research into the effectiveness of individual versus group treatment.

19.1.2 Very low calorie diets

Very low calorie diets (VLCDs) were introduced in the 1970s in an attempt to emulate the impressive weight loss achieved by starvation therapy. Such diets consist of an energy intake of below 2.5 MJ (600 kcal) for several days or weeks, and are usually consumed in a liquid form. High initial weight losses, of greater than 3 kg per week, can be achieved with VLCDs but these losses include considerable amounts of fluid and lean body tissue (Garrow *et al.*, 1989). To reduce potential risks from loss of lean body tissue, the COMA report on *The use of very low calorie diets in obesity* (Department of

Health, 1987) indicated that such preparations must provide a minimum of 1.7 MJ (400 kcal) per day for women and 2.1 MJ (500 kcal) per day for men. This must be accompanied by 40 or 50 g per day of high biological value protein, for men and women respectively. The report also recommends that the vitamin and mineral content should also, at least, meet the UK recommended daily allowances (now known as reference nutrient intakes). The National Task Force on the Prevention and Treatment of Obesity (1993) in the USA defines VLCDs as containing less than 3.4 MJ (800 kcal) and recommends a protein intake of 0.8–1.5 g/kg of ideal body weight and the full complement of recommended daily allowance for vitamins and minerals.

Both COMA (Department of Health, 1987) and the National Task Force on the Prevention and Treatment of Obesity (1993b) recommend that VLCDs should only be used under medical supervision, in obese individuals with a BMI greater than 30, who are refractory to more moderate dietary interventions. There are a number of contraindications, and these are listed in Table 19.3.

Table 19.3 The use of VLCDs in the treatment of obesity.

Contraindications	Relative Contraindications
Cardiac disorders	Abnormal psychological states
Cerebrovascular disease	Diabetes (on insulin or oral hypoglycaemics)
Hepatic or renal disease	Treated hypertension
Gout	Porphyria
Pregnancy	Infants, children, adolescents
	Breast feeding mothers, elderly

The COMA report (Department of Health, 1987) also recommends that VLCDs be used for periods of no more than 4 weeks. Their repeated use is also not encouraged. However, VLCDs have been used in a number of studies for longer periods, in combination with exercise, behavioural modification and nutrition education. There is usually an initial low energy diet for 1–4 weeks, a VLCD phase, a re-feeding phase and a maintenance phase. In the short term, the degree of weight lost compares favourably with that lost on a low energy diet (Wadden *et al.*, 1989; National Task Force, 1993;

Hakala, 1994a), there being an average loss of 1.5–2.0 kg/week in women and 2.0–2.5 kg/week in men (average 20 kg over 12 weeks) compared with 0.4–0.5 kg/week (8.5 kg in 20–24 weeks) on the low energy diet (National Task Force, 1993). It is argued, however, that the analysis of many clinical trials involving VLCDs have not included patients who failed to complete the programme, so biasing the results in favour of greater weight losses (National Task Force, 1993).

The long-term effectiveness of VLCDs is questionable. A study by Wadden *et al.* (1989) considers three treatments: VLCDs, behavioural therapy, or VLCDs and behavioural therapy combined. At the end of a year, the combined approach achieved greater results (4.7 kg, 6.6 kg and 10.6 kg respectively). However, at the 5-year follow-up, it was found that many of the subjects in all three groups had returned to their pre-treatment weight and had received additional weight loss therapy.

19.1.3 Milk diet

This form of diet is used for the treatment of obesity under medical supervision. It consists of around 1.5–2 l of whole cows' milk combined with multivitamins, ferrous sulphate and a non-starch polysaccharide. Patient adherence to the milk diet is dependent upon whether they are able to tolerate such a large volume of milk (Garrow, 1981). There are approximately 5.0 MJ (1190 kcal) and 58 g of protein in 1.8 l of milk, and compliance with the regimen will result in weight loss. A study by Garrow *et al.* (1989), with outpatients, concluded that there was no significant difference between the amount of weight lost on a VLCD and a milk diet. The milk diet, if strictly adhered to, would supply 3.4 MJ (800 kcal) per day; it is obvious that the latter should have produced a greater rate of weight loss and, as it did not, this raises questions about compliance with these diets. In the same study, there was a greater weight loss, in grams of nitrogen per kilogram of body weight on the VLCD, than on the milk diet, when compliance was 'improved' by either an inpatient stay or jaw-wiring. If there is a need to convince an individual that weight loss is achievable on an energy restricted diet, a milk diet may be preferable to a VLCD.

19.1.4 Alternative dietary approaches

There are a number of dietary approaches (Newmark & Williamson, 1983) that do not necessarily promote the dietary recommendations of COMA (Department of Health 1991, 1994, 1998). Examples include food combining diets and one-food diets. Some of the literature promoting these diets suggests that they may affect the body's metabolism, resulting in weight loss, however, often these claims cannot be supported by scientific studies. Any weight loss is usually the result of energy restriction and long-term improvements in eating habits are not usually promoted.

19.2 Factors affecting compliance with a prescribed diet

The psycho-social costs of attempting to follow a weight loss regimen were discussed in Section 18.2. Anyone who wishes to discover how difficult it is only need try it themselves for a few months. Personal experience in this field tends to promote a more sympathetic attitude towards failure in others. However, the sympathy does not protect the obese person from the complications of obesity and failure of compliance is by far the most common reason for diets 'not working'. This is clearly shown by the efficacy of diets at achieving weight loss in a closed metabolic ward and the failure of the same diets in the same patients to achieve as much weight loss as outpatients (Garrow *et al.*, 1989).

Relatively few trials have been done to investigate how greater compliance with a diet can be achieved. Frost *et al.* (1991) calculated compliance by comparing the observed rate of weight loss over 12 weeks among obese outpatients with the calculated weight loss had they strictly complied with the prescribed diet. Patients who were prescribed a diet that supplied 4.6 MJ (1100 kcal) per day should have lost, on average, 17.9 kg in 12 weeks, but actually lost only 2.9 kg. Those on 6.7 MJ (1600 kcal) per day should have lost 10.4 kg and actually lost 3.3 kg. Those on 7.1 MJ (1700 kcal) per day should have lost 8.5 kg and actually lost 5.0 kg. It is interesting to note that as the severity of the energy restriction decreases, compliance improves and weight loss increases. However, the analysis was done retrospectively and the patients were not randomised to the different treatment groups. The authors conclude that prescribing a 'realistic' diet achieves better weight loss than a more severe restriction of energy intake, which results in poor compliance.

Summerbell *et al.* (1998) tested the hypothesis that novelty and simplicity were important factors in obtaining compliance to a weight reduction diet. Obese outpatients were randomly assigned to a conventional 3.4 MJ (800 kcal) diet (control), an iso-energetic diet of milk (milk-only) or a milk diet with, on a single day of each week, a single extra specified food item (milk-plus). The hypothesis was that:

(a) the milk-based diets would gain better compliance than the conventional diets, because they were novel and simple, and
(b) the milk-plus diet would achieve better compliance than the milk-only diet because it was less restrictive and gave the patient better control.

The results confirmed hypothesis (a). Mean weight loss on the control diet was only 1.4 kg after 4 weeks and 2.6 kg after 16 weeks; this was significantly less than on the milk-based diets. However, hypothesis (b) was not confirmed; the weight loss on the milk-only diet was 7.4 kg after 4 weeks and 11.2 kg after 16 weeks. The single extra permitted food provided, on average, an extra 2.6 MJ (628 kcal) per day in the first 4 weeks and 2.4 MJ (568 kcal) per day in weeks 5–16. Over the 16 weeks, compliance was 51% for the milk-only diet compared with 60% for the milk-plus diet, a non-significant difference. With all 3 diets compliance was better during the first 4 weeks than during weeks 5–16, this supports the idea that novelty is an important factor in achieving compliance with a diet. A questionnaire at the end of the study indicated greater satisfaction with the milk-only diet than with the other 2 diets.

Undoubtedly Eyton (1987) is correct in saying that observed weight loss is a powerful factor in persuading the patient to continue with the regimen and the novelty of the treatment is another factor. This is understandable, because the person who has tried and failed to lose weight will be impressed by a novel treatment that achieves the desired effect quickly. In many ways this is unfortunate because the loss of a substantial amount of weight is a long process, as the desirable rate of weight loss is probably initially less than 1 kg per week, and gets slower with time (Section 18.6.2). By the time an obese person has lost, for example, 20 kg, the novelty of the diet has worn off, and the rate of weight loss is much slower than it was initially. This suggests that weight loss should be attempted in a series of steps, with periods of weight maintenance in between. Alternatively, motivation may be maintained by continually changing the mode of treatment in order to maintain the element of novelty. These are theoretical speculations that have not been tested in practice.

19.3 Psychological support and behaviour modification

It is obvious that the obese person trying to reduce weight by dieting is in a psychologically fragile state. As discussed in Section 18.2 they are being asked to 'do violence to all their tastes and habits' with which they became obese in the first place and so far have not managed to reverse this trend. If the effort is to be successful this time, it will probably be because there is better psychological support than on previous occasions. Psychological support (or the reverse) for the obese dieter comes from three main sources:

- the health-care professional who is responsible for their therapy
- other people who are similarly trying to lose weight, and
- their immediate circle of friends, family or peer group.

19.3.1 Support from the therapist

It is well known that some doctors, dietitians or slimming-group leaders are more effective in helping people to lose weight than others who are applying the same regimen. Atkinson *et al.* (1977) report a 9-week double-blind trial of mazindol versus placebo in which the patients were assigned to one of 5 therapists, of whom two were physicians and 3 were not. The trial showed that there were no significant differences between the groups related to mazindol or placebo, or physician versus non-physician therapist. However, the groups with non-physician therapist number 2 and number 4 lost significantly more weight than those with non-physician therapist number 5. It is plausible that the difference lies in the ability of some therapists to provide psychological support better than others do.

In some cases, well-intentioned therapists may undermine, rather than support, the patients attempt to lose weight. Experienced clinicians in this field will be familiar with the 'diet relationship trap' that awaits those who dispense advice on weight-reducing diets (Garrow, 1992). Initially, there is a warm and optimistic relationship between the patient who feels the need of dietary advice, and the therapist who feels able to give it; the former is in the role of victim and the latter is the rescuer. With successive consultations, as long as the advice is followed and weight is lost, these positive feelings persist and strengthen. The testing time comes (as it will come) when the patient returns having gained weight since the last visit and having deviated from the prescribed diet. This is a cause of embarrassment and regret to both parties, indeed the patient may have a sufficiently low self-esteem to not attend the next appointment, as they clearly do not deserve to take up the valuable time of the therapist when they do not even follow the advice given. All this is inevitable and understandable, but the trap is that in this situation the therapist may forget that the relationship is supposed to be a victim–rescuer one. The therapist may become resentful that their advice has been ignored, their time has been wasted, and the patient has not even come for the appointment and so has been shown to be irresponsible and despicable. Those who have not spent hundreds of hours trying to provide support for obese patients, may be amazed that health professionals could behave so unprofessionally, but it is a mistake all too easy to make and in which the patient often actively colludes.

Giving dietary advice is easy, what is difficult is to judge the correct response when the patient defaults from the diet. It is not helpful to berate the patients as this merely does even more damage to the relationship. It is not helpful to be so sympathetic that cordiality is preserved, but on the mutual understanding that dieting is impossible and doomed to failure, as the relationship is then no longer a therapeutic one. The good therapist tries to establish why this failure happened and what can usefully be done to reduce the chance that it will happen again. Techniques by which this may be achieved are discussed in more detail in Chapter 21.

19.3.2 Support from fellow-members of slimming groups

It is plausible that dieters who are managed as groups should draw support from their peers who have similar problems. However, formal assessments of obese patients treated either individually or as groups have failed to show an advantage to those treated in groups (Section Group versus individual therapy). Probably, people in slimming groups are even more diverse than the group leaders, and it will sometimes happen that particularly difficult members will demoralise the whole group. Anecdotal evidence (Bush *et al.* 1988) indicates that it is easier to establish an *esprit de corps* in a group that all enrol at the same time for a course of, for example, 10 weekly sessions, than in a group where members join and leave at irregular intervals. Groups perform a social function in enabling members to meet others from the same neighbourhood and indeed sometimes this is the main motivation for members to attend commercial groups (Eyton, 1987). However, if members of a group find a congenial 'buddy' with whom they can exchange notes, and provide mutual support, this can be very valuable.

19.3.3 Support from family and friends

The tendency of an individual to gain or lose weight is determined by forces shown in Fig. 24.1 (Chapter 24). In other chapters of this book, the influence of the genetic and environmentally determined characteristics of the individual, the health-care professional, the regimen used and of the general environment of the whole system, is considered. The remaining influence is that of the immediate social circle or peer group of the person involved. This is a very difficult field of research, because this peer group is ill defined and will change from time to time. However, it is evident that this is a potentially very important source of psychological support, or sometimes of discouragement. A good therapist or group leader may be excellent at providing support, but contact with this person is once a week or less, whereas contact with immediate family and friends is continuous.

A patient may suffer from an adverse influence at home, such as a spouse who is unsympathetic to the weight-loss objective, especially as it affects the standard of catering in the home. In such a situation, it may be profitable for the dieter to form an alliance with some other family member who will provide support instead of discouragement. Often even a school child may be excellent in this role.

19.4 Does dietary treatment do more harm than good?

It has been argued effectively that treating obesity does more harm than good (Garner & Wooley 1991; Wooley & Garner, 1991) and, therefore, treatments for obesity should not be offered (Wooley & Garner, 1994).

Garner & Wooley argue that weight gain following dietary treatment is inevitable, partly as a result of lowered energy requirements (Garner & Wooley, 1991; Wooley & Garner, 1991). However, many researchers would disagree with this claim. A study by Garrow & Webster (1989) showed that when obese women (mean BMI 38) were placed on a diet of 3.4 MJ (800 kcal) per day, for 3 weeks, they lost an average of 5% of initial weight and reduced their resting metabolic rate by 8.8%. The authors stated that, provided the rate of weight loss is not excessive, the final resting metabolic rate of obese individuals will not be significantly different from individuals of a similar body composition who have not lost weight. They concluded that an obese woman will have reduced her energy requirements for weight maintenance by 15% for a weight reduction of 30%.

De Peuter *et al.* (1992) studied two groups of women; post-obese women who had been weight stable for at least 6 months and women who had no history of weight problems. They compared measurements of post-prandial thermogenesis and the rates of energy expenditure at rest, and during activity. At all levels of activity, the average rate of energy expenditure (expressed per unit of fat free mass) was not significantly different between the post-obese women and lean controls.

Amatruda *et al.* (1993) conducted a prospective study of 18 obese women (before and after reducing to ideal body weight) and 14 women who had never been overweight. The obese women were entered into a weight reduction programme, which was

followed by a weight maintenance phase of at least 2 months. Before weight loss, the obese women had a higher resting and total energy expenditure than did the lean women. However, when total energy intake was corrected for weight and resting metabolic rate for lean body mass, there was no significant difference between the two groups. After the weight loss and maintenance phases, the 'reduced' obese women and the lean women had similar lean body mass and resting metabolic rates (RMR). The RMR and total energy expenditure, when adjusted for lean body mass, fat and age were not significantly different to those of the controls. Fifteen obese women who withdrew from the study had similar measurements of lean body mass, resting metabolic rate and total energy expenditure to those women who completed the study. Ten 'reduced' obese women were followed-up for at least one year after achieving ideal body weight. There were no significant differences in total energy expenditure or resting metabolic rate measured at ideal body weight compared with the weight regain that followed. It was concluded that the inability to maintain weight loss was not the result of lowered energy expenditure.

In lean and obese subjects, Liebel *et al.* (1995) measured total energy expenditure and resting energy expenditure and estimated non-resting energy expenditure at usual body weight and after losing 10–20% of body weight. It was found that, with maintenance of a body weight 10% or more below the initial weight, there was a reduction in total energy expenditure of 25 ± 13 kJ (6 ± 3 kcal) per kg fat free mass and in resting energy expenditure of 13 ± 13 kJ (3 ± 3 kcal) per kg fat free mass, in those subjects who had not been obese. In obese subjects, the corresponding figures were 33 ± 21 kJ (8 ± 5 kcal) per kg and 17 ± 17 kJ (4 ± 4 kcal) per kg, respectively. The authors state that these compensatory changes in energy expenditure may make it more difficult for obese people to maintain a lower body weight. This study may be criticised on the grounds that the permanence of the changes in the rates of energy expenditure was not examined. It was reported that the period of weight loss for the non-obese was 4–7 weeks, resulting in a weight loss of 6.8 kg while for the obese, the period of weight loss was 6–14 weeks, resulting in a weight loss of 18 kg. The rate of weight loss may be a factor in the decrease in resting metabolic rate (Foster *et al.*, 1990).

A meta-analysis by Astrup *et al.* (1997a) focused on published studies of RMR in post-obese subjects and matched controls. It was shown that RMR, adjusted for fat free mass and fat mass, was 3% lower in the post-obese subjects than in the controls. There was a normal distribution of adjusted RMR in the post-obese group. However, there was a sub-group of the controls who had a high relative RMR. A low relative RMR was found in 15.3% of the post-obese subjects and 3.3% of the controls. Astrup *et al.* (1997) concluded that a low RMR, for a given body size and composition, is more common in formerly obese subjects than in controls. Nevertheless, the majority of formerly obese subjects had a normal distribution of RMR. Although the debate on the effects of weight loss on energy expenditure will continue, the evidence does not appear to support the argument of Garner and Wooley (1991) that weight gain after dieting is inevitable because of lowered energy requirements.

Garner and Wooley (1991) state that intermittent or 'yo-yo' dieting leads to an increase in metabolic efficiency, resulting in the ability of the body to store more energy and a lower energy intake. They state that weight loss will result in a lower metabolic rate, making further weight loss and maintenance of weight loss more difficult. Other researchers have disputed this. Liebel *et al.* (1995) found that when obese subjects gained weight, a lower proportion of the weight was fat (adipose tissue) compared with non-obese subjects. Also, when obese subjects lost weight, a higher proportion was fat lost as compared with non-obese subjects. When the subjects returned to their initial weight, there were no significant differences in body composition or energy expenditure. Wadden *et al.* (1992a), have examined the relationship of dieting history with resting metabolic rate, body composition and weight loss. They found no evidence that weight cycling was associated with a reduced resting metabolic rate or an increase in percentage body fat. Prentice *et al.* (1992) also found no adverse effect of weight cycling on body composition. The National Task Force on the Prevention and Treatment of Obesity (1993a) reviewed the literature on weight cycling from 1966–1994. These studies failed to find differences in body composition, body fat distribution or metabolic rate adjusted for lean body mass. Among its conclusions, the Task Force stated that the evidence available regarding increased mortality and morbidity is insufficient to override the benefits of weight loss. However, it was acknowledged that the psychological impact of weight cycling requires further investigations.

Garner and Wooley (1991) also suggest that dietary treatment is inappropriate, because obesity is strongly determined by genetic factors. However, as discussed in Chapter 4, environmental factors make a major contribution. While there may be some evidence for a metabolic predisposition to obesity, a study by Prentice *et al.* (1986) showed that the basal metabolic rates and energy expenditures of obese women were higher than those of lean women. Also, obese women were more likely to underestimate their food intake, compared with lean women. Another study supports the findings that obese subjects eat more and exercise less than they think, and that the failure to lose weight is the result of the difference in energy balance, rather than an abnormality of thermogenesis (Lightman *et al.*, 1992). A further study suggests that obese people tend to under-report their energy intake, especially that arising from fatty foods and foods rich in carbohydrate (Heitmann & Lissner, 1995).

It is claimed that 'dieting' may lead to an increase in eating disorders (Garner & Wooley, 1991; Wooley & Garner, 1994) and in particular binge eating. Marcus *et al.* (1985) found that nearly half of patients wishing to take part in a behaviour programme for obesity treatment had severe problems with binge eating, the severity of which was linked with dietary restraint. Marcus (1993), however, asks for further research to clarify the role that dieting may play in the development and maintenance of binge eating problems in obesity, as the literature suggests that, although obese binge eaters do report following strict diets, they do not necessarily adhere to them. Fairburn *et al.*(1993) suggest that using a cognitive behavioural therapy approach, which concentrates on gaining control on overeating before losing weight, will have a more successful outcome in the treatment of binge eaters.

19.5 Should dietary treatments continue?

The benefits to health of weight loss have already been discussed (Goldstein, 1992; Stamler *et al.*, 1980; Kanalay *et al.*, 1993; Wood *et al.*, 1988). It is estimated that in Britain, obesity directly or indirectly costs the NHS in excess of £165 million

(Office of Health Economics, 1994). The incidence of obesity continues to increase and if clinical treatments are not available, individuals will continue to seek help elsewhere in types of programmes, the effectiveness of which may not have been evaluated. In 1987, Bennett stated that 'nothing in the chronicle suggests that worthwhile progress has been made by pursuing efforts to teach people more effective ways to restrict their food intake'. The same could be said today. It is, therefore, important that effectiveness of dietary treatments continue to be evaluated. The question should not be 'should dietary treatments continue' but 'can dietary treatments be improved?'

It is surprising that despite recommendations that obese individuals should lose no more than 0.5–1.0 kg per week (Garrow, 1981, 1991a,b) to prevent excessive loss of lean body mass and the fact that this can be achieved by an energy intake just 2.1–4.2 MJ (500–1000 kcal) per day below energy expenditure, many studies require their obese subjects to adhere to diets which result in a greater energy deficit. The results from many of the studies suggest that compliance is not high. Lean and James (1986) recommend that energy requirements should be estimated and that the energy content of the diet be based upon this. This approach has been used by Frost (1989) and Frost *et al.* (1991), and has been shown to be more effective in achieving weight loss. The long-term results are not known.

Increasing the percentage of energy derived from carbohydrate and decreasing the proportion derived from fat may aid dietary compliance by increasing satiety (Lawton *et al.*, 1993). In many studies, the expected weight loss, for the degree of fat and energy restriction, is not seen. It may be that individuals find that they are unable to make, and maintain, the amount of dietary changes that are required. For instance, Shah *et al.* (1994) asked obese women to reduce their fat intake to 20 g/d. Although the reported intake at 6 months showed a significant decrease in the percentage energy from fat, the reduction to 20 g/d was not achieved. Weight loss was, however, associated with the change in percentage fat contribution to energy. Jeffery *et al.* (1995) gave the subjects of the study a target of 20 g/d of fat, however, at 6 and 12 months the fat intake was 43 g/d and 47 g/d, respectively. The 2.1 kg reduction in weight achieved in this study over a period of 12 months is low for a reported energy intake of less than 6.7 MJ (1600 kcal) per day. It is known that obese subjects underreport their energy intake, especially from fatty and carbohydrate rich foods (Heitmann & Lissner, 1995) and this may be the explanation for the low level of weight reduction.

Among obese women, Lyon *et al.* (1995) assessed compliance with advice to increase the percentage of energy provided by carbohydrate to 55% and to decrease the percentage energy from fat to 30%, without restricting their energy intake. Compliance was measured by enriching meals with ^{13}C glucose and measuring $^{13}CO_2$ in expired air. The mean dietary compliance was $60 \pm 8\%$ (range 20–93%) and the degree of compliance correlated positively with loss of fat mass. The degree of fat restriction was less than in other studies (Björvell & Rössner, 1985, 1992) (a decrease to 51g, 31% of energy) which may have aided compliance in some individuals. Astrup *et al.* (1997b) have evaluated six low fat intervention studies in overweight and obese people. They suggest that a reduction in dietary fat from 40% to 30% of energy will result in an average weight loss of 5 kg in obese patients. It may be that this degree of fat reduction is a more realistic and achievable goal than very low fat diets. More research is necessary into the effects of a gradual reduction in percentage energy from fat, without a large restriction on the quantity of food (Goodrick & Foreyt, 1991).

Many studies expect obese patients to change overnight from an energy intake that either matches, or is in excess of, their energy expenditure, to one that is lower than their expenditure. Prochaska (1991) recognised the need for assessing the stage of change that the individual is at, as there may be an improvement in results for those individuals 'ready for action' or 'in action'. Assuming that the patient is at the correct stage of change, i.e. they are prepared to make change, it may be tempting to dictate the diet on the basis of the changes that they should make. Rollnick (1996) emphasises that there should be an interaction between the professional and the patient, identifying a range of options that could be followed. This could allow for small dietary changes, e.g. eliminating food items totalling 0.4 MJ (100 kcal) per day (Marcus, 1993), thereby reducing energy intake by 0.4 MJ (100 kcal) per day. Alternatively, there could be a gradual reduction in fat intake, as suggested previously. However, the important difference between this method and others, is that it allows the individuals to choose the options that suit them. The Health Education Authority (1997a) has adopted a programme based on stages of change, (see Fig. 18.1) and this needs further exploration in the context of obesity treatment. Ni Mhurchu *et al.* (1997) suggest that the stages of change model needs to be adapted to cope with a complexity of dietary changes.

It is evident that some individuals are successful at losing and maintaining weight; however, it is difficult to predict which individuals will be successful. The measurement of the stage of change that the individual is at may be one predictor of success, in that those individuals who are 'precontemplative' or 'contemplative' are less likely to succeed (Prochaska, 1991). Rodin *et al.* (1977) found that those individuals, who believed that their diet had a role in the development of obesity, were more likely to succeed.

The rate of initial weight loss may also be a factor. Björvell and Rössner (1992) showed a significant correlation between weight loss at 10–12 years of follow-up and the weight loss after a 2-year treatment period and 4-year follow-up. Wadden *et al.* (1992) found that the weight loss during the first month of treatment was the best predictor of weight loss at the end of treatment and at follow-up, one year later. Hakala *et al.* (1993), Hakala (1994a,b) also showed that the best long-term results were seen with those individuals who had the greatest weight losses during treatment.

Perri *et al.* (1989) found that extending the length of treatment results in greater weight losses. Wolfe (1992) suggests that low success in weight maintenance may partially result from the cessation of treatment before subjects reach their desirable weights. She suggests that if obese subjects perceive that the treatment was unsuccessful, in that they have not achieved their desired weight, then their motivation to continue falls. Clients who had attended a commercial weight loss programme were surveyed. Information was gathered on their initial weights and one-year post treatment. She found that 82.4% of the subjects had maintained their weight when the criterion of success was maintenance of weight within 10% of their self-selected goal weight. Success in such treatment programmes may be improved by helping individuals set realistic weight goals (Fairburn *et al.*, 1993; Fairburn & Cooper, 1996). There should also be a focus on weight maintenance after a 10–15% weight loss (Fairburn & Cooper, 1996; Wadden *et al.*, 1996).

Brownell *et al.* (1986) discuss the fact that post-treatment strategies must be developed that help prevent relapse. Post-treatment programmes that have included maintenance programmes are more likely to result in successful outcomes (Perri *et al.*, 1984, 1988).

Within weight loss programmes, although the overall group results may not be impressive, it is clear that within the groups, some individuals do well, suggesting that some types of treatment are more suitable for some individuals than for others. Hakala *et al.* (1993), for instance, found that men achieved better results with individual counselling rather than group counselling. Schwartz & Brownell (1995) surveyed obesity experts for their views on various treatments. Of 170 different characteristics listed as being indications or contraindications for the various treatments, only five achieved agreement from over 50% of the experts.

- mild to moderate obesity as indication for dieting on one's own,
- virtually everyone should exercise, barring medical contraindications,
- moderate to morbid obesity is necessary to justify VLCD,
- psychiatric disturbance suggests individual counselling,
- massive to morbid obesity is necessary to justify surgery.

While the weight ranges were agreed upon for the extremes of treatment, there was little agreement about the weight range for commercial and behavioural programmes. Further studies that match the person's characteristics, e.g. weight history, past dieting success, reason for weight gain, to treatment programmes will help develop approaches for treatments of individuals (Schwartz & Brownell, 1995). Treatments that are tailored to the needs of individuals may improve the overall success. Obese binge eaters, for instance, may have more success with a cognitive behaviour therapy approach (Fairburn *et al.*, 1993).

Weight loss programmes have been criticised for

not meeting ethical standards (Lustig, 1991) and focusing on short-term weight loss (Robison *et al.*, 1995). It is suggested that information should be available about the safety and outcomes of treatment (Institute of Medicine, 1995). The success of the programme may be evaluated on the following information.

- the percentage of participants who complete the programme,
- the proportion of those who complete the programme and their degrees of weight loss,
- the proportion of weight loss that is maintained at 1, 3 and 5 years,
- the percentage of participants who experience adverse physiological or medical effects.
        (NIH Technology Assessment Panel, 1992)

As the maintenance of weight loss is an important feature, it has been suggested that weight loss programmes become weight management programmes. These programmes should be judged not only on the effects on weight loss, but on the effects on the overall health of the individual (Institute of Medicine, 1995; NIH Technology Assessment Panel, 1992).

19.6 Summary

- Dietary treatment is fundamental to the management of obesity, but unless the obese person is willing and able to make long-term changes in lifestyle (of which diet is the most important aspect) treatment will fail. However, merely 'going on a diet' for a finite period (weeks or months) may cause temporary weight loss, but this weight will be regained when the 'diet' is abandoned.

- Dietary treatment presents two interrelated problems as follows.

- To design a diet that is nutritionally sound, but deficient in energy, so the patient's fat tissue (but not too much lean tissue) is burned off to meet this energy deficit.
- To make it as easy as possible for the patient to comply with this dietary design. It is to achieve this second objective that the skill of the therapist is mainly required. Patients differ in their energy requirements, and in the dietary restrictions that they find acceptable, so there is no all-purpose diet that works for everyone. It may be necessary to switch diets for an individual patient from time to time in order to maintain compliance.

- Compliance with a diet depends on factors other than the actual composition of the diet. Support from therapists, family and friends may be at least as important. This support is especially important during the phase of weight maintenance after the excess weight has been lost.

- High carbohydrate, low fat diets may help weight reduction and weight maintenance.

- A reduction of energy intake to 2.1–4.2 MJ (500–1000 kcal) per day below energy expenditure will in the long term cause a loss of 0.5–1.0 kg/week.

- Appropriate weight loss causes a reduction in energy requirements of about 0.07 MJ (16 kcal) per day per kg in man and 0.05 MJ (12 kcal) per day per kg in women. Unfortunately, commercial diets are often promoted on claims that they achieve the most rapid weight loss. Total starvation achieves the most rapid weight loss, but too much of the weight lost is lean tissue and, therefore, there is an excessive reduction in energy requirements.

- Dietary weight-loss programmes should include long-term support for maintenance of weight loss.

20
Treatment of Obesity III: Physical Activity and Exercise

The definitions of exercise and physical activity are given in Section 15.1.1. Traditionally, exercise has not been given priority in obesity treatment programmes or commercial weight loss programmes for people who are overweight. This is probably because evidence indicates that exercise adds only small amounts of weight loss, when accompanying dietary treatment and a general belief that it is difficult to achieve either short- or long-term exercise adherence in obese or overweight people. A broader perspective of treatment, which takes into account health risk, psychological well-being and long-term weight management success, reveals that exercise should be considered a critical part of treatment, particularly with the overweight or mild to moderately obese individual.

20.1 Exercise and weight loss

There have been several recent reviews of studies that have investigated the effect of exercise on weight loss and body composition change (Garrow, 1986; Segal & Pi-Sunyer, 1989; King & Tribble, 1991; Fox, 1992; Blair, 1993; Stefanick, 1993; Wilfley & Brownell, 1994; DiPietro, 1995). Results from studies vary considerably and it is rare that sufficient information is provided to judge fully the nature of the exercise programme. Few appear to comply with current recommendations aimed at improving health and long-term exercise adherence. Two meta-analyses have recently been conducted that produced comparisons between diet only and diet plus exercise weight loss treatments. Ballor & Poehlman (1994) reviewed the effect of adding

exercise to 46 dietary-based weight loss programmes reported between 1964 and 1991. Although results from studies varied considerably, overall there was no significant difference in the amount of body weight, or fat mass, lost between diet only and diet plus exercise groups. Garrow and Summerbell (1995) conducted a similar meta-analysis on studies conducted specifically on overweight and obese subjects. They calculated that over 30 weeks, exercise added an extra 3 kg of weight loss in men and, over a 12-week period, women lost an extra 1.4 kg with exercise. This is in agreement with several other reviews and well-controlled studies (e.g. Wood et al., 1991) that conclude that the expected weight loss, as a result of exercise, is in the region of 2–3 kg. A typical three or four session-a-week aerobic exercise/walking programme expending 2.1–4.2 MJ (500–1000 kcal), would produce this degree of weight loss. Where energy intake is severely restricted, as with VLCD, exercise does not increase weight loss or preserve fat free mass (for example, Phinney et al., 1988).

Ballor and Poehlman (1994) and Garrow and Summerbell (1995) also found evidence for an effect of exercise on greater loss of fat mass and conservation of fat free mass, although the degree to which this is because of preservation of muscle tissue remains unclear. More intensive exercise, such as resistance training, can significantly increase fat free mass and reduce weight loss or even increase body weight. Fat mass may, however, still be reduced (Walberg, 1989) and a recent study using magnetic resonance imaging indicated no loss of muscle tissue during weight loss in obese women undergoing a resistance exercise programme and diet (Ross *et al.*, 1995). There is also some indication that exercise for longer periods is more likely to rely on fat oxidation and may be quite effective for maximising fat loss when accompanied by a fat restricted diet (Tremblay & Beumann, 1995). There is currently no substantial evidence to indicate that exercise has a specialised function in the reduction of visceral fat in the obese (Kopelman, 1997).

The addition of more incidental physical activity to daily routines, such as household chores and walking to the shops, may have a significant effect on weight loss over longer periods. However, epidemiological studies have generally failed to show a strong relationship between energy expended through physical activity and BMI. This may be because of the difficulties of questionnaire-based recall of incidental physical activity. Decreases in the amount of time engaged in sedentary mode may also play a role in weight reduction. Time spent watching television, videos, or using computers has increased (Office of Population Censuses and Surveys, 1990) and several studies have indicated a positive relationship between fatness and television viewing in adults and children (Dietz & Strasburger, 1991). It is proposed that, not only do inactive leisure pursuits reduce time for physical activity, they are associated with eating high energy density snacks such as crisps and biscuits. It is likely that a reduction of the amount of time devoted to inactive leisure pursuits may offer an important strategy for long-term weight management.

In summary, it is clear that aerobic exercise cannot compete with dietary methods for rapid weight loss. However, it should be considered as an accompaniment to a moderate dietary regime, as it will usually increase the amount of weight lost in both men and women. Furthermore, it is likely that more of the weight lost will be fat. The degree to which muscle tissue is preserved, or even supplemented, through exercise requires further research but exercise may have important consequences for sustained weight loss. Resistance training may have an important effect on conservation of muscle tissue and has been found to be an acceptable mode of exercise in overweight and obese individuals. Increases in lifestyle activity and reductions in sedentary pursuits may also play a vital role in an overall behaviour change programme. Exercise is more likely to play a critical role for weight loss in the overweight and mildly obese individuals (Fig. 20.1), as the severely obese find difficulty in achieving levels of exercise that substantially modify energy balance. Current recommendations for the appropriate amount of activity for health are shown in Table 20.1.

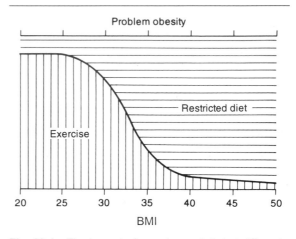

Fig. 20.1 The impact of exercise and diet at different BMI levels (from: Garrow, 1986, reproduced with permission).

20.2 Exercise and sustained weight loss

Ensuring sustained weight loss remains the major challenge in obesity treatment. Although dietary-based programmes and surgical treatments have been successful in reducing weight to healthier levels, recidivism remains disappointingly high. King & Tribble (1991) reviewed the long-term effects of programmes with follow-up measures of at least six months. The average sustained weight loss was 4.0 kg in four diet-only programmes, 4.9 kg in five exercise-only programmes and 7.2 kg in three diet and exercise programmes.

One of these exercise studies (Pavlou *et al.*, 1989) demonstrated convincingly that exercise was important for long-term weight loss. Overweight Boston policemen (160) were randomly assigned to one of four 12-week diets. Half of each group were given 90 minutes of supervised exercise, which included warm up and stretching, followed by moderate to vigorous aerobics and callisthenics three times per week. There were minimal differences in weight loss among the groups at the end of

Table 20.1 Recommendations for appropriate amount of activity for health.

Health Education Authority (Killoran *et al.*, 1995)

- People should take 30 minutes of moderate intensity physical activity, such as a sustained brisk walk, on at least five days of the week
- Ideally these 30 minutes should be one period of sustained activity, but shorter bouts of 15 minutes are also beneficial

Centres for Disease Control and Prevention (Pate *et al.*, 1995)

- Every US adult should accumulate 30 minutes or more of moderate-intensity physical activity on most, preferably all, days of the week.

Quebec Consensus Conference (Blair & Hardman, 1995)

For good health, physical activity should:
- Involve large muscle groups
- Impose more than a customary load
- Require a minimum total of 700 kcal/week
- Be performed regularly, if possible daily

(In practice, sustained rhythmic exercise such as brisk walking for 20–30 minutes would fulfil this requirement in most adults.)

the treatment, but only exercising groups were successful in sustaining weight loss at 8 and 18 months (Fig. 20.2). Regardless of their group, participants who did not continue to exercise were not successful in maintaining their weight loss. These results are supported by further studies involving women (van Dale *et al.*, 1990; Kayman *et al.*, 1990), showing that only a small percentage of non-exercisers are able to sustain weight loss. In a more recent study, Svendsen *et al.* (1994) re-assessed

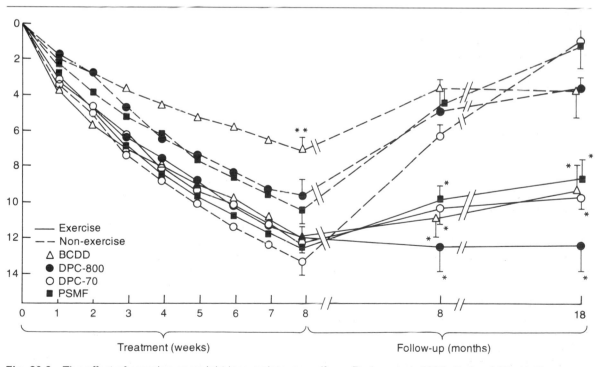

Fig. 20.2 The effect of exercise on weight loss maintenance (from: Pavlou *et al.*, 1989, © *Am J Clin Nutr*).

randomised diet, diet and exercise, and control groups at six months, following a 12-week programme. Women from the diet and exercise group who were still exercising had sustained significantly greater weight loss (10.9 kg versus 6.6 kg) and fat mass (10.0 kg versus 5.4 kg). They also had a greater increase in resting metabolic weight (11.1 kJ (3 kcal) per kg per day versus 1.1 kJ (0.3 kcal) per kg per day) when compared with non-exercisers from the same group. Examples of a healthy package of moderate physical activity are shown in Table 20.2.

The mechanisms for this effect remain unclear. The additional energy expenditure through exercise will contribute and the maintenance or increase in lean tissue and its effect on basal metabolic rate may also be influential. There is a strong suggestion from participants, practitioners and some researchers (Wilfley & Brownell, 1994) that psychosocial mechanisms, such as mastery and empowerment as a result of improved confidence, body image and self-esteem, are also involved.

20.3 Physical activity and health in the obese

Active living could be regarded as the normal state of existence and perhaps we should not be surprised that long periods of sedentary living can lead to loss of functional capacity and serious health problems. Substantial evidence now exists to support this. Inactive living carries an independent twofold risk for all-cause mortality. This is similar to the risk associated with hypertension and hyperlipidaemia and is not far behind the risk of smoking (Powell *et al.*, 1987) (Fig. 20.3). Furthermore, several epidemiological studies with a range of populations have indicated that the relationship follows a dose response pattern, with increasing activity providing greater protection from disease and mortality (Fig. 20.4). This relationship has been established in the overweight as well as the normal weight population (Fig. 20.5). Longitudinal data now demonstrates that increases in fitness and activity improve subsequent relative risk (Blair *et al.*, 1995). People who become more active and improve their fitness also improve their risk profile substantially.

The accumulated epidemiological and experimental evidence is now sufficiently strong to have convinced the major medical authorities worldwide that physical inactivity should be regarded as a **fourth** primary risk factor for coronary heart disease and stroke. This suggests that inactivity should be vigorously treated in its own right. This is particularly the case for obese people as the incidence of sedentary living in this group is high.

Physical activity can also have a positive effect on other risk factors and diseases in the obese population. It can assist in favourably modifying blood

Table 20.2   Examples of a healthy package of moderate physical activity (modified from: US Surgeon General's report on physical activity and health).

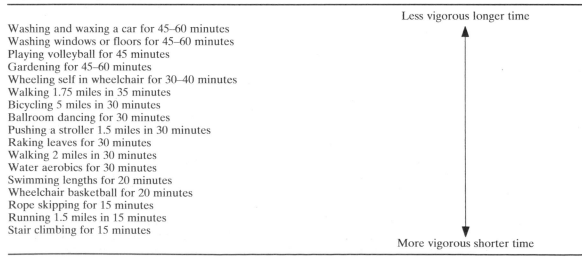

Washing and waxing a car for 45–60 minutes
Washing windows or floors for 45–60 minutes
Playing volleyball for 45 minutes
Gardening for 45–60 minutes
Wheeling self in wheelchair for 30–40 minutes
Walking 1.75 miles in 35 minutes
Bicycling 5 miles in 30 minutes
Ballroom dancing for 30 minutes
Pushing a stroller 1.5 miles in 30 minutes
Raking leaves for 30 minutes
Walking 2 miles in 30 minutes
Water aerobics for 30 minutes
Swimming lengths for 20 minutes
Wheelchair basketball for 20 minutes
Rope skipping for 15 minutes
Running 1.5 miles in 15 minutes
Stair climbing for 15 minutes

Less vigorous longer time

More vigorous shorter time

Note: If performed daily, the energy equivalent is 4.2–6.3 MJ (1000–1500 kcal) per week for overweight people.

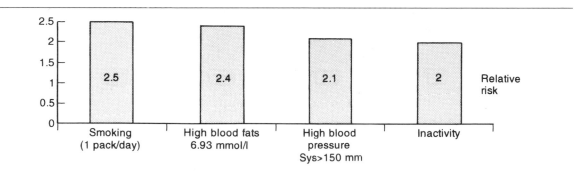

Fig. 20.3 Physical inactivity as a fourth primary risk factor (data from Powell *et al.*, 1987).

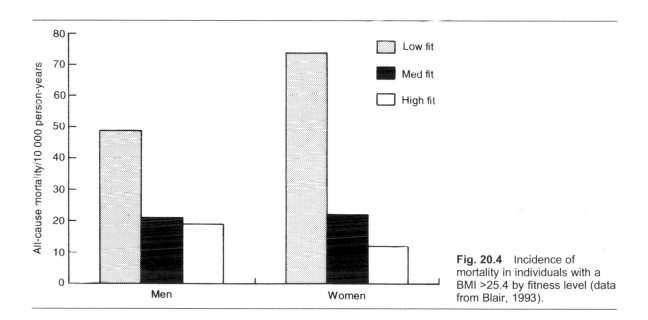

Fig. 20.4 Incidence of mortality in individuals with a BMI >25.4 by fitness level (data from Blair, 1993).

lipids, particularly HDL cholesterol, in overweight men and women (Wood *et al.*, 1991). In a study by Krotkiewski *et al.* (1979), blood pressure was reduced in obese exercisers, even in the absence of weight loss. Additionally, exercise has been established as an important adjunct to the treatment of diabetes, as it increases insulin sensitivity, glucose transporter-4 concentration and glucose disposal (Helmrick *et al.*, 1991). Other important benefits of exercise for obese people include improved functional capacity, which is low in those who are obese. Exercise has also been shown to be effective in the reduction of mild and clinical depression (Martinson & Morgan, 1997) and anxiety (Raglin, 1997), which are more common in obese people. Exercise

has also been shown to improve self-esteem and general psychological well-being.

In summary, overweight and obese people are even more likely to be inactive and unfit than the normal weight population. Consequently, increased activity, in its own right, should be judged as a key outcome of obesity treatment programmes, as a key risk factor is directly eliminated. In addition, exercise will help modify other risk factors, and improve functional capacity and psychological well-being in the obese. To support this, recent evidence, Barlow *et al.*, 1995 and Lee *et al.*, 1998 demonstrates that those people who are overweight and mildly obese, but are also active, are at much reduced overall risk for mortality and morbidity than those who are

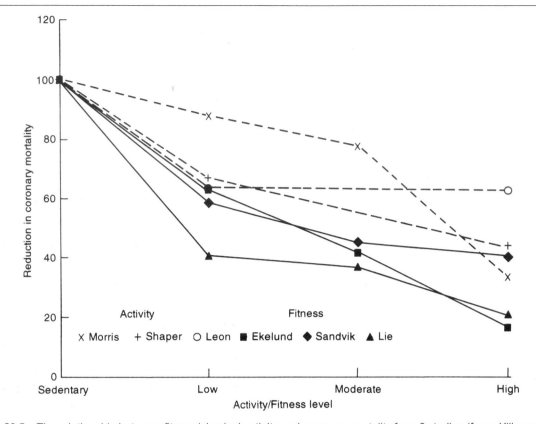

Fig. 20.5   The relationship between fitness/physical activity and coronary mortality from 6 studies (from: Killoran *et al.*, 1995).

obese and inactive. In addition to helping people lose weight and sustain weight loss, exercise is critical to improving the overall health profile in obese people and should be considered an essential part of treatment.

20.4 Considerations for treatment

20.4.1 Objectives of the exercise component

The overall goal of the programme should be to produce long-term changes in exercise habits at a level commensurate with maximising health and wellbeing.

20.4.2 Exercise for optimising health

In the 1970s, the American College of Sports Medicine (ACSM) provided guidelines for exercise

for the improvement of aerobic fitness. The recommendation of aerobic exercise, 3–4 times per week at 60–80% of maximum heart rate for at least 20 minutes, became widely accepted as a standard formula for practitioners. It is now clear that this prescription is not appropriate for health contexts and, in particular, is too demanding for overweight or obese individuals. Examination of the epidemiological evidence clearly shows that the greatest gains in public health are to be made by moving the sedentary sector of the population to moderate levels of activity (Fig. 20.6). The US Centre for Disease Control and Prevention, in collaboration with ACSM (Pate *et al.*, 1995), the Health Education Authority (Killoran *et al.,* 1995) and the Quebec Consensus Conference on Physical Activity and Health (Blair & Hardman, 1995), after thorough reviews of existing evidence, independently produced similar new guidelines for activity

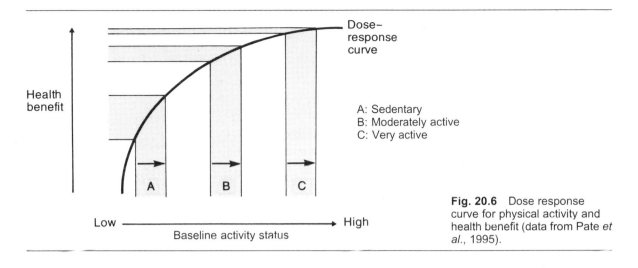

Fig. 20.6 Dose response curve for physical activity and health benefit (data from Pate *et al.*, 1995).

promotion that are more appropriate for those who are overweight and obese.

Every adult should accumulate 30 minutes of moderate intensity physical activity, equivalent to brisk walking, on at least 5 days per week (Table 20.3 for alternatives). The intensity, duration and frequency of such a programme is sufficient to improve fitness and metabolic profile, commensurate with improved health status in those who were previously sedentary or who were largely inactive (Haskell, 1994). Additionally, for overweight and obese people, it will increase energy expenditure above baseline by over 4.2 MJ (1000 kcal) per week. For very overweight people who achieve this level of activity, energy cost will be even higher owing to the increased load involved in moving their extra body weight.

20.4.3 Exercise for optimising total energy expenditure

The achievement of energy balance, through increased energy expenditure, is even more critical in obese people. Consideration should be given to each of the following.

- Any movement expends energy. However, exercise using large muscle groups, such as the legs and arms, uses most energy, particularly when used to move body weight. Additional energy is used when moving weight up slopes or stairs.

- Time spent in sedentary activities such as watching TV is lost time for movement.

- Unlike vigorous exercise, which depletes carbohydrate stores and encourages re-feeding, light to moderately intense activity maximises lipid utilisation as an energy source and encourages lipid deficit and use of fat stores, particularly when accompanied by a low fat, energy reduced diet.

- As activity increases in duration, it draws upon fat as a source of fuel to a greater degree.

This suggests that overweight and obese individuals should focus on three energy expenditure targets:

(a) more weight bearing movement as part of the daily routine,
(b) less time spent in sedentary pursuits,
(c) bouts of longer periods of exercise, sustained for 40 minutes or more.

In addition, they should avoid vigorous activity.

Figure 20.7 graphically demonstrates comparisons between a sedentary individual, one who seeks opportunities for physical activity in the daily routine and one who performs a bout of vigorous activity during leisure time to make up for an otherwise sedentary routine. Even though activity of low intensity is slower in expending energy, it is likely to occur more frequently and accumulate significantly over weeks and months to make a

Table 20.3 Energy expenditure by body weight for selected activities (adapted from McArdle *et al.*, 1991).

Activity	kcal/min^1/kg^{-1}	71 kg (157 lb) kcal		80 kg (176 lb) kcal		92 kg (203 lb) kcal		98 kg (216 lb) kcal	
		1 min	30 min	1 min	30 min	1 min	30 min	1 min	30 min
Sedentary									
Sitting	0.021	1.5	45	1.7	51	1.9	57	2.1	63
Standing	0.025	1.8	54	2.0	60	2.3	69	2.5	75
Household									
Cleaning	0.062	4.4	132	5.0	150	5.7	171	6.1	183
Cooking	0.045	3.2	96	3.6	108	4.1	123	4.4	132
Shopping	0.062	4.4	132	5.0	150	5.7	171	6.1	183
Scrubbing	0.109	7.7	231	8.7	261	10.0	300	10.7	321
Occupational									
Digging	0.145	10.3	309	11.6	348	13.3	399	14.2	426
Painting	0.077	5.5	165	5.9	177	7.1	213	7.5	225
Exercise									
Cycling 5.5 mph	0.064	4.5	135	5.1	153	5.9	177	6.3	426
Cycling 9.4 mph	0.100	7.1	213	8.0	240	9.2	276	9.8	294
Running 11.5 min/mile	0.135	9.2	276	10.9	327	12.5	375	13.3	399
Running 9 min/mile	0.193	13.7	411	15.4	462	17.8	534	18.9	567
Swimming crawl slow	0.128	9.1	273	9.8	294	11.8	354	12.5	375
Swimming crawl fast	0.156	11.1	333	12.5	375	14.4	432	15.3	459
Walking easily	0.080	5.7	171	6.4	192	7.4	222	7.8	234
Walking briskly	0.120	8.5	255	9.6	288	11.0	330	11.7	353
Weight training	0.116	8.2	246	9.3	279	10.6	318	11.4	342
Leisure									
Badminton	0.097	6.9	207	7.8	234	8.9	267	9.5	285
Social dancing	0.051	3.6	108	4.1	123	4.7	141	5.0	150
Gardening (mowing)	0.112	7.6	228	9.0	270	10.3	309	11.0	330
Gardening (raking)	0.054	3.8	114	4.3	129	5.0	150	5.3	159
Golf	0.085	6.0	180	6.8	204	7.8	234	8.3	249
Table tennis	0.068	4.8	144	5.4	162	6.3	189	6.7	201
Tennis	0.109	7.7	231	8.7	261	10.0	300	10.7	321

difference in long-term energy balance. Ideally, the obese person should increase incidental daily movement **and** incorporate an extended session of exercise, such as brisk walking, each day.

Table 20.3 provides examples of the energy expenditure for a range of physical tasks by body weight, which might be incorporated into lifestyle. Similarly, Table 20.4 shows the energy expended by walking at different body weights for different frequencies on the basis of one week.

20.4.4 Optimising initiation and adherence to exercise in the obese

Little is gained unless long-term changes in exercise and physical activity patterns are established, and this has to be the overall objective of this aspect of treatment. Information regarding exercise behaviour change in obese people is sparse and there is a general belief that physical activity promotion for such individuals in the obese is futile. The degree of overweight has been a predictor of early dropout from exercise classes and programmes with general adult populations. However, several studies have shown that some obese people have been successful in maintaining an exercise programme for up to 18 months (Gwinup, 1975; Hill *et al.*, 1989; Pavlou *et al.*, 1989). Programmes have generally been driven by physiological rather than psychological principles, often with exercise prescription that is inappropriate for obese people with insufficient physical and psychological preparation.

A good deal of progress has been made in the field of motivational psychology regarding the fac-

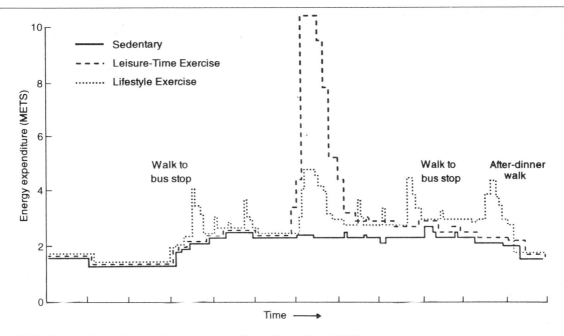

Fig. 20.7 Contrasting patterns of energy expenditure (from: Blair, 1992).

Table 20.4 Walking, energy expenditure and potential weight loss (calculated using values from Ainsworth *et al.*, 1993).

30 minute sessions of brisk walking per week	63 kg (140 lb)		76 kg (168 lb)		88 kg (196 lb)		101 kg (224 lb)	
	kcal/week	lb fat/year	kcal/week	lb fat/year	kcal/week	lb fat/year	kcal/week	lb fat/year
1	160	3	190	3	222	3	255	4
3	480	7	570	9	666	10	765	12
5	800	12	950	14	1110	17	1275	19
7	1120	17	1330	20	1554	23	1785	27

Note: Figures assume energy intake remains the same.

tors concerned with behaviour change and its application to the exercise setting (Biddle, 1994; Dishman, 1994).

Techniques such as cognitive behaviour therapy (Fox, 1992) (many of which have been outlined in Chapter 21) have been applied to dietary change, motivational interviewing (Rollnick, 1996), activity counselling and contracting (Fahlberg & Fahlberg, 1990), but have not been used systematically. Yet, it appears from research focusing on the exercise psychology of obese people that such individuals have misconceptions about the type and amount of activity required, they lack self-confidence in their ability to exercise and do not have self-regulatory and exercise behaviour management skills. Many also need motivational and social support through regular contact. Many of these approaches have been used with some success in changing other health behaviours. Treatments involving a systematic support system for exercise behaviour, based on motivational principles, sound educational policy and featuring counselling and sensitive leadership, have potential for greater long-term success than has typically been reported to date. For example, a group exercise programme specifically for overweight women that focused on peer support, has reported attendance rates of over 90% (Gillett, 1988). As with other behaviours, long-term adherence also depends on opportunity for sustained contact (Perri *et al.*, 1986).

In addition to relying on changes in individual motivation, it is critical that the environment is made more conducive to exercise (Chapter 17). Alliances are needed between transport, environment, leisure and health agencies, and local authorities to facilitate walking, cycling and active play and leisure.

20.4.5 Agencies for treatment

Exercise is probably best placed as a component in a multidisciplinary and staged approach to obesity treatment, which in the UK has not been widely developed. The primary care setting has largely reached capacity but, with extra resources, could provide clinics to assist in treatment. Leisure centre based exercise prescription schemes have flourished in the UK in the past five years (Fox *et al.*, 1997). Although their effectiveness in long-term increases in exercise promotion has yet to be fully established, they offer potential as a site for structured exercise programmes and counselling for obese people. The corporate setting remains relatively undeveloped. Commercial weight loss programmes are currently heavily patronised and, with a closer partnership with the scientific community, may develop effective and accessible programmes, particularly for the overweight or mildly obese individual. Because children's behaviour is largely determined by family and school environments, parents and schools should be involved in interventions, and family-based programmes appear to be most successful (Epstein, 1996).

20.5 Summary

- Physical activity is a useful adjunct to dietary restriction for weight loss and seems to be very important for successful long-term maintenance of a healthy weight. Furthermore, inactivity is a primary risk factor for mortality and morbidity and should be targeted in its own right, but the benefits are potentially even greater for obese people, than for the normal weight population.

- Activity also carries many additional benefits, including improved functional capacity and psychological well-being.

- Physical activity should be included as an essential part of obesity treatment, with patients supported in their efforts to steadily build up a daily routine involving moderately intense exercise, such as brisk walking, more incidental or opportunistic movement and physical work, and reduced time spent in sedentary pursuits.

- For some obese individuals, substantial programme support will be required, particularly in the early stages. Such programmes could be designed and offered in primary or secondary health care settings, leisure and community centres, or commercial and corporate settings.

- Physical activity recommendations for obese people are as follows.
  - Build up slowly to walking for 30 minutes per day on at least 5 days per week. Walk at a pace that achieves mild breathlessness. Two 15-minute sessions are almost as good.
  - Eventually consider extending some sessions to 40 minutes or more to encourage fat burning.
  - Increase the amount of activity in the daily routine, such as housework or shopping.
  - Reduce the amount of time spent in activities that involve sitting down such as watching television.
  - Consider resistance training to conserve muscle mass and maintain resting metabolic rate.
  - Try to find ways to make exercise enjoyable.

- Physical activity programme recommendations for obese people are as follows.
  - Consult the doctor if there are any pre-existing symptoms of disease.
  - Look for opportunities for individual counselling and/or group therapy featuring education, behaviour change strategies, social support and motivational interviewing techniques.
  - Look for opportunities for structured exercise sessions, specifically designed for obese individuals, conducted by sensitive leaders who focus on gradual individual improvement.
  - Maintain long-term contact with a professional.
  - Aim for maximum enjoyment of exercise.

- Environmental changes to encourage activity among obese people could be:
  - (a) traffic free cycling and walking routes to schools, shops and work,
  - (b) greater access to parks, leisure centres and other sports facilities,
  - (c) reward systems to substitute walking and cycling for the car, e.g. for shopping, or journeys to school or work,
  - (d) attractive alternatives to escalators and lifts.

21
Treatment of Obesity IV: Behavioural Treatment

21.1 Background

Behavioural treatments for obesity originated with the idea that an 'obese eating style', either innate or acquired, was the cause of obesity. Behavioural treatment would, it was argued, extinguish the abnormal eating behaviours and allow body weight to return to a 'normal' level (Ferster *et al.*, 1962). In the event, the existence of the obese eating style proved hard to demonstrate outside of the laboratory. The weight of the evidence suggested that any eating abnormalities were more likely to be the result of prolonged dieting than to be the underlying cause of the disorder (Nisbett, 1968). In the meantime, behavioural techniques such as self-monitoring and stimulus control already looked promising, so they were incorporated as adjuncts to dietary treatment, intended to help obese people to change their eating behaviour for the better regardless of the origin of any abnormality (Brownell & Kramer, 1989). As in other areas of behaviour therapy, the basic behavioural programmes were later modified to include a cognitive therapy component, which involved identifying and changing negative thoughts (Meichenbaum, 1977). This combined treatment approach has now been used widely for over 30 years under the general heading of cognitive behaviour therapy (CBT).

21.2 Efficacy of cognitive behavioural treatment

In 1967, Richard Stuart published the results of a case series of obese patients treated with the then new behavioural techniques, which demonstrated impressive weight losses. Since that time, many reviews have confirmed the efficacy of CBT (in its various manifestations) in comparison with no treatment, or minimal interventions (Wilson, 1993; Bennet, 1986; Brownell & Kramer, 1989). However, the initial optimism has been succeeded by a more sober evaluation of treatment efficacy, in the light of the results from longer-term follow-up studies (Brownell & Wadden, 1992; Wilson, 1994). Overviews of CBT outcomes show that weight loss is usually modest, averaging little more than 5–10% of initial weight, and rarely persists once the active treatment phase is ended. Longer-term follow-up studies show a tendency for a gradual return to the original weight over subsequent years, such that any advantage of CBT over dietary treatment has disappeared by five years. Nevertheless, most authorities agree that the combination of CBT with advice on nutrition and on exercise, offers the most consistently effective results, apart from surgical treatments, and probably represents the state-of-the-art in obesity treatment at present (Council on Scientific Affairs, 1988; Rossner, 1995).

21.3 Developments in cognitive behavioural treatment

In recent years, there have been a number of developments in the practice of CBT aimed at increasing weight loss during the active treatment phase and improving weight maintenance. Evidence has accrued suggesting that longer treatment programmes produce more weight loss, and typical treatment programmes now average 16 weeks, compared with 10–12 weeks for the earlier ones (Brownell & Jeffrey, 1987). Stricter dietary regimens, such as very low calorie diets (VLCD), also produce more initial weight loss, so some programmes combine VLCD with CBT (Wadden *et al.*, 1989). Behavioural techniques are increasingly being applied to participation in physical activity, in the light of finding that higher activity levels are associated with better long-term weight maintenance (Wood *et al.*, 1991). Finally, attention is being paid to health risks and psychological well-being as important outcomes. Treatment programmes that improve health and quality of life for the chronically obese patient are now recognised as valuable, even when weight loss is modest or minimal.

21.4 The elements of cognitive behavioural treatment

21.4.1 Self-monitoring

In CBT programmes, an eating diary is an important element of both the assessment and the treatment. During the assessment phase, patients are asked to record their food intake, along with information on the setting of consumption (e.g. mood, speed of eating, situation), and the events subsequent to the meal. This record provides the data for a 'functional analysis', which identifies the factors that might be cueing or reinforcing eating. One common problem with dietary diaries is that the recorded food intake is lower than the predicted energy intake (Prentice *et al.*, 1989). Discussing the patient's inability to remember or record what they have eaten, can be an important step in helping them to acknowledge their problem. Adherence to self-monitoring can also serve as a simple compliance indicator. If the patient who alleges his or her commitment to lose weight fails to keep a food record, then there are motivational conflicts to be tackled before treatment is likely to be worth pursuing.

In the treatment phase, the diary is used to record progress towards behavioural goals and highlight new problems. The self-monitoring process, in itself, has also been found to be beneficial in reducing food intake, albeit in the short term. Few people, whether they are of normal weight or obese, keep a good mental account of what or when they eat, so a written record provides a much better basis for planning and monitoring change.

Over the longer term, the habit of keeping food records appears to be associated with better weight maintenance (Baker & Kirschenbaum, 1993). Whether diary recording actually promotes control, or is a reflection of a general pattern of compliance, remains to be established.

21.4.2 Setting behavioural goals

Obesity treatment programmes traditionally define outcome in relation to weight loss, with the ultimate goal being a weight (or BMI) within the normal range. Current evidence on treatment outcomes has led some authorities to question the practice of setting the goal of 'normal weight', when it is manifestly unachievable. Setting an unrealistic goal predisposes to failure and may lead the patient to attribute the failure to his or her personal shortcomings rather than the real problems with treatment. Unrealistic goals can also lead patients (and health professionals) to undervalue modest weight losses, and to eschew treatment approaches which claim only modest outcomes, despite the fact that a small weight loss can have significant health benefits (Goldstein, 1992). The consensus now is that weight goals should reflect the reality that weight losses are unlikely to exceed 5–10% of initial body weight. The process of accepting a realistic goal could itself be therapeutic, encouraging the patient to acknowledge the chronicity and challenge of weight control, rather than continue to search for a magical solution.

While the goal of obesity treatment is weight loss, the reasons for weight loss are to reduce cardiovascular and metabolic complications of obesity and to improve body satisfaction. Weight loss offers the ideal, but not the only solution. Cardiovascular and metabolic risks are susceptible to changes in dietary quality and physical fitness, and many treatment programmes are moving towards including these as independent indicators of clinical success. Patients who have shown a consistently poor treatment response (e.g. little or no weight loss) and, especially, those whose weight has been steadily rising, would benefit from achieving weight stability combined with lower CVD risk, even if weight loss were minimal.

CBT programmes also include specific behavioural goals reflecting the changes in eating behaviour or activity, which are targeted over the treatment period. Specific behavioural goals allow the patient and the therapist to monitor progress, and the achievement of short-term goals can sustain motivation when progress towards long-term goals is slow. The process of negotiating and agreeing goals can also serve as a form of behavioural rehearsal, and contribute directly to a positive treatment outcome.

21.4.3 Stimulus control

Stimulus control is one of the central elements of behavioural treatment. It derives from the idea that eating is triggered by a range of external or internal cues, such as being in an environment where eating usually occurs. The triggering process could be an innate response to food cues, or learned as a result of repeated associations between particular stimuli and eating, or be part of a coping repertoire, e.g. to ameliorate negative moods. Controlling eating at the final stage of this chain is known to be difficult, but regulating exposure to cues earlier in the chain should be easier. In other words, stimulus control is substituted, in part, for self-control.

The basic approach consists in identifying the chain of events leading up to problem eating, and developing strategies to modify exposure early on in the chain. One of the simplest examples would be to avoid buying highly palatable foods, or if this is impossible, to store them so that they are not easily on view. Stimulus control methods can also be adapted to help increase activity and decrease sedentary behaviour. Simple re-organisations of homes and workplaces (e.g. moving commonly used equipment further away) can increase the levels of activity involved in daily living.

21.4.4 Learned self-control

The stimulus-control approach is based on reducing exposure to the stimuli that trigger eating. In the longer term, the obese person may wish to try to eliminate the associations between such stimuli and the urges to overeat.

Exposure and response prevention is a well-recognised behavioural technique for modifying learned responses. It depends on prolonged exposure to the eliciting cues, without performance of the behaviour, which extinguishes the conditioned responses. This method has been used successfully with bulimic patients to help them learn to look at, or taste, binge food without having a binge (Fairburn & Wilson, 1993). It can be adapted to help the obese person develop control over situations that normally trigger abandonment of the diet. At first, exposure induces a dramatic increase in the urge to eat, but this reduces over 5–30 minutes providing a vivid experience of the development of control. Systematic exposure to emotional cues is more difficult, but one possibility is to use imagined mood stimuli, combined with real food exposure. Alternatively music or films can be used to arouse emotions, combined with exposure to increasingly 'difficult' food. In 'homework' assignments the patient can follow a self-exposure programme with problem foods or situations, progressing through a hierarchy of situations which vary in difficulty level.

21.4.5 Modifying self-defeating cognitions

Many obese people appear to have ways of thinking about weight and weight control that compromise their motivation and self-efficacy. With the development of cognitive approaches to therapy, the investigation and modification of negative thoughts came to be an accepted part of behavioural programmes. Mahoney & Mahoney (1976) were among the first to describe the ways of thinking which compromise treatment compliance in obesity. Examples include 'all or nothing' thinking (e.g. if I cannot diet properly, I might as well give up entirely) and 'catastrophising' (my failure to lose weight last week means that the programme is useless). The usual technique is to ask patients to recall or record their thoughts about their eating (and activity) behaviour. This record is discussed in the treatment sessions to give the patient the chance to consider the evidence for and against the ideas that they have recorded. They can then develop arguments against some of the negative thoughts and practise challenging the thoughts at the times that they occur in everyday life. There have not been any systematic comparisons of behaviour therapy with and without the cognitive approach, but clinical experience suggests that for some patients it is very helpful and for many it has the advantage of being a novel addition to the methods of self-control which they usually use.

21.4.6 Improving body image

Body dissatisfaction has in the past been considered to be an inevitable reaction to obesity and has rarely been targeted in treatment programmes (Rosen *et al.*, 1991). There is now increasing recognition that dissatisfaction contributes to low self-esteem and self-efficacy, and could compromise compliance with treatment. Given that most obese adults will still be well above 'normal weight' after the treatment programme has ended, a focus on improving body image may be valuable. Body dissatisfaction is also associated with avoidance of physical display, especially activities such as sports which require self exposure. Modifying body image could improve adherence to activity recommendations.

The literature relating to body image disturbance among patients with bulimia nervosa or normal weight women provides some guidance (Butters & Cash, 1987), but in these conditions body shape is essentially normal and body dissatisfaction is considered to be part of the psychopathology, a form of 'dysmorphophobia'. This is not true for obese people, since they really are much fatter than is generally thought to be attractive. Significant prejudice against obese people has been thoroughly documented and they suffer teasing, insults and outright discrimination (Allon, 1982). For an obese person, a better body image necessitates learning self-acceptance despite an appearance which falls short of cultural ideals of beauty, as well as learning to cope with the stigma of overweight (Sobal, 1991). The key changes towards a better body image are cognitive and behavioural. They include dissociating appearance from self-esteem (a cognitive change) and not allowing body appraisal to influence choices of activity (a behavioural change). Clinical experience suggests that a group-based treatment programme has many advantages in helping obese adults to develop more 'weight-blindness' in their evaluation of themselves and their future plans.

21.4.7 Modifying disordered eating patterns

Patterning of eating has attracted only limited attention in obesity management, although the 'night eating syndrome' was described by Stunkard many years ago (Stunkard, 1959). However, many obese patients report some degree of disturbance of eating patterns. Most commonly, this involves an eating pattern which varies considerably from day to day; it may also involve long periods of restriction and other phases of frequent excessive consumption. From the patient's perspective, the restriction may be seen as a desirable compensation for periods of overeating, but the irregularity of this pattern may compromise regulatory processes.

Animal studies suggest that eating (and the anticipatory physiological changes) can be conditioned to environmental cues, thus hunger develops when mealtime cues are present. Likewise, meal size is controlled by the (learned) interval between eating and the next meal, consequently animals tend to eat larger meals in anticipation of a longer meal-to-meal interval. If normal human eating operates on similar lines, an irregular meal pattern prevents the conditioning of hunger to mealtime cues, or meal-size to the usual inter-meal interval. This suggests that a regular meal pattern should be established early on in treatment, perhaps even before implementing caloric restriction.

In the draft criteria for the DSMIV, a 'new' disorder, Binge Eating Disorder (BED) has been defined, it is characterised by episodes of binge eating at least twice a week for six months, involving eating to uncomfortable excess and being distressed (Spitzer *et al.*, 1993). The binge eating problem can be assessed through an interview (Marcus & Wing, 1987) or with a formal measure, such as the Eating Disorder Examination (Fairburn & Cooper, 1993). In the past, patients with binge eating have been treated identically with obese non-binge eaters. However, some authorities now recommend that binge eaters should be offered help in developing normal eating patterns and regaining control over eating. Modifications of the programmes used for bulimia nervosa provide one model for treatment (Porzelius *et al.*, 1995), but there is no agreement as yet, over whether these should be introduced before, after or in parallel with weight control. It is also not clear whether strict dieting would be contra-indicated in BED as it is in bulimia nervosa. A conservative approach might start with an emphasis on regular meal patterns, reduction of restraint and strategies to reduce binge frequency (stimulus control, stress management and exposure as appropriate). This could be followed by advice on improving dietary quality and increasing physical activity. Finally, more restrictive dietary advice could be cautiously considered.

21.4.8 Stress management

The place of stress in the control of diet or weight is poorly understood. Stressful life events have sometimes been linked to weight gain (Van Strien *et al.*, 1986a), dieters themselves often attribute their problems of dietary control to stress, and stress is widely believed to induce a preference for high fat or 'comfort' foods. However, the literature on the effects of stress on diet suggests more complex effects (Greeno & Wing, 1994). Animal studies indicate that 'anorexia' is a more common reaction to stress than 'hyperphagia' (Robbins & Fray, 1980). Human studies also identify extreme stress (and distress) with loss of appetite and weight, but lesser degrees of stress have variable effects. Variation in the response may depend on the individual, the type and amount of stress, and the availability of other coping resources such as social support. Clinically, it is possible to establish whether or not stress is associated with poorer dietary control by keeping a stress record in parallel with the dietary record. If stress appears to be a factor in loss of dietary control, then training in stress management could be useful. This chapter is not the place for a detailed description of stress management. The principal features are, however, early identification of sources of stress, the use of relaxation and positive self-talk to mitigate the acute stress responses, and development of appropriate resources to manage both the source of stress and the persistence of the stress response, problem-focused and emotion-focused coping (Woolfolk & Lehrer, 1984).

The other reason for considering stress management is that recent research developments have suggested that stress could play a part in promoting abdominal fat storage (Björntorp, 1996). At present, this is largely limited to observations that abdominal obesity is linked with life stress in epidemiological studies (which does not necessarily indicate a causal effect) and to some suggestions that there are biochemical pathways which could account for the effect (Rebuffe-Scrive *et al.*, 1992).

Nevertheless, these observations strengthen the case for either including an element of stress management in obesity treatment programmes or recommending stress management to obese patients with demonstrable problems in stress-induced eating.

21.4.9 Improving long-term maintenance

Short-term weight loss appears to be considerably easier than long-term maintenance of loss. Several different procedures have been tried as a means of reducing relapse, including booster sessions and relapse training (Perri, 1992). The principle is that the patient is encouraged to acknowledge the likelihood of relapse and either return to treatment, or have strategies to deal with dietary lapses to avoid them becoming relapses. This latter approach usually calls on the model developed in the management of alcoholism, where the 'abstinence violation effect' has been identified as a factor in relapse (Berkowitz, 1994). The therapeutic strategy is principally cognitive, challenging the thought processes which otherwise lead from 'I've failed' to 'I might as well give up trying'. Unfortunately, there is no clear evidence that either relapse training or booster sessions, make a substantial difference in the long term, but this is undoubtedly an area for development and innovation.

There is a growing emphasis in obesity treatment research on the need for permanent lifestyle changes, although this is not yet reflected in commercial programmes, which still promise rapid weight loss and neglect the longer term. Patients themselves may prefer the short-term perspective and find it hard to face up to the obvious conclusions that must be drawn from their personal histories of weight loss and regain. In this context, education about the genetic contribution to obesity (Sorensen, 1995) may be helpful, since it could reduce the sense that weight control difficulties are entirely attributable to failures of self-control. A different illness model, which acknowledges the biological underpinnings and the chronicity of the obese condition, may assist patients in recognising the need to make permanent lifestyle changes and making the appropriate long-term commitment. The obese individual needs to weigh up the advantages and disadvantages of making such significant long-term changes. They should feel able to reach a decision that is informed by an understanding of the medical perspective, but free from coercion by healthcare professionals.

21.5 Indications for cognitive behavioural treatment

The question of which patients would benefit most from behavioural treatments has never been addressed empirically, although it is widely suggested that a stepped care model be applied, related to the degree of overweight. In this model, patients who are only mildly overweight would simply be offered dietary advice; the moderately obese would be referred for CBT with dietary advice, while the severely obese would be recommended for pharmacological or surgical treatment (Brownell & Wadden, 1992). The rationale for this would seem to be that the slightly overweight would not require such intense treatment, while the severely obese are unlikely to achieve enough weight loss, given the modest clinical outcomes of CBT. However, it is possible that CBT would be well suited to providing overweight patients with skills that would prevent the otherwise, almost inevitable, weight gain, i.e. preventively. It is also possible that the severely obese would gain some benefit from CBT if surgery cannot be used. Alternatively, CBT combined with pharmacotherapy, may provide a useful treatment option at some point in the future.

Behavioural treatment may also be specifically indicated where the obese person has an eating disorder. Significant minorities of obese patients have serious problems of control over eating, of which the most significant is probably binge eating disorder. In these cases, there is a real question over the appropriateness of providing simple dietary advice, and a growing interest in developing some of the CBT methods to focus on the specific difficulties of the obese binge-eater.

21.6 Summary

• It is now recognised that obese people do not have an 'eating style' that is characteristically different from normal weight people. Nevertheless, weight loss can be achieved by self-monitoring, stimulus control and changing self-defeating thoughts about dieting, collectively this is called cognitive behaviour therapy (CBT).

• There was initially optimism that the weight loss achieved by CBT, although usually modest, would be long lasting, as it would permanently alter the patient's attitude to food. In fact, longer-term studies show that the effect of CBT alone disappears by five years after therapy. Current research seeks to combine the merits of CBT in preventing weight regain, with greater weight loss achieved initially with restrictive diets and exercise.

• CBT may contribute to the well-being of obese people by effects that do not depend on weight loss. Thus, improvement in body image and self-esteem, control over disordered eating patterns and management of stress are themselves valuable outcomes.

22
Treatment of Obesity V: Pharmacotherapy for Obesity

Pharmacological treatment of obesity is still regarded with suspicion and scepticism by some medical practitioners, who are unconvinced about the dangers of excessive body weight and concerned about perceived dangers of 'slimming drugs'. Any strategy for the use of an anti-obesity drug should take this into account, by ensuring that such drugs are used with the high expectation of medical benefit for a particular patient. The emergence of new drugs for the treatment of obesity and the increasing number of published trials examining the longer-term use of drugs are likely to lead to a gradual change of attitude within the medical profession. At the present time, licensing authorities restrict the use of anti-obesity drugs to patients with a BMI of 30 or greater, on the basis of epidemiological evidence that shows a dramatic increase in the mortality ratio above this level. It seems unlikely that this BMI cut-off point will be lowered until there is additional published information about efficacy and safety of anti-obesity drugs for patients with a BMI of less than 30 who have significant co-morbidities. It is important for physicians to respect licensing recommendations, given the current climate of opinion that does not favour the use of such drugs.

22.1 Indications for anti-obesity drug treatment

The accepted first-line strategy for weight reduction and weight maintenance is a combination of diet, physical activity and behaviour modification. The primary goal for treatment is a 10% weight loss. It may be appropriate to consider drug therapy for those patients with a BMI of 30 or greater who have failed to lose this amount of weight, or whose weight is no longer decreasing after at least 3 months of structured dietary management. Before commencing drug treatment for obesity the following points need to be addressed.

- Initiation of drug treatment will depend on the clinician's judgement about the risks to an individual from continuing obesity.

- Drug treatment may be particularly appropriate for patients with co-morbid risk factors or complications from their obesity.

- A drug should not be considered ineffective because weight loss has stopped, provided the lowered weight is maintained. Continuation of the drug should depend on the balance between the health benefits of maintained weight and the potential adverse effects of the drug.

22.2 Types of drug treatment for obesity

There are currently two categories of anti-obesity drugs; those that act on the gastrointestinal system (bulk-forming agents and pancreatic lipase inhibitors) and those that act on the central nervous system to suppress appetite.

22.2.1 Drugs acting on the gastro-intestinal system

(a) Bulk forming agents

There is no published evidence to suggest that bulk forming agents (e.g. methyl cellulose) have any beneficial long-term action for weight reduction.

(b) Pancreatic lipase inhibitors

Orlistat inhibits pancreatic and gastric lipases, thereby decreasing ingested triacylglycerol hydrolysis. It produces a dose-dependent reduction in dietary fat absorption that is near maximal at a dose of 120 mg three times daily. These actions lead to weight loss in obese subjects (James *et al.*, 1997). Adverse effects of orlistat are predominantly related to its gastro-intestinal action owing to fat malabsorption. These include loose or liquid stools, faecal urgency and oily discharge and can be associated with fat-soluble vitamin malabsorption. As the consumption of a high-fat meal will inevitably lead to severe gastro-intestinal symptoms, it is possible that some of the weight loss with orlistat treatment results from an 'antabuse effect', enforcing behaviour change. Orlistat is not itself absorbed from the bowel.

22.2.2 Centrally acting anti-obesity drugs

Drugs that act on the central nervous system can be divided into three groups.

- those acting via serotoninergic (5-HT) pathways, e.g. fenfluramine and dexfenfluramine,
- those acting via catecholamine pathways, e.g. phentermine,
- those acting via serotoninergic and noradrenergic pathways, e.g. sibutramine.

(a) Drugs acting on serotoninergic pathways

The two drugs from this category, fenfluramine and dexfenfluramine, have recently been withdrawn by the manufacturer, because of concerns about their safety. As a consequence, they will not be considered further, although reference will be made to the published information about the use of dexfenfluramine because this is of considerable relevance to the use of any anti-obesity agent.

(b) Drugs acting on catecholamine pathways

Phentermine is a phenylethylamine derivative with minor sympathomimetic and stimulant properties. Given as an oral sustained release resin complex, it is well absorbed from the small intestine, producing peak plasma concentrations within 8 hours of administration and therapeutic concentrations persisting for at least 20 hours (Silverstone, 1992). Although phentermine has mild stimulant properties, its abuse potential appears to be low. The dose of phentermine is 15–30 mg before breakfast. The use of phentermine is not currently recommended for beyond 12 weeks' treatment.

(c) Drugs acting on noradrenergic and serotoninergic pathways

Sibutramine promotes a sense of satiety through its action as a serotonin and noradrenaline re-uptake inhibitor. In addition, it may have an enhancing effect on thermogenesis through stimulation of peripheral noradrenergic receptors. Sibutramine is well absorbed following oral ingestion and undergoes extensive first pass metabolism in the liver to produce two pharmacologically active metabolites that have long elimination half-lives of 14–16 h. This enables sibutramine to be given once daily, to achieve steady blood concentrations. The ultimate elimination of the two active metabolites is to inactive conjugated products, which are excreted mainly in the urine. Sibutramine (10 mg daily) results in a comparable weight loss to that seen with a twice daily dose of dexfenfluramine over a 12-week period (Lean, 1997). Adverse effects include nausea, insomnia, dry mouth, rhinitis and constipation. However, the noradrenergic actions of the drug may cause an increase in blood pressure and heart rate in some individuals, or prevent the expected fall in these parameters with weight loss. In hypertensive patients sibutramine should be used with caution.

22.3 Do patients become dependent on anti-obesity drugs?

There is no published literature to suggest that the use of any of the cited anti-obesity drugs results in drug dependence.

22.4 Drugs not appropriate for the treatment of obesity

Diuretics, human chorionic gonadotrophin (HCG), amphetamine, dexamphetamine and thyroxine **are not** treatments for obesity and **should not** be used to achieve weight loss. Under no circumstance should thyroxine be prescribed for obesity in the absence of **biochemically proven** hypothyroidism. Metformin and acarbose may be useful in the management of the obese non-insulin-dependent diabetic patient; they have no proven efficacy for obesity alone and are not licensed for such use.

22.5 For how long is it appropriate to prescribe an anti-obesity drug?

The experience from the use of dexfenfluramine for patients during a 12-month randomised controlled treatment trial, provides clues to identifying obese subjects who may benefit from longer term treatment (Guy-Grand *et al.*, 1989). In this study, approximately 30% of the dexfenfluramine-treated group responded to the compound, as judged by a 10% reduction in body weight from their index weight, which was maintained throughout the 12-month study period. This 10% weight loss occurred in the 'responder' group within 3 months. Published reports of longer-term trials involving sibutramine and orlistat suggest similar 'responder' groups (Guy-Grand *et al.*, 1989). A 12-week interval may be used as the time period when 'responders' to drug treatment can be identified and the decision taken to continue the medication.

22.6 Appropriate prescribing

It seems appropriate, on the basis of this evidence, to prescribe a compound for no longer than 12 weeks in the first instance, and then to assess the weight loss. It will be advisable to stop the drug in those patients who have not achieved 10% weight loss from the start of the episode of managed care, because the published evidence suggests that they will not respond to its action in the longer term. In contrast, if a 10% weight loss is achieved, the drug may be continued beyond this initial period as long as the weight is continually monitored. The drug **should not** be continued if there is a subsequent maintained weight regain of >3 kg.

22.7 Selection of an appropriate anti-obesity drug

This will be largely dependent on the experience of the prescriber in using one or another agent. However, patients who confess to difficulties in controlling their eating may be better suited to sibutramine, while patients who deny such a problem may benefit more from orlistat. Failure to achieve satisfactory weight loss with one agent may indicate a trial of an alternative compound at a later stage. There is no information at the present time as to whether patients who are 'non-responders' to one drug will also be non-responsive to another drug.

Combination therapy of two compounds cannot be recommended until efficacy and safety data have been published from long-term trials.

22.8 What criteria should be applied to judge the success of anti-obesity drugs?

Health risks of obesity are related to the degree of overweight and any weight loss is, therefore, likely to reduce this risk. A decrease in body weight of 10% of the initial followed by weight maintenance, can therefore have a major effect on risk factors.

- The objective for treatment should be a weight loss of 10% or more of the initial body weight (observed from the start of the episode of managed care) that is maintained for at least 12 months. If this weight goal is achieved then a new weight loss target should be agreed with the patient.

- A drug should not be considered ineffective because weight loss has stopped, provided the lowered weight is maintained. Continuation of the drug should depend on the balance between the health benefits of maintained weight and the potential adverse effects of the drug.

- The results from short-term (12 weeks or less) studies of drug therapy demonstrate rapid weight relapse after discontinuation of the drug. It seems inappropriate to stop an anti-obesity drug after such a time period if the drug is successful in assisting weight loss.

22.9 What are the concerns about long-term anti-obesity treatment?

These concerns relate to efficacy, safety and cost.

- There is considerable published evidence to support the efficacy of anti-obesity drugs **when**

prescribed for selected patients in an appropriate setting.

- Safety is crucial. Adverse effects associated with the presently and imminently available drugs are usually minor and transient and do not warrant their discontinuation. However, this is largely based on short term (3–6 month) use; there have been relatively few longer-term studies (12 months or longer) of the use of such agents. These concerns have been strengthened by the association between the use of some centrally acting agents and the development of primary pulmonary hypertension and the finding of cardiac valve abnormalities in patients treated with fenfluramine and dexfenfluramine (Abenhaim *et al.*, 1996; Connolly *et al.*, 1997). When assessing the suitability of a patient for treatment with an anti-obesity drug, it is important to consider the likely benefit from the use of a drug. The risk from any drug will be extremely small, provided that the medical benefits from moderate weight loss are high. This underlines the importance of the selection of appropriate patients for treatment.

- Cost is of obvious importance. Drugs are expensive and the cost of treatment of obesity could be large. This must be counterbalanced by the likely decrease in morbidity and premature mortality, and the consequent saving of health-care resources. No direct data are available at present to compare costs, although several estimates have been published.

22.10 What are the appropriate arrangements for the continuation of treatment of a patient with a prescribed anti-obesity drug?

The following points should be considered.

- Programmes for weight management must include clearly defined procedures for monitoring of progress. These will include recording of body weight and changes in any allied conditions.

- Documentation of the issue of prescriptions, to identify misuse or poor compliance or unduly protracted therapy, and a clear record in the case notes detailing, with dates, previous treatment with an appetite suppressant drug.

- It is advisable that patients prescribed anti-obesity drugs are supervised at least at monthly intervals and a record of body weight, blood pressure and any other appropriate measures for the individual is entered in the case notes.

- Written notification should be sent to the patient's general practitioner, if another physician initiates the prescription, which details the reasons for treatment, the dose and its intended duration and alerts the doctor to possible untoward effects. The letter should also include details of the proposed follow-up, and subsequent correspondence should include further information about progress. Such information is in line with the recommendations of the General Medical Council's standards for good practice (General Medical Council, 1995).

- Once a weight loss target has been achieved, there should be an opportunity for re-negotiation of a new target, if considered appropriate, and/or long-term monitoring with reinforcement. Studies confirm that weight loss maintenance programmes require frequent contacts with programme providers. This is consistent with the view that obesity is a chronic condition that requires continuous ongoing care for obese (or formerly obese) patients from those professionals providing the treatment.

A system of regular medical audit should be a pre-requisite of a weight management programme, with a record of results and audit action. The audit should consider not only absolute weight loss but also alterations in co-morbid conditions. The results of the audit should be available to an external reviewer if requested.

22.11 'Over the counter' therapies for obesity

Numerous compounds available over the counter or through mail order, are promoted as weight loss remedies. Examples of these include herbal remedies, fat magnets and slimming patches. Many claim rapid and substantial loss of fat tissue but such claims are not supported by published scientific evidence nor the results from randomised, controlled trials. Furthermore, the rate of weight loss promoted as a possible consequence of the use of certain compounds is medically undesirable. Many healthcare professionals consider that the medicinal claims for these compounds should require them to be evaluated and licensed as a medicine, prior to their being made available to the public.

22.12 Summary

- The first line strategy for weight loss and its maintenance is a combination of supervised diet, physical activity and behaviour modification. This approach must be pursued throughout, even when adjunctive therapies are used.

- Anti-obesity drugs may be justified in adult patients at medical risk from obesity (body mass index of 30 or greater) where dietary methods have been unsuccessful in achieving a 10% weight reduction after a period of at least three months from the start of the episode of care.

- An anti-obesity drug should not be prescribed for longer than three months, in the first instance. After three months, weight loss should be assessed. It is advisable to stop the drug in those obese patients who have not achieved a 10% reduction from the start of the episode of managed care. If a 10% weight loss is attained, the drug may be continued beyond this initial period, provided that body weight is continually monitored and weight not regained. The drug should not be prescribed beyond the period stipulated by its product licence.

- The absence of extensive safety data means that the use of anti-obesity drugs must be closely monitored, with patients being subject to very regular medical review.

- There should be written notification to the patient's general practitioner when another physician initiates a prescription for an anti-obesity drug. There is an ethical duty of the prescribing doctor, if he or she is not the general practitioner, to inform the patient of the importance of notifying the patient's general practitioner. The potential dangers of conflicting treatments and misdiagnosis should then be made clear to the patient if the general practitioner is not informed.

23
Treatment of Obesity VI: Surgical Treatments

23.1 Introduction

The essential difference between medical and surgical treatments for obesity concerns the extent to which control passes from the patient to the doctor. In medical treatment the patient is advised to alter behaviour, usually relating to diet and/or physical activity. Ability to comply with this advice may be enhanced by drug treatment, but ultimately the control remains with the patient, who at any stage can elect to stop the behavioural change, or stop taking the drug. In contrast, with surgical treatments the patient surrenders a large measure of control. Usually the patient will have a general anaesthetic and after recovery from the operation, something has changed, which the patient cannot reverse. Some fatty tissue may have been excised, or there may have been a change in the patient's ability to eat a meal of a normal size, or absorb the food that has been eaten. Of course the patient initially consented to this operation, but having done so the change is permanent, unless in some instances the surgeon is willing to perform a second reversal operation. From the patient's viewpoint this transfer of control has advantages and disadvantages. The advantage is that to a large extent the responsibility for the outcome now lies with the surgeon; the patient expects that, without effort on their part, their excess weight will be reduced. However, this also brings a disadvantage. For example, in the case of gastric restriction or malabsorption operations, the patient finds that they have to adopt a restricted diet in order to avoid vomiting

or diarrhoea. It may, however, be possible to avoid these side effects by taking a high proportion of their energy intake as alcohol, which easily passes restrictions in the bowel, and is easily absorbed without the action of digestive enzymes. However, a high-alcohol diet is not the intended outcome of these operations, so responsibility is again thrown back on the patient to exercise some dietary restraint.

23.2 Excision of fatty tissue

23.2.1 Apronectomy

Massively obese patients accumulate large amounts of fat in the anterior abdominal wall, the weight of which causes the abdominal wall to stretch and hang down like an apron on the thighs of the patient. An operation to remove this extra skin and fat is technically quite easy, and may help to relieve the respiratory problems of such patients and improve them cosmetically. It does not affect the great majority of excess fat and, therefore, is not a treatment for obesity.

23.2.2 Liposuction

It is possible to introduce a trochar under the skin and suck out fatty material. This is favoured by some plastic surgeons who seek to respond to the patient's desire for local removal of fat, but the total weight of fat that can be safely removed by this procedure is trivial and so it is not a treatment for obesity.

23.3 Malabsorption techniques

23.3.1 Jejuno–ileal bypass

Payne & De Wind (1969) reported a series of 80 patients who had end-to-end anastomosis of the first 35 cm of jejunum to the last 10 cm of ileum. The rationale was that food leaving the stomach would be incompletely digested during its rapid passage down the small bowel, now reduced to only 45 cm in length. As a result, the patient would be able to eat an unrestricted diet, but still lose weight. Initially, the patients had a mean weight of 141 kg. In the first year, after operation, they lost 44 kg, in the next year 25 kg and in the third 12 kg. There were, however, many complications, some of which did not become evident until years after the operation, e.g. the formation of oxalate stones in the kidney. Much litigation ensued and the operation was abandoned by about 1980.

23.3.2 Gastric bypass

The operation of stapled gastroplasty, pioneered by Mason in Iowa, replaced jejuno–ileal bypass as the most generally used operation for severe obesity (Section 23.4.2). However, some surgeons favour an operation that gives a combination of malabsorption and restricted intake, such as that shown in Fig. 23.1 (Kral, 1995). The advantage is that it provides greater and more prolonged restriction of food intake (because a large meal causes 'nimiety' or discomfort), without causing the disastrous malabsorption states which occurred with the jejuno–ileal bypass operation. The disadvantage is that the more complicated system of anastomoses requires greater surgical skill and the malabsorption state requires medical monitoring for life and may entail multiple hospital admissions in the first two post-operative years.

23.4 Techniques to restrict intake

23.4.1 Jaw wiring

Wiring the jaws together is a standard procedure in the treatment of fractures of the lower jaw, or when a part of the lower jaw has been removed in the treatment of a tumour. The patient can then drink, but not chew, and usually loses weight. Garrow (1974) suggested this procedure as an alternative to

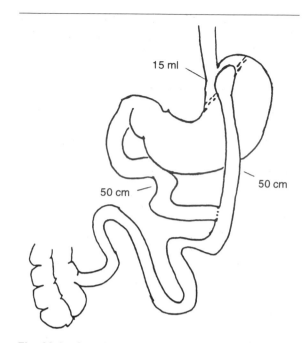

Fig. 23.1 Gastric bypass excluding most of the stomach, the duodenum, and a 40–50 centimetre segment of proximal jejunum (from Kral, 1995).

the then-prevalent jejuno–ileal bypass for severely obese patients who were unable voluntarily to restrict their food intake. The dental technique that was used needed to be modified because strong fixation is required to resist the strains of coughing or sneezing in subjects with healthy jaws and facial muscles. Rodgers *et al.* (1977) reported a series of 17 patients, initially twice their ideal weight, who lost a median of 25.3 kg in 6 months without serious complications. The lost weight was, however, rapidly regained at an unusual rate when the wires were removed. Subsequently, Garrow & Gardiner (1981) suggested fitting a waist cord when the wires were removed. Garrow & Webster (1986) reported a series of 35 patients who were offered jaw wiring combined with a waist cord. Of these, 9 dropped out during the jaw wiring phase and another 12 during the waist-cord follow-up (mainly because they moved away or became pregnant). The remaining 14 (who were initially 54.1 kg overweight) on average lost 42.4 kg during 11 months of jaw wiring. There was a regain of 9.6 kg during the waist-cord phase, which resulted in an average weight loss of 32.8 kg over 3 years. This procedure has not been tested in a randomised-controlled trial, but these results compare well with other surgical procedures, with a much lower cost or morbidity.

23.4.2 Stapled gastroplasty

This operation, devised by Mason (1982), divides the stomach by means of a line of staples into a small upper pouch with a capacity of about 15 ml, which communicates with the main body of the stomach by means of a stoma about 9 mm in diameter (Fig. 23.2) When the patient eats or drinks, the pouch rapidly fills and stops further ingestion because, until the pouch has emptied through the small stoma, any additional food would reflux up into the oesophagus. This procedure is highly effective in limiting intake of solid food, but liquids can be taken fairly easily. In time, the pouch tends to stretch, thus permitting intake of greater quantities of food. The procedure is relatively simple and safe, because the bowel is not cut open, and the food that trickles through the stoma is subsequently normally digested and absorbed. The average weight loss (28.8 kg at one year) is less than in gastric bypass (43.9 kg) but with fewer complications. The relative merits of the two

types of operation are being investigated in the ongoing Swedish Obese Subjects (SOS) study (Lindroos *et al.*, 1996).

23.4.3 Extra-gastric banding

Techniques are being developed by which the capacity of the stomach can be reduced by wrapping inextensible material around the outside of the stomach. In some cases, it is possible to do such operations by laparoscopic techniques. There is not yet sufficient long-term follow-up data to evaluate these procedures, which may prove to be safer and cheaper than operations that involve opening the abdominal cavity.

23.4.4 Artificial bezoar

The objective of reducing gastric capacity might be achieved if an inert mass (such as a liquid-filled balloon) was introduced into the stomach by means of a gastroscope. However, such devices have not proved useful; they did not cause substantial or sustained weight loss and frequently caused ulceration of the gastric mucosa.

23.5 Long-term results of gastric surgery for obesity

The best source of information about the effects of surgical treatments on the health and well-being of severely obese patients comes from the SOS study. This is an ongoing study in which it is intended to enrol 2000 cases treated by surgery and 2000 controls, who are treated by 'conventional' means, i.e. dietary advice. The study is not randomised, since the 'controls' declined to have surgery and hence may be different from those treated surgically. In particular, the controls are initially somewhat less obese than those treated by surgery (BMI lower by about 2 in controls, compared to surgical patients). Despite these limitations, it is the best study available to answer many important questions about the effect of surgical treatment. The weight loss after 2 years was typically 30 kg after gastroplasty and 40 kg after gastric bypass (Sjöström *et al.*, 1995).

The effect of this massive weight loss on health-related quality of life (HRQL) has recently been reported by Karlsson *et al.* (1998). Of the 487 patients reported on, 65% had gastroplasty, 28%

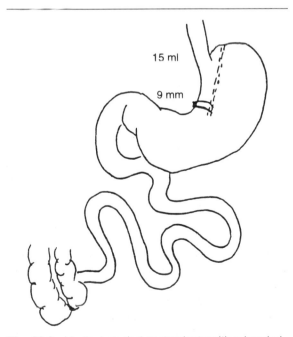

Fig. 23.2 Vertical stapled gastroplasty with a banded outlet from the 15-millilitre pouch (from Kral, 1995).

had gastric banding, and 7% had gastric bypass; this indicates the relative use of these types of operation among participating surgeons in Sweden. On average, the results showed that during the first six months after surgery, male patients lost 29.1 kg and females lost 26.0 kg. In the second six months there was a weight loss of 3.5 kg, and in the second year a weight regain of 2.5 kg occurred. After two years the average weight of male patients decreased from 130.8 kg (BMI 40.8) to 100.6 kg (BMI 31.5), and for female patients the corresponding figures were 115.1 kg (BMI 42.3) and 88.4 kg (BMI 32.5). The average control weight loss was only about 1 kg in two years in both genders.

HRQL improved dramatically in the surgical patients compared with the controls. However, the improvement in HRQL was related to the magnitude of the weight loss, as shown in Fig. 23.3. Those who lost >40 kg showed a striking improvement in obesity-related psychosocial problems (OP) which occurred mainly in the first six months after operation, increased still further for the next six months and then remained constant up to two years. However, those who lost <10 kg after operation had a smaller immediate improvement, which was not sustained after the first six months. These data strongly suggest that the OP of severely obese patients are related to the degree to which they are overweight, and can be relieved by weight loss. It also suggests that the small weight losses that have been shown to confer large metabolic benefits (Section 18.3) may not be enough to correct the OP of severely obese patients.

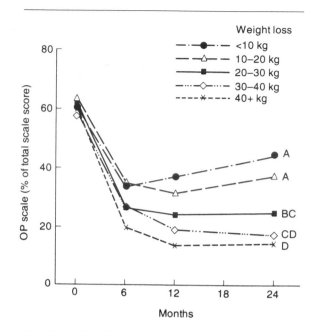

Fig. 23.3 Obesity-related psychosocial problems (OP) in everyday life before and after gastric restriction surgery, by weight reduction two years after intervention. Mean level at baseline and at 6, 12 and 24 months after treatment are plotted for five groups of patients differing in the amount of weight loss: <10 kg (n = 38), 10–20 kg (n = 114), 20–30 kg (n = 136), 30–40 kg (n = 88) and >40 kg (n = 101). OP scale scores are transformed into a 0–100 scale, that is, raw scores are divided by the highest possible score and multiplied by 100. High scores represent dysfunction. Groups with different letters are significantly different at two-year follow-up (P<0.05; Turkey's range test) (from: Karlsson *et al.*, 1998).

23.6 Summary

- In severely obese Swedish patients, gastric surgery causes massive weight loss, maximal at about one year after operation, and this greatly improves the health and quality of life compared with weight-stable obese controls.

- Weight loss of this magnitude, attained by non-surgical methods, confers similar benefits to weight loss attained by surgical methods. However, few patients achieve this level of weight loss, even with the assistance of drugs. The place of jaw wiring with a waist cord has not been effectively researched. The effect of gastric balloons has been disappointing.

- In view of these findings expert committees evaluating the cost-effective options for the treatment of severe obesity in the US (Institute of Medicine, 1995) and the UK (Anon, 1997) have endorsed the use of surgical treatments, subject to the provisos in the NIH Consensus Statement (Consensus Statement, 1991).

- Essentially these are that surgical procedures should be reserved for those who are severely obese (BMI >40), who have failed non-surgical treatment, and who have consented after a realistic briefing on the likely complications. Experienced surgeons in special centres should perform the operations, and lifelong monitoring is required post-operatively.

24
Treatment of Obesity VII: Resources and Evaluation

24.1 The economic cost of obesity

It is clear that a reduction in the prevalence of obesity in this country will require a concerted programme, not only involving healthcare professionals, but also organisations that most affect the social environment. These include government ministries and companies involved in the production and distribution of food, the provision of transport and leisure facilities, and those who educate schoolchildren and adults about diet and health. Such changes will have an economic cost, which it is beyond the scope of this Task Force to calculate. However, calculations have been published which attempt to put an economic cost on the present burden of obesity and overweight. Accordingly, an effective programme to control obesity would have potential economic savings, as well as savings in human life and disability.

Seidell (1997) reviewed the economic costs in several countries under three headings.

(1) direct cost involved in the diagnosis and treatment of disease directly related to obesity,
(2) indirect costs related to the loss of productivity by absenteeism, disability pensions and premature death,
(3) personal costs, since obese people generally earn less than their lean counterparts.

Usually the data are not available to make accurate estimates of the economic costs under headings 2 and 3, but the healthcare costs under heading 1 are quite well documented. However, in Finland, records of the social security system are linked to health records and it is, therefore, possible to calculate the proportion of disability pensions that are attributable to obesity. After adjustment for age, geographical region, occupation and smoking, the relative risks of work disability for women and men with BMI >30, compared with BMI <22.5, were 2.0 (1.8–2.3) for women and 1.5 (1.3–1.7) for men (Rissanen et al., 1990). About 25% of all disability pensions from cardiovascular and musculoskeletal causes in women and about 13% in men, could be attributed to overweight (BMI >25) alone. The authors comment that the similarity in other industrialised countries with living conditions and prevalence of overweight in Finland suggests that similar financial burdens are caused by overweight in countries such as the UK.

It should be noted that the rates of pensionable work disability in women increase from 6.3 per 1000 at a BMI of 22.5, to 12.2 per 1000 at a BMI of 30. Among men, over the same weight range, the increase is from 9.2 per 1000 to 12.4 per 1000. Therefore, it is overweight (Grade 1) as shown in Fig. 2.1 that is responsible for this striking increase in disability over a range in which the mortality rate is hardly affected. Among Finnish people who are obese (Grade II or III), the rate of disability is even higher.

In terms of healthcare costs of excess weight, mortality is the least useful indicator, since chronic non-fatal disease is a far greater burden than premature mortality, and overweight is a far greater burden than obesity. This is because far more people are involved. These relationships are illustrated in Table 24.1 (Seidell, 1995).

Table 24.1 Costs of healthcare provision for overweight in the Netherlands (millions of Dutch guilders) (from: Seidell, 1995).

Service	Cost of overweight (BMI>25)	Cost of obesity (BMI>30)
General practitioners	101	27
Medical specialists	82	30
Hospital admissions	496	178
Medication	549	147
Total	1228	382

The costs shown in Table 24.1 are derived by estimating the economic costs of different diseases, ascribing a proportion of this cost to obesity and summing the obesity-related portions. The estimated costs therefore depend on the total cost of the health services and assumptions about the proportions of disease costs attributable to obesity. Table 24.2 shows the proportions of the costs of various diseases that were attributed to obesity by Lévy *et al.* (1995). The conclusion was that the direct cost of obesity to the French healthcare system in 1992 was 11.89 billion French francs (FF), with a further 0.6 million FF in indirect costs. Note that since the risk of hip fracture is less in people with a BMI of >27, there is a small economic saving in healthcare costs of obesity in this respect.

Similar calculations have been done by Colditz (1992) for the economic costs of obesity in the USA

Table 24.2 Proportion of various diseases attributable to obesity (BMI >27) (from: Lévy *et al.*, 1995).

Disease	Relative risk	Attributable proportion (%)
Obesity	–	100.0
Hypertension	2.9	24.1
Myocardial infarction	1.9	13.9
Angina pectoris	2.5	20.5
Stroke	3.1	25.8
Venous thrombosis	1.5	7.7
NIDDM	2.9	24.1
Hyperlipidaemia	1.5	7.7
Gout	2.5	20.0
Osteoarthritis	1.8	11.8
Gallbladder disease	2.0	14.3
Colorectal cancer	1.3	4.7
Breast cancer	1.2	3.2
Genitourinary cancer	1.6	9.1
Hip fracture	0.8	−3.5

(here defined as BMI >27.8 in men and BMI >27.3 in women). He calculated that in 1980 there were around 34 million obese adults in the USA. Costs were ascribed (in 1986, US $) to NIDDM as 57% of the total cost for NIDDM, which comes to $11.3 billion. Gall bladder disease was costed at 30% of total costs, i.e. $2.4 billion, cardiovascular disease at 19% costs, i.e. $22.2 billion, hypertension at 77% costs, i.e. $1.5 billion, colon and breast cancer at 2.5% costs, i.e. $1.9 billion. These partial costs sum to $39.3 billion, which were about 5.5% of the total healthcare costs in the USA in 1986.

Estimated economic costs of obesity vary in different countries, at different times and depending on cut-off used to define obesity, but all available estimates conclude that somewhere between 1–5% of total healthcare costs are attributable to overweight and obesity. Authors of various economic analyses comment that their estimates are conservative, as there are several items for which no costing is available. It is also obvious that, with increasing prevalence of obesity in all affluent countries, the total burden on the healthcare budget is always increasing. We can, therefore, safely conclude that there are massive economic savings to be made in healthcare costs, apart from any other benefits to well-being, if the prevalence of obesity is reduced.

24.2 Professions involved in the treatment of obesity

It has been shown in this Task Force report that obesity in an individual, or in a population, arises when the interaction between the characteristics of that individual, or population, and their environment gives rise to a prolonged positive energy balance. Figure 24.1 is an attempt to describe this graphically. The individual (A) is at the centre, with whatever characteristics he or she has acquired from genetic or environmental sources. Immediately surrounding the individual is a shell (B) of people, usually family and friends, who help to shape the opinions and behaviour of the individual on all matters, including healthcare.

We know that over the past two decades in the UK, as in other affluent countries in the world, the prevalence of obesity has been markedly increasing, so the typical individual in Fig. 24.1 is travelling towards the left of the diagram. This trend cannot

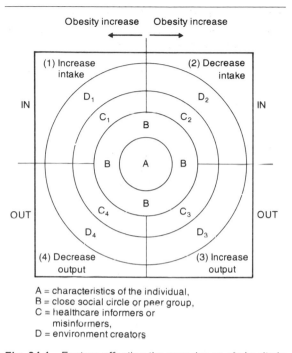

A = characteristics of the individual,
B = close social circle or peer group,
C = healthcare informers or
    misinformers,
D = environment creators

Fig. 24.1 Factors affecting the prevalence of obesity in a population.

be dependent to any significant extent on a change in the genetic make-up of the population, because that can only change with succeeding generations. It must, therefore, be the interaction between this genetic constitution and the environment, which has changed. To find a cause for the change, or the potential to reverse it, we must examine the outer shells in Fig. 24.1, which contains the healthcare informers and environment-creators. For convenience the outer shells have been divided into quadrants relating to energy intake (above) and energy output (below).

The obvious targets for blame for the increased prevalence of obesity in the UK are either the individual (A), because increasing obesity always arises as a result of what the individual does or does not do; or else the healthcare professionals in C2 and C3 who have failed to persuade the individual to decrease energy intake and/or increase energy output. This obvious response is unhelpful and inaccurate, since the point of Fig. 24.1 is to indicate that the energy balance of individuals or populations is a result of a very large number of influences,

some of which have no obvious relationship to healthcare. Thus, the inventor of a better computer game or the sponsor of a charity fun-run, may affect the balance of energy output, and the recipes advocated by a television chef or the pricing policy of a supermarket manager may affect the balance of energy intake. In Chapter 26 the recommendations of this Task Force are put in the context of the components of our society who are likely to affect the success of attempts to prevent or treat obesity in our population. This section aims to show that virtually every profession and occupation, to a greater or lesser degree, has a role in one or more of the segments of Fig. 24.1.

24.2.1 Healthcare informers and misinformers

Dietitians and other healthcare workers are trained to advise people on diet, of which energy intake is one aspect. The number of trained dietitians in relation to the size of the general population is very small, so the majority of the population receives their advice on diet through mass-media channels rather than by individual tuition. Attempts are being made to improve the teaching of nutrition to schoolchildren and their teachers, and to healthcare workers such as doctors, nurses and care assistants, but this is a slow process and it operates against a background of misinformation, which will be discussed later. Furthermore, reduction in energy intake is not necessarily the most important message to transmit, especially to schoolchildren, who require a good level of nutrition to grow and develop normally, and who may be too easily led into inappropriate search for thinness. Health education literature therefore must steer a careful line between advice to those who need to reduce their excessive fat stores and those who do not, and the compromise that results is often very ineffective.

Misinformation about diet is very prevalent, as it is commercially very profitable. Especially in the early months of the year, when many people have resolved to lose weight, there is a spate of books and magazine articles promoting this or that magical weight-loss remedy which removes the tedium of dieting. They are written by skilful journalists who do not know, or do not care, about the principles of energy balance, but who present very plausible regimens with touching testimonies to their efficacy by satisfied disciples. Why should anyone undergo the costs of dieting (Section 18.2) if the results can easily be achieved by wearing underclothes with special thermogenic properties, or rubbing in lotion which will dissolve underlying fat, or carrying a talisman which will realign their energy meridians to form a slimmer persona?

Concerning energy output, there is a similar balance of healthcare informers and misinformers (C3 and C4 in Fig. 24.1). For a person of given age, height and gender, virtually the only way in which energy output can be altered is by altering the amount and nature of physical activity. Chapter 20 provides information about the changes in the amount and nature of exercise, which are feasible and desirable. Again, the proportion of trained exercise physiologists and physical educationists is very small in relation to the total population, so the message is transmitted (and often distorted) by the mass media. There are also many sources of misinformation concerning ways in which energy expenditure can be increased without effort. Advertisements depict smiling slim women reclining gracefully while electrodes stuck to the skin are said to be exercising their muscles. In fact, the amount of muscular work that can be induced in a normal person by surface electrodes is very slight, and will have no significant effect on total energy expenditure, or physical fitness. 'Nutritional supplements' are advertised which are said to inhibit the absorption of fat or carbohydrate from the diet and thus increase energy losses from the body, but these are ineffective (and would be potentially harmful if they had the claimed effect). Other 'natural' supplements are said to speed up the metabolism, but this is not true to any significant degree.

24.2.2 Environment creators

Probably the most powerful force behind the increased prevalence of obesity in affluent countries has been the changing environment, which promotes a positive energy balance (i.e. an excess of energy intake over energy output). Taken individually these technological changes are most welcome. We want food and drink to be inexpensive, palatable and easy to prepare. We want labour-saving devices which perform tiring chores without much physical effort by the human operator. We want to be able to watch our favourite sport from the comfort and safety of our own homes and to have mechanical transport that will take us easily, and quickly wherever we want to go. It is one of the rewards of civilisation that such advances have rescued us from the drudgery of the subsistence farmer in under-developed parts of the world. However, the penalty which goes with this reward is an environment which promotes obesity.

The big commercial gains go to those in sections D1 and D4 of Fig. 24.1; there are profits to be made if people can be persuaded to buy more food and drink, and exert themselves less. The commercial forces in sections D2 and D3, which need strengthening, are relatively small. Certainly, there is profit in slimming clubs, and in sport or gymnasium facilities, but these cater for the higher socio-economic groups in society, who are anyway less prone to obesity. Facilities for physical activity in population centres occupy valuable space, which could more lucratively be used for other types of development. The public highway, which is a potential source of outdoor physical activity by walking, jogging or cycling, is under ever-greater pressure to provide for mechanical transport.

24.3 Evaluation of effectiveness and efficiency of treatment programmes

Cochrane (1972) distinguished two different measures of the usefulness of healthcare procedures. He used the word 'effectiveness' in relation to research results, as opposed to the results when a therapy is used in routine clinical practice in a defined community, which was its 'efficiency'. There can be few areas of healthcare in which the difference between these two measures is so clearly shown as in the treatment of obesity. For example, a balanced reducing diet designed to provide 3.4 MJ (800 kcal) daily was effective in causing a patient to lose 227 kg, reducing in weight from 315 kg to 85 kg over a period of 723 days in a metabolic ward. This must be a world record for weight reduction by any method (Bortz, 1969). Yet, the efficiency of exactly the same diet in achieving weight loss in an outpatient setting is miserable, e.g. a mean loss of 2.64 kg in 16 weeks (Summerbell *et al.*, 1998). The difference between the two measures is related to differences in compliance, which is discussed in Chapter 19.

24.4 Maintenance of weight loss

Weight loss is the easiest, but not the only, measure of success in the treatment of obesity. The objectives are also to achieve indefinite maintenance of a healthy weight after weight loss, and maintenance of normal self-esteem in the formerly obese person (Section 18.1). On these criteria, Bortz's treatment was not efficient, because on discharge from hospital this patient spectacularly failed to maintain the progress he had made in hospital, either in terms of weight or psychological status.

Anything that causes a negative energy balance, whether it is a low-energy diet or increased energy expenditure by exercise or any other method, is an effective treatment for obesity. The physical principles of energy balance have been shown to be totally reliable when calculating the change in energy stores in human subjects in a metabolic ward. Excess weight in obese people has an energy value of approximately 29.4 MJ (7000 kcal) per kg, so an energy deficit of 4.2 MJ (1000 kcal) per day will cause a weight loss of 1 kg/week. This proviso is necessary because changes in weight occur as a result of changes in body glycogen and water, which is a small and very labile component of the energy stores of the body (Garrow & Webster, 1989).

However, it is clear that the efficiency of weight control measures in the UK over the past two decades has been very poor because in practice, the prevalence of obesity has greatly increased (see Section 4.1.2) In Cochrane's terminology, we have effective treatments but they are not efficient.

24.4.1 Systematic reviews of effective treatment and prevention of obesity

A systematic review of the methods for prevention and treatment of obesity has been published by Glenny *et al.* (1997). They comment on the generally poor quality of randomised controlled trials (RCT) in this field. More specifically, although they had identified 97 RCT, in only 10 were the methods of randomisation explained; in most trials the sample size was small (less than 30 per treatment group); and the drop out rate was often high or was not stated. They decided to exclude all studies that did not have a minimum of one-year observation of the participants. Their tentative conclusions are that, for obese children, family therapy and lifestyle modification appears to be effective in prevention and treatment, respectively. For adults, 'behavioural therapy and multicomponent strategies may be useful', as is 'continued therapist contact', and perhaps drug treatment up to nine months. Surgery 'appears to be effective in the morbidly obese'.

This raises the question of why is the research in this field of such poor quality? Obesity is a common and important problem for which effective treatments are available, so why is there not a plethora of well-controlled long-term RCTs, as there is for most of the important diseases such as cancers, heart disease or arthritis? The explanation may lie in the nature of the clinicians that deal with obesity (who may not be of scientific orientation) or in the nature of the disease and those who suffer from it, or at least of those who are willing to be enrolled in an RCT of obesity treatment. A patient with cancer, heart disease or arthritis will probably be referred to a hospital specialist, who can offer treatment that would not otherwise be available to the patient. If the patients have confidence in the line of treatment proposed, it is unlikely that they will drop out of treatment, or dabble in alternative treatments from time to time.

The situation with obese patients is quite different. In the single-centre trial described by Summerbell *et al.* (1998) there were initially 64 patients who met the entry criteria, recruited over a period of six months. Of these, 19 declined to be randomised to one of the three diet groups and of the 45 who were randomised, another 15 either dropped out or did not provide the data required for completion of the 16-week trial. The final results were obtained on 30 patients divided between three treatment arms. In drug trials, in which there is a greater incentive to participate, there are similar drop-out rates. For example, in the huge multi-centre trial of dexfenfluramine (Guy-Grand *et al.*, 1989) there were 822 patients recruited from 24 centres in 9 European countries, each centre was asked to provide at least 20, but no more than 42 patients. By the end of the trial (at 12 months) there remained only 63% of those on the drug and 54% of those on placebo. It is evident, therefore, that to achieve a two-arm drug trial with 30 completers in each group at 12 months, it is necessary to recruit about 170 eligible patients, assuming that about 30% of those eligible will decline to be randomised.

24.4.2 Steps towards more efficient treatment of obesity

Much of this Task Force report has been concerned with the influences which prevent treatments that work in metabolic ward conditions from being equally effective in the real world of free-living individuals. These influences are to be found in the obese person, in the healthcarer professionals who treat obesity, and in the general social environment. It is noteworthy that the 'behavioural' treatments, which are identified by the review of Glenny *et al.* (1997) because they 'appear to be effective' are not in themselves primary treatments. They do not directly affect energy balance, but they help the patient to comply with those aspects of treatment that do affect energy balance. For patients who have previously been unable to adhere to a low energy diet; behavioural therapy, continued therapist contact, and medication with anorectic drugs are all strategies that may be useful, and may help to make an effective treatment more efficient. Surgery is a special case because its characteristic is that it largely removes from the patient the need to comply voluntarily with a diet, the diet is effectively enforced by blocking the ability to eat a normal amount of food (Chapter 23).

However, this may have its disadvantages in the long run because the inhibition of food intake achieved by surgery or drugs will become less strong as time passes, and the ability to exert cognitive control may be less than it would have been without the 'helpful' treatment. The 2-year follow-up of cases treated by surgery shows a slight weight regain from the minimum weight at 12 months after the operation (Section 23.5). Although the patients on dexfenfluramine lost more weight than those on placebo during the 12-month trial reported by Guy-Grand *et al.* (1989), three years after the end of the trial at least one sub-group had regained all the weight lost, whereas the placebo group was still below the baseline weight (Pfohl *et al.* 1994). This certainly does not show that drug treatment is worse than placebo treatment in the long term, because these follow-up results were obtained from only a sub-group of 22 patients out of the 34 who completed the drug therapy part of the trial. However, it must warn us that, just as effective treatments may fail for lack of compliance, so also aids to compliance may fail with the passage of time. Perhaps the most important lesson we can learn is that, so long as the environmental pressures depicted in Fig. 24.1 tend to push individuals in the direction of increasing obesity, it is likely that even the best strategies for preventing and treating obesity will not be fully efficient.

24.5 Summary

- The professions involved in the treatment and prevention of obesity are, to varying degrees, virtually everyone in the population, since the equilibrium represented in Fig. 24.1 is affected by everything which affects our lifestyle.

- The professions most involved are those in healthcare who are able to offer reliable information about diet and physical activity, and in some cases treatment of obesity by psychological, pharmacological or surgical methods.

- The effectiveness of these health informers is limited by the activities of health misinformers, and by those who alter our environment in ways which usually favour the development of obesity.

- A solution to the problem requires concerted action by all these professions, as well as by the politicians and journalists who must try to balance the pressures of commercial interests with countervailing pressures that tend to shift the equilibrium in Fig. 24.1 towards the right. Specific suggestions about how this might be achieved are given in Chapter 26.

- Evaluations of treatment programmes with long follow-up data are biased towards certain types of treatment, which require less lifestyle change from the patients. Patients treated by surgery need lifetime follow-up for their own safety and drug trials are funded so as to permit effective follow-up and low drop-out rates. In contrast, it is very difficult to obtain good long-term follow-up for treatments based solely on lifestyle change (diet, exercise and CBT).

- Novel and simple diets gain better compliance than conventional diets that have been tried (and failed) on previous occasions. However, a novel diet will, in the long term, cease to be novel. There is probably a case for rotating lifestyle-based treatments every few months so as to preserve the effect of novelty.

- There is a conflict between those who try to treat and prevent obesity and those powerful interests whose livelihood depends on promoting 'obesogenic' features in the environment. It requires government action to tilt the balance in favour of those who seek to improve public health.

25
Suggestions for Further Research

25.1 Introduction

- Obesity is now a major public health problem in the UK. As far as possible, research in a particular specialist field should not be considered in isolation, but should be conceived, and assessed, in the wider context.

25.2 Health risks of obesity

- There is strong epidemiological evidence that obesity is associated with the health risks described in Chapter 2 and that the greater the degree of obesity and the younger the person, the greater is his or her risk, relative to normal-weight controls. However, there are many aspects of this relationship about which we need more detailed information.

- The association between obesity and mortality and morbidity is highly confounded by other factors such as cigarette smoking, alcohol intake, physical activity and diet. These are also correlated: for example, smokers are more likely to have a high alcohol intake and low intake of dietary antioxidants. As far as possible epidemiological studies on obesity should provide data on the smoking habits, alcohol intake, physical activity and diet of the subjects studied.

- For given disabilities, how much risk should be ascribed to total body fat, and how much to intra-abdominal body fat? It is, therefore, important that future studies should include a measure of abdominal fat, i.e. a measurement of waist circumference, as a minimum.

- Do the risk factors that are associated with obesity have the same effects as the same risk factor in a non-obese person? For example, does the risk associated with a given degree of hypertension in an obese person present the same threat to health as that degree of hypertension in a lean person?

- There is epidemiological evidence that substantial weight gain during adult life carries health risks not explained by the degree of obesity achieved. This observation needs to be confirmed and explained.

- Much more information is required about the subsequent health risks in obese children and adolescents.

- Health education programmes to limit obesity have been strikingly unsuccessful, possibly because there is anxiety about inducing eating disorders by excessive anti-obesity propaganda. More information is needed about the role (if any) of health education messages about obesity in causing eating disorders and on the social stigmatisation of obesity.

25.3 Clinical assessment of obesity

- It would be valuable to have an accurate marker for total body fat. This might be a substance produced by adipocytes in relation to their weight (e.g. leptin, see Section 6.5.1 and 6.5.2). Alternatively, it might be a tracer that mixes rapidly with fat (as labelled water does with body water, see Section 3.1.2) or a scanning technique that is not expensive in terms of time and money (see Section 3.2). This would enable workers to study the effect of treatments on fat loss, rather than merely on weight loss.

- There is evidence that different fat depots have different functions: for example, intra-abdominal fat versus subcutaneous fat (see Section 2.5). Also, fat on the hips and thighs of adult women may be a special store to provide energy for lactation (see Section 7.5.2). There may be other examples of fat depots with specialised functions. It would be useful to be able to identify and measure the size and activity of such depots, easily, in living subjects.

25.4 Epidemiology

- The increasing prevalence of obesity in the population makes it vital that regular surveys continue to be conducted in order to monitor trends and aid in the prediction of health service needs.

- There have been very few repeat cross-sectional surveys of children and young adults. These are essential in order to monitor trends in the prevalence of obesity and to aid in the prevention of obesity in adulthood.

- There is a need for more longitudinal studies, particularly among children and young adults.

- There have been very few studies of obesity among ethnic groups in the UK. There is, therefore, a need for more data on BMI and central adiposity, and also for research assessing the effects of obesity on morbidity and mortality in these groups.

- More research is needed among vegetarians to ascertain the reasons for their lower prevalence of obesity compared with that for omnivores.

25.5 Aetiology of obesity I

- The greatest need is for a reliable measure, among free-living people, of their habitual energy intake from food and drink.

- There is need for better understanding of the relationship between macronutrient balance and energy balance (see Chapter 9).

- A more detailed knowledge of the different phenotypes of obesity will allow a more precise

understanding of the factors leading to obesity in different individuals and hence to tailor treatments more appropriately.

25.6 Aetiology of obesity II: genetics

- The comments in Section 25.1 apply in particular to research on the genetics of obesity. The lay public equate the discovery of an obesity-related gene to a discovery that obesity is totally determined by inheritance and hence is untreatable. We endorse the suggestion of Allison & Faith (1997) that there is need for a simple model, comprehensible to the lay public, which explains the practical consequences of estimated heritability in a given population.

- Research on rare genetic causes of extreme obesity is moving very rapidly. These are extremely helpful in providing 'proof-of-principle' knowledge about fundamental principles of energy regulation.

- The possibility of gene therapy in some of these rare monogenic disorders looks increasingly likely, but will bring benefit to a very few people.

- There is a need to keep these rare monogenic disorders in perspective with regard to the developing epidemic of overweight and obesity, in which genetic effects are much subtler in creating a susceptibility to the fattening effects of the modern environment.

- The prevalence of obesity in a population changes much more quickly than the genetic makeup of the population. This suggests that the genes confer susceptibility to environmental influences. More research is needed to clarify these genetic–environmental interactions.

- The frequent call for research on gene–environment interactions is probably more relevant to obesity than to any other disease. In the post-genome era this will require integrated studies from the molecular, through the physiological, to the environment.

25.7 Aetiology of obesity III: critical periods for obesity development

- In a sense, every stage of growth is a critical period for obesity development, as subsequent stages start where the previous stage left off, not at a neutral baseline. However, it is evident that there is no critical period, in the sense that we could say: 'If a person is/is not obese at age *x* years, that is how it will be ever after'. Obesity can appear, or disappear, at any age, but the rate at which it will do so is slower in old people than young ones.

- Young adulthood is an age that has so far received little attention. The predisposing factors appear to be more environmental and beha-vioural than physiological. They are, therefore, amenable to intervention.

- The optimum means of preventing excess weight gain in childhood and adolescence (without precipitating eating disorders) is poorly resear-ched so far and should be a matter of high priority.

- For further understanding of critical periods we need longitudinal measurements in representa-tive samples of individuals (not groups) over the whole life span.

25.8 Aetiology of obesity IV: metabolic factors

- A clear picture of the metabolic features of lean and obese people has emerged from modern techniques for measuring body composition, and metabolic rate at rest and during various activi-ties (Sections 3.6, 5.3 and 8.2). The main area which still needs clarification concerns the influence of different lifestyles on energy expenditure, and the mechanism by which energy expenditure and energy intake are coupled (see also research suggestions in 25.5, 25.9 and 25.10).

- The possible role of gene variants in UCP2, UCP3 and β-$_3$ receptors in determining indivi-dual variations in metabolic rate is an area of current interest that should be resolved soon.

- Low levels of habitual energy expenditure undoubtedly contribute to obesity at a popula-tion level. It would be of value to determine whether genetic susceptibility to obesity is mediated through individual preferences in activity patterns and to determine whether these

are influenced by physiological factors (e.g. muscle fibre types and endorphin responses to exercise), or whether they are entirely socio-behavioural phenomena.

25.9 Aetiology of obesity V: macronutrient balance

- A more detailed understanding of the effects of specific dietary components (e.g. certain fatty acids, and slow versus fast-release proteins and carbohydrates) would be desirable.

- Most research to date has investigated the effect of macronutrients on energy expenditure (ther-mic effect of feeding or 'specific dynamic action'). In general, the macronutrient balance of isoenergetic diets has little effect on energy output.

- More information is needed on the effect of macronutrient balance on energy intake, and timing of meals.

- Is the oxidative hierarchy for macronutrients important? Is it immutable, or does it change with different diets, or different levels of physical activity?

- For practical reasons, many human studies are limited to a rather short time frame. Longer studies are desirable wherever possible. It is important to perform such studies in conditions that mimic a realistic environmental setting.

25.10 Aetiology of obesity VI: appetite control

- In spite of a significant body of existing research, there are still many gaps in our understanding of appetite regulation within the context of normal living. Studies have tended to adopt simple paradigms in which covariables are held con-stant. This limits the applicability of some of the findings.

- There is a need to integrate research from neu-roendocrinology, physiology and psychobiology. Modern brain imaging procedures offer oppor-tunities for a fresh approach to understanding human appetite control.

- The causes of aberrant appetite drives in eating

disorders (with particular reference to causes of bingeing) remain an important area for future research.

25.11 Aetiology of obesity VII: endocrine causes

- It is difficult to suggest definite research questions in this field at present. There are many endocrine changes in obesity, most of which prove to be consequences, rather than causes of obesity, since they revert towards normal when body composition normalises. The hottest topic at present is leptin, for which the role in energy balance in man is unclear. Gut hormones play a part in regulating food intake, but again the control system is so confounded by interaction between systems that a good research question is difficult to define. The suggestions for further research listed in Section 25.10 apply equally to the endocrine research agenda.

25.12 Aetiology of obesity VIII: psychological factors

- Every clinician in this field is aware that psychological distress is a feature of patients who seek treatment for obesity. However, there are equally obese people who are evidently not distressed, and do not seek treatment, so clinic populations are biased in this respect. It is virtually impossible to design a study which will show which psychological problems predispose to obesity, and which are a consequence of obesity or attempt to treat the obesity. As with endocrine changes (Section 25.11) this extensive confounding makes research questions difficult to define.

25.13 Aetiology of obesity IX: diet and epidemiology

- One of the most intriguing, but unexplained, associations with obesity concerns gender, education and social class (Sections 4.2 and 4.3). Obesity is associated more strongly with lower socio-economic class in men than in women, but this varies between countries. Level of education is negatively associated with obesity, especially with respect to risk factors such as parity.

Plausible hypotheses to explain these associations are that poorer, less educated people have a diet which is more likely to promote obesity, or that they have less effective cognitive control of excess weight, but there is no evidence to support either speculation. More research is required in this area.

25.14 Aetiology of obesity X: food choice, food policy and eating patterns

- There is a need for better understanding of the nature and importance of heightened responsiveness to external cues and 'palatability' and their relationship to food choice, initiation of eating, and long-term energy balance.

- There is a need to establish the importance and implications of restrained eating and/or dieting in the development or control of compulsive eating, eating disorders and obesity.

- There is a need for a better understanding of the influences of specific tastes, flavours, and textures which may contribute to 'fat' preferences, the potential influence of these sensory responses on food selection, and their associations with energy balance and weight status.

- The possible relationships of specific food or food group selections and nutrient sources to variability in dietary fat intakes, energy density and body weight status need to be clarified.

- There is a need for a better understanding of the acquisition and modification of food preferences in general, including the role of energy density, food structure and composition, and psychobiological effects (e.g. mood, satiety), and improved understanding of the nature and role of food 'cravings'.

- The relationships of hedonic value or specific sensory characteristics of foods and meals to energy intake, post-prandial satiety and metabolism need to be determined.

- More research is needed into the physiological, cognitive, and behavioural responses to the availability and consumption of macronutrient-replaced and/or reduced-energy food products.

- Social and psychobiological influences on uptake

and long-term compliance with public guidance on diet and lifestyle, including communication strategies need to be determined.

- The effects of changes in eating patterns, particularly the timing of insertion of extra eating events ('snacks'), and their composition, on satiety, compensatory eating, and long-term energy balance needs to be critically evaluated.

25.15 Aetiology of obesity XI: physical inactivity

- Further studies are needed on the mechanism and extent to which various levels of exercise are related to subsequent energy and macronutrient intake.

- Just as we need to know why people comply to varying extents with dietary advice that they know to be beneficial, we need similar information about physical activity.

- Research indicates that it is more effective to encourage children not to be very inactive, than directly to encourage them to be active. Research is needed to explain this finding, and to see if it applies also to adults, and to obese adults.

25.16 Significance of within person weight variation

- Existing databases should be examined to see if the characteristics of weight variability or stability are constant within individuals, or if people switch from one category to another; and if so, what causes them to do so.

- There is a need to obtain better data on the magnitude of the variation, and the extent to which this variation decreases the estimated association between obesity and health risk.

25.17 Prevention of obesity

- We need to know why obesity is not seen as a health hazard by most of the public and the media, despite the evidence available.

- There appears to be an opportunity to prevent obesity in primary schoolchildren. Pilot schemes are required to see if this can be used in practice.

- The SIGN guidelines for secondary prevention of obesity by general practitioners provide an opportunity to study the efficacy of this approach.

- The problem of prevention of obesity is essentially the same as the problem of maintenance of weight loss (see Chapter 17). Therefore, similar research objectives apply.

25.18 Treatment of obesity I

- Research is needed to identify individuals, e.g. those with intra-abdominal fat, who would particularly benefit from losing weight. This would enable resources to be used more effectively.

- Research is needed to improve weight loss outcomes in those individuals who are resistant to treatment.

- Setting a series of small weight goals, rather than a larger final weight target, may be seen as more achievable by patients and increase success. Research is needed in this area.

- Further exploration into the treatment of obesity using motivational interviewing and the 'stages of change model' is needed.

25.19 Treatment of obesity II: dietary treatment

- There is a need to know more about the potential benefits of high carbohydrate, low fat diets *ad libitum* versus restricted diets in weight loss and weight maintenance programmes.

- Further research is needed in the area of energy prescribed diets, i.e. those that result in a negative energy balance of 2.1–4.2 MJ (500–1000 kcal) per day.

- Further research is needed into the effectiveness of group versus individual therapy.

25.20 Treatment of obesity III: physical activity and exercise

- The mechanisms by which exercise is associated with long-term sustained weight loss have not been determined.

- The ideal combination of aerobic and resistance training, and their relationship with macro-nutrient intake and body composition change during weight loss, have not been established.

- Programme and individual factors associated with early dropout or reluctance to take up exercise among obese people have yet to be established. This information is necessary for individual tailoring of programmes.

- Programme and individual factors associated with successful maintenance of exercise routines in obese people have not been fully determined.

25.21 Treatment of obesity IV: behavioural treatment

- The value of CBT in achieving more prolonged weight loss has been established (Chapter 21). Future research needs to clarify how CBT can best be combined with other types of treatment to achieve the best overall results with maximum economy of time and resources.

- Much research on CBT has been conducted on middle-class patients who are willing to pay for such treatment. More information is needed about the extent to which these techniques can be used effectively in poorer and less well-educated people.

- CBT has been successful in treating disabilities associated with obesity (e.g. low self-esteem, negative body image). Follow-up research is needed to see if removing these disabilities helps or hinders weight loss and hence what effect it has on long-term weight-related complications such as diabetes, hypertension and osteoarthritis.

25.22 Treatment of obesity V: pharmacotherapy for obesity

- This is the area of obesity research that is best funded and most active, as there are huge profits to be made from an effective and safe anti-obesity drug. There is no need to suggest further research in this area.

25.23 Treatment of obesity VI: surgical treatments

- The efficacy of gastric surgery in causing weight loss is clearly established and the SOS study in Sweden shows that massive weight loss in severely obese people confers substantial benefits in health and quality of life. Further research is needed on the category of obese people who would benefit from surgical treatment and the long-term costs as well as benefits of providing lifetime monitoring for such patients.

- Further research is needed on less invasive methods of treatment, such as jaw wiring and waist cords.

25.24 Treatment of obesity VII: resources and evaluation

- More research on the cost-effectiveness of procedures to prevent and treat obesity is essential if public funding is to be obtained for the recommendations in Chapter 26. The problem of circularity is a familiar one, funds for programmes depend on showing cost-effectiveness, but to show cost-effectiveness requires funds for programmes.

- The solution to this vicious circle is to ensure that whenever programmes are set up the resources are carefully defined, and there is proper provision for evaluation of the outcome.

- There is urgent need for better studies on lifestyle-based treatment programmes, to balance the publications on surgical or drug treatments.

26
Recommendations of the BNF Task Force on Obesity

We believe that to reverse the current trend towards increasing obesity it will be necessary to obtain consensus on four key issues, on which action must be taken by various groups of people. Changes are needed both in people and in the social and economic environment in which they live. The key issues are as follows.

I.   Obesity is a serious health hazard to an increasing proportion of the population. Action is needed now to prevent the spread of the problem to epidemic proportions.
II.   Part of the solution involves a change in the national diet towards inclusion of more foods of low energy density, such as fruit and vegetables.
III. Another part of the solution involves a change in national lifestyle to involve a higher level of physical activity.
IV.   Strategies are needed both for prevention and for treatment of obesity, but one strategy cannot be expected to be effective for both objectives.

There is nothing impossible or contradictory about these issues, and if II and III were grasped it would confer great benefit to the general health of the public, in addition to the specific effect in controlling obesity. The groups within the population who need to grasp these issues are again four, but many individuals will fall into more than one group. The groups to whom our recommendations are addressed are as follows.

A: Policy makers
B: Those who can contribute to the prevention of obesity
C: Those who can contribute to the treatment of obesity
D: Communicators and educators who can influence the attitudes of the public and/or healthcare professionals towards obesity

The recommendations set out below are very brief statements showing how the understanding and actions of these groups may work together to achieve effective action of the key issues. It does not lie within the power of any single group to achieve the overall objectives: concerted action is needed. The evidence on which the recommendations are based is given within the text of the book and will not be repeated here. However, reference is made to the important sections where evidence to support the recommendations can be found.

A. To policy makers

Government, local authorities and health authorities.

Action on issue I

As the prevalence of obesity has increased so dramatically in the last few years, the explanation for this change must lie in environmental rather than genetic factors, and so in principle must be reversible (Chapters 2 and 6). Policy makers are the group who are best placed to alter these environmental factors by example, by regulation, and by showing that they take the problem seriously. If policy makers are not seen to recognise the importance of the 'obesogenic' environment, there is little hope that the situation will improve.

Action on issues II, III and IV

Commercial slimming clubs can provide a valuable service. Local health authorities should consider a system of endorsement of those clubs which provide a good service, based on sound principles for the appropriate achievement and maintenance of weight loss in overweight people.

The work of responsible healthcare workers in the field of obesity management is undermined by irresponsible claims for weight loss cures for which there is no evidence of efficacy. Although medicinal claims for pharmaceutical preparations are tightly regulated, the control of charlatans in the weight loss field is very loose. Sanctions, such as prosecutions under the Trade Descriptions Act, put the burden on the local authority to show the claims are false, rather than on the advertiser to show that they are true. We believe that it is in the public interest that this burden of proof should be shifted onto the advertiser, prior to the publication of the advert.

Action on issue III

To change the national level of activity requires facilities which the individual cannot provide: it requires action from central government, local authorities and health authorities to provide recreational facilities and public highways that are safe and convenient places in which to take more physical activity (Chapters 15 and 20). Transport policy should aim to provide positive incentives to walk or cycle at least part of the way to work, rather than to rely on motorised transport.

B. To those in a position to help to prevent obesity

Public health directors, general practitioners, dietitians, practice nurses and other healthcare professionals, schools, teachers, parents and carers, slimming clubs and the diet, food and fitness industry.

Action on issue I

This group can contribute to the general recognition of the range of weight-for-height at which health risks become significant, so that people entering this range can seek to control their weight gain (Chapter 2).

Action on issue II

The food and catering industry could continue to develop and promote foods of lower energy density, and ensure that these are readily available and attractively presented (Chapter 18).

Action on issue III

A more physically active lifestyle should continue throughout life from childhood to old age (Chapters 15 and 20). This requires action from school authorities and from policy makers to provide opportunities for safe, enjoyable and affordable physical activity for all members of the population.

Action on issue IV

Prevention of weight regain in obese people who have lost weight is of paramount importance: this area is considered below.

C. To those who treat obese people

General practitioners, dietitians, exercise specialists, practice nurses and other healthcare professionals, local health authorities, slimming clubs, and the diet industry.

Many members of this group are also in group B. Their role in treatment will be considered here.

Action on issue I

Healthcare professionals with one-to-one contact with the public are especially well placed to explain to overweight people the relation of their weight to their disabilities (Chapter 2) and the benefits that weight loss might bring (Chapter 17).

Action on issues II and III

It is probably worse to treat obesity inadequately than not to try to treat it at all. To provide adequate treatment it is necessary to have an understanding of the physiological, social and psychological bases of obesity, and to be able and willing to provide accurate information and long-term support for the obese person. This report tries to set out clearly current knowledge on these topics. The chances of controlling the obesity problem in the UK would be greater if those health care professionals who do not possess, and do not intend to acquire, the necessary skill and concern for obese people would refer them to other health care professionals who are better equipped. Local health authorities need to ensure that such people are available.

Action on issue IV

Successful management of obesity is never a quick or simple process. It is not possible to summarise briefly the complexities of treatment programmes, which are described in detail elsewhere in this report, but the essential steps are as follows.

(a) To clarify, by discussion with the obese individual, the cost/benefit of losing weight, or not, and to decide if treatment is likely to bring net benefit to him or her (Chapter 17). In particular to agree if his or her present weight represents a health hazard and, if so, what magnitude of weight loss would reduce this hazard to an acceptable level.

(b) To choose, depending on the circumstances of the individual and the treatment facilities available, the treatment modes that appear most likely to achieve the desired result (Chapters 18 to 22 for treatment modes, and Chapter 17 for treatment objectives).

(c) To ensure that a competent and sympathetic healthcarer is available to review progress at appropriate intervals (normally every 1–4 weeks). To provide encouragement if progress is good, and to troubleshoot (and if necessary change the treatment option) if it is not. Whatever happens, those involved should strive to retain the victim/rescuer rather than the prosecutor/defaulter relationship (Section 19.3).

(d) To refrain from making exaggerated claims for the efficacy or rapidity of weight-loss programmes, because these undermine the efforts of those who are providing a reliable but less spectacular service (Chapter 18).

(e) To provide an indefinite after-weight-loss service on which the formerly obese person can call if they experience unwanted weight regain. This might be integrated with the services designed to prevent obesity described above.

D. To communicators who shape the public and healthcare professionals' attitudes to obesity and weight loss

Journalists/editors/producers in both print and broadcast media, and health educators, the medical royal colleges.

Action on issue I

The Task Force believes that the public attitude to obesity is a major contribution to the increasing prevalence of the condition, and for this the media must bear some responsibility. There is great public interest in news items about a 'breakthrough' in the field of obesity, followed later by an exposé of the flaws in any previous claims. It is difficult to produce punchy copy which distinguishes between those who are of normal weight and inappropriately want to lose weight, and those who would benefit from weight loss but do not realise this. However, the media should refrain from suggesting that there are conflicts of scientific opinion in areas where they do not exist.

The work of a journalist in the healthcare field is made easier by a constant flow of 'press releases' from public relations companies extolling the virtues of particular therapies or products, especially in the field of weight loss. If the press release copy is published uncritically this publication is then used as an endorsement of the therapy or product, which may be seriously misleading to the public. Journalists have a responsibility to check the validity of claims that they quote.

The questions asked by medical journalists' associations (Appendix 1) indicate an interest in the causes of obesity and in methods of achieving (preferably rapid) weight loss. This is understandable, but it would be encouraging if obesity was regarded primarily as a public health problem rather than a cosmetic one.

The Royal Colleges responsible for standards of professional education among healthcare professionals (doctors and nurses) need to ensure that their examinations look for a proper understanding of the causes, consequences and management of obesity among the professionals whom they license.

Appendix:
Answers to Questions from
Medical Journalists

The Task Force secretariat asked the Medical Journalists Association (MJA) and the Guild of Health Writers (GHW) to send in a list of the questions about obesity that most concerned their members. We are very grateful to John Illman (MJA) and to Jean Williams and Claire Crowther (GHW) for responding with the questions that are set out below, with consensus answers from the Task Force. The questions are grouped under headings, in the same order as in the Task Force report.

(a) Definition of obesity

Q. I've always been a bit on the plump side, but how can I tell if I'm really overweight, or just a bit chubby?

A. An operational definition of obesity in adults, based on risk to health, is set out in Chapter 2. Briefly, a body mass index (BMI) of 20–25 is OK and one above 30 is obese. If you are in the range 25–30 your health risk will be determined by such factors as a family history of heart disease or diabetes and the distribution of your body fat, but in any case you should not let your weight creep up into the obese range. More muscular individuals may have a slightly higher BMI without necessarily being overweight. Waist circumference is also thought to be important in determining health risk. There is an increased risk to health associated with a waist circumference of over 94 cm (34 in) in men and over 80 cm (32 in) in women. A substantial risk to health is associated with a waist circumference of over 102 cm (40 in) in men and over 88 cm (35 in) in women.

(b) Epidemiology of obesity

Q. Will giving up smoking make me gain weight?

A. Stopping smoking will not make you gain weight, but it is a danger period, which requires vigilance (see Section 4.4). Even if you gain a few pounds, it is healthier to stop smoking. The health risk of smoking 20 cigarettes a day is equivalent to the health risk of being 20 kg (44 lb) overweight and it is highly unlikely that you will gain that much weight.

Q. Where does Britain stand in the obesity league in the Western World?

A. The proportion of the population with obesity in the UK is intermediate, being below the levels in the USA, Australasia, south and east Europe, and above Scandinavia and Japan. In all developed countries, and in many developing countries, obesity is increasing, which means there are no grounds for complacency.

Q. Why do people become obese at age 30–50 years? To what extent are lifestyle stresses precursors to obesity, for example divorce, bereavement and job loss?

A. There is no simple answer to this question (see Chapters 5–14). Many people increase in weight steadily throughout life and as a result become obese in middle-age. An important factor is decreasing physical activity (e.g. giving up sport participation in late 20s) without a corresponding decrease in energy intake.

Q. Does HRT make you gain weight?

A. No.

Q. Is it true that obese people have a lower metabolic rate and really do not eat any more than those of normal weight?

A. No. On average, obese people have higher energy expenditures than lean people of the same age, height and gender. They must therefore eat more to maintain their extra weight, but many obese people sincerely believe that they eat less than normal. For years scientists have been looking for obese people with very low metabolic requirements, but when they are tested in a metabolic ward the error lies with the obese person's estimation of their diet, rather than with their metabolism.

Q. Does obesity run in families?

A. Yes, but both cultural and genetic effects (see Chapter 6) can influence this. There is a strong interaction between the genetic pre-disposition and the environment. Obesity is rarely seen in cultures where energy expenditure is high and the energy density of the diet is low, even though these are the conditions in which a 'thrifty gene' would confer a survival advantage.

Q. Is obesity really a result of simple overeating?

A. Yes, but overeating is not 'simple' (see Chapters 9, 10 and 13).

Q. Why do we eat less fruit and vegetables in the UK compared with the French or Greeks? Is it availability or culture? Is it easier for the food industry to produce high-fat than low-fat foods?

A. The lower consumption of fruit and vegetables in the UK probably has historical and agricultural explanations (see Chapter 14) which have shaped the national cuisine to value meat and dairy

products. Repeated consumption of high fat foods can potentially reinforce the liking for these foods.

The food industry produces a wide variety of products ranging from those containing no fat (e.g. many breakfast cereals) to those that are completely comprised of fat (e.g. cooking oils). Complex meal products produced commercially have a composition that is not necessarily much different from their traditional counterparts prepared in the home. There is no special value to the food industry selling fat over other ingredients (Section 14.3), but it is difficult to significantly alter the composition of many foods without changing their sensory acceptability or functionality. Thus, while there have been tremendous efforts to market reduced-fat or reduced-energy versions of traditional foods, these have met with mixed success with consumers.

Q. To what extent does our current lifestyle (e.g. more use of convenience foods versus less home cooking) contribute to the increased prevalence of obesity?

A. While diet composition is undoubtedly important, Chapter 14 points out that changes in diet composition or marketing in the UK and other western nations do not logically explain the marked rises in obesity observed over the past two decades, which probably more closely parallel changes in physical activity.

Q. Is it true that inactivity is contributing to obesity in children? What can be done about it? Should children take more exercise or eat differently?

A. Very few studies show any relationship at all between activity and body fat in children and adolescents, partly because habitual activity is difficult to measure. For general health reasons, all children should be active (see Chapter 15), but some children need to be much more active than they are. It is the amount of time spent in inactive pursuits (e.g. television watching and computer games) that is most critical to weight gain or loss in children.

Q. Do psychological factors (e.g. comfort eating) sometimes result in obesity?

A. Yes, some people become fat because a psychological disturbance causes them to dramatically overeat (see Chapter 12), but this is not the main reason for the increased prevalence of obesity.

Q. Is there any problem with eating between meals? If so, does it depend on the behaviour pattern, or on the choice of foods eaten?

A. Section 14.4 clearly documents that, at a given total energy intake, the typical frequency or pattern of eating across the day makes little difference to energy balance. Indeed, people with high energy requirements (e.g. athletes) tend to eat frequently, but are lean. However, the composition of foods is important, with high-fat, energy-dense foods likely to be more problematic for weight control, whether eaten within or between main 'meals'. Irregular eating patterns may also create more difficulties for personal efforts to control intake and weight.

Q. Are children eating breakfast less often than in previous years? Is this resulting in a greater intake of high-fat foods from the tuck shop?

A. A recent survey, published by Gardner Merchant (1998) *What are today's children eating?* found that just 6% of 8- to 16-year-old children leave for school with nothing to eat or drink. This figure, however, rises to 12% in those aged 15–16 years and to 18% for girls in the same age group. There is no reliable data on the influence of high-fat foods from tuck shops on consumption patterns and nutritional intake of children.

(c) Treatment of obesity by diet and slimming products

Q. Is yo-yo dieting really bad for you?

A. Yes, it is disheartening to regain lost weight, and it would be better to aim to lose more slowly and maintain the loss. There is no evidence that yo-yo dieting causes a decrease in metabolic rate. Weight variability is associated with health risk (see Chapter 16) but it is not clear if the health risk is caused by the weight variation.

Q. Why do I lose weight quickly in the first few weeks of dieting, and then find it so hard to shift the extra pounds after this?

A. There are two main reasons:

• When you start to diet, you lose glycogen and the water associated with it. For every 1000 kcal energy deficit, you would use up 1 kg of this glycogen and water mixture. When this supply runs low, the energy is drawn mainly from adipose tissue; for a deficit of 1000 kcal you would use up only 140 g of adipose tissue. Therefore, the rate of weight loss for a given daily energy deficit decreases when the energy reserve being used by the body switches from mainly glycogen to mainly fat.

• When people start on a diet they are enthusiastic to lose weight and are careful to keep to the diet, but after a week or so they become somewhat bored and are not so strict, so extra food is consumed.

It is important to aim for an appropriate rate of weight loss (see Chapter 18).

Q. I want to lose weight before my holiday in a month's time. Is crash dieting harmful?

A. If 'crash dieting' means having less than 3.4 MJ (800 kcal) per day it is harmful, because in total starvation about half the weight lost is lean tissue and half fat, so crash dieting over a month would cause too large a loss of lean tissue. Also, when you went on holiday and ate normally you would experience a rapid weight regain, as your glycogen stores refilled (see Chapter 18).

Q. How can I tell how many calories a day I should be eating if I want to lose weight?

A. If you eat 1000 kcal/day less than you expend you will (in the long run) lose 1 kg/week. There are formulae to predict energy expenditure (based on weight, height, age, gender and level of activity) but these are not particularly helpful to the would-be dieter, because it is so difficult to calculate accurately how many calories your diet supplies. In practice it is better to use the rate of weight loss over several weeks as a guide: if you are losing more than 1 kg/week your diet is too restricted: if you are not losing weight at all it is not restricted enough.

Q. Do slimming products really help you to lose weight?

A. Use of slimming products does not guarantee weight loss, if you eat twice as much of a calorie-reduced food as you would have done for the normal food it is unlikely you will lose weight. However, if using low-calorie foods as part of a calorie-controlled diet helps you to reduce your total energy intake such foods will help you to lose weight.

Q. Is there a problem with obesity in older people – do they reduce their activity and not reduce their food intake to compensate? How should diet change with age?

A. Both inactivity and obesity are most prevalent in people who are 55–64 years old. Ironically, activity has the greatest potential to benefit older people who lose physical and social independence if they are inactive. They should maintain activity to preserve lean tissue, and to be able to eat sufficient food to maintain nutrient intake.

Q. Does the food combining diet help you to lose weight?

A. Any regimen in which you must follow rules about what you can and cannot eat will probably cause weight loss, at least for a few weeks, because you will reduce your total energy intake. However, there is no scientific foundation for the idea that you will gain weight if, for example, you eat protein and carbohydrate together, or fruit with meals instead of separately. The weight loss on a diet depends on the energy value of the diet, not at all on the sequence or combinations in which food items are eaten.

Q. Are low-fat diets appropriate for everyone who wants to lose weight?

A. Yes, usually, but it depends on just how low in fat they are. We need small amounts of fat to remain healthy, oily fish, for example, gives some

protection against heart disease. Also, very low-fat diets are difficult to keep to. It takes more than simply reducing fat intake to lose weight, it takes a reduction in total calorie intake and/or increase in energy expenditure through physical activity.

Q. Does exercise really help you to lose weight?

A. Yes, although exercise has a weaker effect on weight loss than dieting, it has a strong effect on general health. Everyone should, therefore, exercise whether they are overweight or not. People who need to lose weight should combine dieting and exercise, but the more overweight they are the more they will have to rely on dieting (see Chapters 15 and 20).

(d) Treatment of obesity by drugs

Q. I've tried all sorts of diets without success over the years, could anti-obesity drugs help me?

A. Anti-obesity drugs may cause short-term weight loss in conjunction with a diet (see Chapter 21). A well-designed diet is more effective in the long run, and only 'fails' if you do not keep to it or have unrealistic expectations (see Chapter 19).

Q. Will there ever be a pill to prevent obesity?

A. Probably not. It would have to reduce energy intake and/or increase energy expenditure (see Chapter 5) and be taken for life by practically everyone, because most of the population is susceptible to obesity (see Chapter 16). It would also have to be taken before full adulthood is reached and it is unlikely it would be cost-effective or safe in these conditions.

Q. Are drug treatments a good way forward, or will drugs treat the symptoms rather than the cause? Is cultural therapy a better answer than drug therapy?

A. The requirements for an effective drug therapy are set out in the previous answer, and for a cultural therapy in Chapters 17–21. Drugs will be useful to the extent that they make lifestyle changes easier to achieve, provided that they are cost-effective and safe.

(e) Maintenance of weight loss

Q. What's the best way to keep weight off for good? I have successfully lost pounds on diets in the past, but they always creep back on again and it is so demoralising. Is there a way around it?

A. Weight maintenance is not automatic; it requires vigilance (see Section 18.4). Some people rely on a regular brisk walking routine for 30 minutes a day, increasing to 45 or 60 minutes a day. The best way around it is to continue to practice, to some degree, those steps that led to the weight loss in the first place.

(f) Obesity management in childhood

Q. Should overweight children be put on diets?

A. No, the objective is not to lose weight, but to control weight gain (see Section 18.1.1). Children should be encouraged to eat healthier meals along with their families and to be active rather than watching TV.

Q. Are we educating children in schools about obesity/food and nutrition?

A. Not enough, but this is an area in which the British Nutrition Foundation (BNF) teaching packs have been very well received. Further information about BNF resources can be found on the BNF website (www.nutrition.org.uk). Education for exercise and healthy nutrition should be (but is not) a compulsory part of the curriculum.

Q. Is there a particular danger age, e.g. if obese by 15 obese for life?

A. This is discussed fully in Chapter 7. In general the longer children remain fat, the more likely they will be fat for life. The best opportunity to prevent obesity in children is probably between the ages of 5 and 12 years (see Chapter 18.1.1).

(g) Obesity in pregnancy

Q. Should you diet in pregnancy if you are overweight at the start?

A. Not to lose weight, but to limit weight gain (see Section 18.1.2).

Q. What is the best way to lose weight after a baby?

A. Breast feeding uses some of your excess body fat to feed the baby (and has other advantages for the baby). Make sure you are being active: 30–45 minutes of pram pushing on as many days as possible, and specific muscle toning exercises for the abdominal and hip region. Make sure you are eating regularly and healthily.

(h) Who should treat obesity, and how?

Q. Should GPs be doing more about obesity? Do they need to know more about nutrition?

A. Yes, to both questions (see Chapter 24). Attempts are being made to improve the situation (e.g. Scottish Intercollegiate Guidelines Network, 1996) but change will take time.

Q. What is the best medical practice in the treatment of obesity?

A. Weight loss followed by a weight maintenance programme. For details see Chapters 16–25.

Glossary

Adipocyte: A mature fat cell.

Adipogenic: The potential to increase adiposity.

Adipostat: A physiological mechanism which contributes towards control of body fatness.

Alleles: Alternative forms of a gene found at the same locus on homologous chromosomes.

Apoptosis: Programmed cell death.

Appetite: The drive to eat, especially related to food with specific sensory qualities (see also **Hunger**).

Apronectomy: Surgical removal of extra skin and fat from the abdomen.

Association: In relation to genetics, association is the occurrence of a particular allele in a group of subjects more often than can be accounted for by chance.

Bardet Biedl syndrome (BBS): An autosomal recessive condition that results in mental retardation, retinitis pigmentosa, polydactyly, hypogonadotrophic hypogonadism and obesity.

Basal metabolic rate (BMR): Energy expended on the fundamental 'running costs' of an organism; including respiration, circulation, cellular homeostasis and cellular repair. Measured 12 hours after a meal in a thermo-neutral environment, at rest.

Binge eating disorder (BED): Consumption of objectively large amounts of food with a subjective loss of control, at least twice a week. Diagnosis requires the problem to have been present at least 6 months and to cause marked distress.

Body Mass Index (BMI): (see also **Quetelet's Index**) An index used to assess the degree of overweight or obesity; calculated using the equation: weight (kg) ÷ (height (m))^2. In this book, a BMI of over 25 is considered overweight and a BMI of over 30 is considered obese.

Brown adipose tissue (BAT): Highly vascular tissue with a specialised function of generating heat to maintain the body temperature of small mammals when the ambient temperature is low.

cDNA: Single stranded DNA complementary to a messenger RNA (mRNA).

Chromosomes: Thread-like bodies situated within the nucleus and composed of DNA and protein.

Clones: Cells derived from a single cell by repeated mitoses and all having the same genetic constitution (see also **Mitosis**).

Codon: A sequence of 3 adjacent nucleotides, which code for 1 amino acid or the end of an amino acid chain (a peptide or protein).

Cohen's syndrome: An autosomal recessive condition resulting in learning difficulties, a typical facial appearance, small hands and feet, short stature and truncal obesity.

Cushing's syndrome: A condition that occurs as a result of excess corticosteroid secretion from the adrenal gland. Progressive central obesity is common.

Dietary induced thermogenesis (DIT): Obligatory energy expended in the digestion, absorption, transport and metabolism of recently ingested food. Also known as post-prandial thermogenesis; the term Specific Dynamic Action is now obsolete.

Epidemiology: A study of the distribution and determinants of disease within and between populations.

Epistasis: Effects of the alleles at one locus may depend on which alleles are present on another locus.

Exercise: (see also **Physical activity** and **Sport**) A component of physical activity, which is volitional, planned, structured, repetitive and aimed at improving or maintaining health.

Fat free mass (FFM): The sum of all tissues in the body, minus fat.

Gamete: Cell containing one set of chromosomes.

Gene: A part of the DNA molecule that directs the synthesis of a specific polypeptide chain. It is composed of many codons.

Genotype: Genetic constitution of an individual.

Homologous chromosomes: Chromosomes that pair during meiosis and contain identical loci (see also **Meiosis**).

Hunger: Drive to eat resulting from an energy intake inadequate to maintain energy balance (see also **Appetite**).

Insulin dependent diabetes mellitus (IDDM): An endocrine disorder caused by insulin deficiency. Treatment requires the regular injection of insulin.

LGA (large for gestation age): LGA babies are above the 90th centile for weight at birth.

Leptin: A protein that is thought to act on the central nervous system to inhibit food intake and regulate energy expenditure.

Linkage disequilibrium: The association of two linked alleles more frequently than would be expected by chance.

Lipase: An enzyme that breaks down fat, to produce fatty acids and glycerol.

Lipectomy: Surgical removal of fat.

Liposuction: The sucking out of fat from under the skin.

Locus: The site of a gene on a chromosome.

Macrosomia: Reflects the enlargement of all organs, except the brain and kidneys, in newborn babies. Cellular hyperplasia and hypertrophy of tissues occur due to the effects of insulin.

Meiosis: A process of cell division, resulting in the formation of gametes.

Metabolic equivalent (MET): The energy required to perform an activity, expressed as a multiple of energy requirement at rest, or RMR.

Mitosis: Division of a cell nucleus that results in the formation of two cells, each with the same number of chromosomes as the parent nucleus.

Myocardial infarction: A heart attack; occurs when an artery to the heart muscle is blocked.

Non-insulin dependent diabetes (NIDDM): A metabolic disorder, which occurs as a result of insensitivity to the action of insulin. Often associated with overweight or obesity, treatment is by diet and/or oral hypoglycaemic agents.

Northern blot: Technique for transferring RNA fragments from an agarose gel to a nitro-cellulose filter on which they can be hybridised to complementary DNA.

Obesity: A BMI of over 30 in adults.

Overweight: A BMI of between 25 and 29.9 in adults.

Oxidation: In the context of use of fuel in the body, oxidation is the process of adding oxygen to release energy.

Phenotype: Appearance (physical, biochemical or physiological) of an individual which results from the interaction of the environment and genotype.

Physical activity: The integrated sum of all minor physical movements, together with all gross muscular work involved in moving the body or in performing physical work.

Physical activity level (PAL): Total energy expenditure divided by BMR.

Physical fitness: A multidimensional indicator of several functional capacities, e.g. cardiovascular endurance, muscular strength and/or mobility.

Polycystic ovarian syndrome (PCOS): The association of hyperandrogenism with chronic anovulation in women. Obesity is commonly, but not universally present.

Post-prandial thermogenesis (PPT): See DIT.

Prader–Willi syndrome: A rare genetic disorder that results initially in neonatal hypotonia, feeding difficulties and failure to thrive. By 2–3 years of age, it results in insatiable food seeking behaviour, weight gain and obesity.

Quetelet's index: Alternative name for BMI, named after the Belgian researcher who first proposed this index.

Respiratory quotient (RQ): The ratio of the amount of carbon dioxide produced to the amount of oxygen consumed. Lower quotients indicate a greater use of fat as a source of fuel and higher quotients indicate a greater use of carbohydrates.

Resting metabolic rate (RMR): The metabolic rate in an individual at rest. In contrast to BMR, RMR can be measured within a shorter interval from the last meal.

Restriction fragment polymorphism (RFLP): Polymorphism due to the presence or absence of a particular restriction site within DNA. A restriction fragment is a DNA fragment generated by a restriction endonuclease.

Seasonally affected disorder (SAD): A disorder characterised by atypical depressive episodes, which tend to occur seasonally.

Segregation of genes: The segregation of alleles during meiosis so that each gamete contains only one member of each pair of alleles.

Social class: Categorised according to the *Standard Occupational Classification*, Volume 3, OPCS. London:HMSO. The classification is as follows:

I	professional (e.g. accountants, engineers, doctors)
II	managerial and technical/intermediate (e.g. marketing and sales managers, teachers, journalists, nurses)
III non-manual	skilled occupations – non manual (e.g. clerks, shop assistants, cashiers)
III manual	skilled occupations – manual (e.g. carpenters, goods van drivers, joiners, cooks)
IV	partly skilled (e.g. security guards, machine tool operators, farm workers)
V	unskilled occupations (e.g. labourers, cleaners)

Social mobility: A change in social class from childhood to adulthood.

Sport: Physical activity that involves structured competitive situations governed by rules.

Stapled gastroplasty: An operation that divides the stomach by means of a line of staples into a small upper pouch with a capacity of about 215 ml. Used in the surgical treatment of obesity.

Stop codon: One of three codons that cause termination of protein synthesis.

Total energy expenditure: The total amount of energy expended by an organism; includes BMR and also physical activity

Triacylglycerol: Neutral fat consisting of a molecule of glycerol combined with three fatty acids. Also called triglyceride.

Uncoupling protein: A mitochondrial protein unique to BAT, responsible for the capacity of BAT for heat production.

Waist circumference: A useful measure of health risk in relation to obesity. A waist circumference of over 94 cm (34 in) in men and over 80 cm (32 in) in women is thought to be associated with an increased health risk. A substantial risk is associated with a waist circumference of over 102 cm (40 in) in men and over 88 cm (35 in) in women.

Waist-hip ratio (WHR): The ratio of waist size to hip size, calculated by dividing the waist measurement by the hip measurement. A high waist to hip ratio would indicate a central fat distribution, a low waist to hip ratio would indicate a peripheral fat distribution.

References

Aaron JI, Mela DJ, Evans RE (1994) The influences of attitudes, beliefs and label information on perceptions of reduced-fat spread. *Appetite,* **22,** 25–37.

Abenhaim L, Moride Y, Brenot F *et al.* (1996) Appetite-suppressant drugs and the risk of primary pulmonary hypertension. *New England Journal of Medicine,* **335,** 609–16.

Abrams B (1993) Prenatal weight gain and post-partum weight retention: a delicate balance (Editorial). *American Journal of Public Health,* **83,** 1082–83.

Acheson KJ, Ravussin E, Wahren J *et al.* (eds) (1984) Thermic effect of glucose in man: obligatory and facultative thermogenesis. *Journal of Clinical Investigation* **74,** 1572–80.

Adamson A, Rugg-Gunn A, Butler T, Appleton D, Hackett A (1992) Nutritional intake, height and weight of 11–12 year old Northumbrian children in 1990 compared with information obtained in 1980. *British Journal of Nutrition,* **68,** 543–63.

Agras WS, Telch CF, Arnow B *et al.* (1994) Weight loss, cognitive-behavioral, and desipramine treatments in binge eating disorder. An additive design. *Behavior Therapy,* **25,** 225–38.

Ahlborg G, Felig P, Hagenfeldt L *et al.* (1974) Substrate turnover during prolonged exercise in man. Splanchnic and leg metabolism of glucose, free fatty acids and amino acids. *Journal of Clinical Investigation,* **53,** 1080–90.

Ainsworth BE, Haskell WL, Leon AS *et al.* (1993) Compendium of physical activities: classification of energy costs of human physical activities. *Medicine and Science in Sports and Exercise,* **25,** 71–80.

Allison DB, Faith MS (1997) A proposed heuristic for communicating heritability to the general public, with obesity as an example. *Behavioural Genetics,* **27,** 441–5.

Allison DB, Kaprio J, Korkeila M, Neale MC, Hayakawa K (1996) The heritability of body mass index among an international sample of monozygotic twins reared apart. *International Journal of Obesity,* **20,** 501–6.

Allison DB, Paultre F, Heymsfield SB, Pi-Sunyer FX (1995) Is the intrauterine period really a critical period for the development of obesity? *International Journal of Obesity,* **19,** 397–402.

Allon N (1982) The stigma of overweight in everyday life. In: *Psychological Aspects of Obesity* (ed. B.B. Woman) pp. 130–74. New York: Van Nostrand Reinhold.

Almeras N, Llavallie J, Despres JP, Bouchard C, Tremblay A (1995) Exercise and energy intake: effect of substrate oxidation. *Physiology & Behaviour,* **57,** 995–1000.

Amatruda JM, Statt MC, Welle SL (1993) Total and resting energy expenditure in obese women reduced to ideal body weight. *Journal of Clinical Investigation,* **92,** 1236–42.

Anderson AO, Gatenby SJ, Walker AD, Mela DJ, Southon S (1995) Dietary patterns in healthy adult volunteers: A preliminary investigation. In: *Proceedings of the Second International Conference on Dietary Assessment Methods,* Abstract No. 6. Boston: Harvard School of Public Health.

Anderson H, Leiter LA (1996) Sweeteners and food intake: relevance to obesity. In: *Progress in Obesity Research 7,* (eds A Angel, H Anderson, C Bouchard, D Lau, L Leiter, R Mendelson) pp. 345–9. London: John Libbey.

Andres R, Elahi D, Tobin JD, Muller DC, Brant L (1985) Impact of age on weight goals. *Annals of Internal Medicine,* **103,** 1030–33.

Anon (1997) The prevention and treatment of obesity. *Effective Health Care,* **3,** 1–12.

Armstrong N, Balding J, Gentle P, Kirby B (1990) Patterns of physical activity among 11–16 year old British children. *British Medical Journal,* **301,** 203–5.

Arnow B (1995) The emotional eating scale: the development of a measure to assess coping with negative affect by eating. *International Journal of Eating Disorders,* **18** (1), 79–90.

Ashwell M, Durrant M, Garrow JS (1978) Does adipose

tissue cellularity or the age of onset of obesity influence the response to short-term inpatient treatment of obese women? *International Journal of Obesity*, **2**, 449–56.

Ashwell M, North WRS, Meade TW (1978) Social class, smoking and obesity. *British Medical Journal*, **277**, 1466–7.

Astrup A (1996) Obesity and metabolic efficiency. *Ciba Foundation Symposium*, **201**, 159–68.

Astrup A, Gøtzsche P, Toubro S *et al.* (1997a) A low resting metabolic rate in formerly obese: a meta-analysis. *International Journal of Obesity*, **21** (Suppl 2), S19.

Astrup A, Toubro S, Raben A, Skou AR (1997b) The role of low fat diets and fat substitutes in body weight management: what have we learned from clinical studies? *Journal of the American Dietetic Association*, **97** (7), 582–7.

Astwood EB (1962) The heritage of corpulence. *Endocrinology*, **71**, 337–41.

Atkinson RL, Greenway FL, Bray GA *et al.* (1977) Treatment of obesity: comparison of physician and non-physician therapists using placebo and anorectic drugs in a double-blind trial. *International Journal of Obesity*, **1**, 113–20.

Atwater WO, (1902) On the digestibility and availability of food materials. *Agricultural Experiment Station 14th Annual Report.* Connecticut, Storrs.

Australasian Society for the Study of Obesity (1995) *Healthy Weight Australia: a national obesity strategy.* Sydney: ASSO.

Axelsson I, Jakobsson I, Raiha N (1988) Formula with reduced protein content: effects on growth and protein metabolism during weaning. *Pediatric Research*, **24**, 297–301.

Baeke JAH, Van Staveren WA, Burema J (1983) Food consumption, habitual physical activity and body fatness in young Dutch adults. *American Journal of Clinical Nutrition*, **37**, 278–86.

Bahary N, Siegel DA, Walsh J *et al.* (1993) Microdissection of proximal mouse chromosome 6: identification of RFLPs tightly linked to the *ob* mutation. *Mammalian Genome*, **4**, 511–15.

Baird DT (1978) Polycystic ovary syndrome. In: *Advances in gynaecological endocrinology. Proceedings of the Sixth Study group of the Royal College of Obstetricians and Gynaecologists.* (ed. HS Jacobs) pp. 289–300. London: Royal College of Obstetricians and Gynaecologists.

Baker LC, Kirschenbaum DS (1993) Self-monitoring may be necessary for successful weight reduction. *Behavior Therapy*, **24**, 377–94.

Balding J (1997) *Young People in 1996.* Exeter: Schools Health Education Unit, University of Exeter.

Ballor DL, Poehlman ET (1994) Exercise-training enhances fat-free mass preservation during diet-induced weight loss: a meta-analytical finding. *International Journal of Obesity*, **18**, 35–40.

Bandini LG, Schoeller DA, Dietz WH (1990) Energy expenditure in obese and non-obese adolescents. *Pediatr. Res.* **27**, 198–203.

Barasi ME, Phillips KM, Burr ML (1985) A Weighed Dietary Survey of Women in South Wales. *Human Nutrition: Applied Nutrition*, **39A**, 189–94.

Barker DJP (1995) Fetal origins of coronary heart disease. *British Medical Journal*, **311**, 171–4.

Barker ME, McClean SI, McKenna PG, Reid NG, Strain JJ, Thompson KA (1989) *Diet, Lifestyle and Health in Northern Ireland.* Northern Ireland: University of Ulster.

Barlow CE, Kohl HW, Gibbons LW, Blair SN (1995) Physical fitness, mortality and obesity. *International Journal of Obesity*, **19** (Suppl 4), S41–S44.

Basdevant A, Craplet C, Guy-Grand B (1993) Snacking patterns in obese French women. *Appetite*, **21**, 17–23.

Baucom DH, Aiken PA (1981) Effect of depressed mood on eating among obese and non-obese dieting and non-dieting persons. *Journal of Personality & Social Psychology*, **41**, 577–85.

Beales PL, Kopelman PG (1996) Obesity genes. *Clinical Endocrinology*, **45**, 373–8.

Beaton GH, Tarusak V, Anderson GH (1992) Estimation of possible impact of non-caloric fat and carbohydrate substitutes on macronutrient intake in the human. *Appetite*, **19**, 87–103.

Beaudoin R, Mayer J (1953) Food intake of obese and non-obese women. *Journal of the American Dietetic Association*, **29**, 29–33.

Beazley JM, Swinhoe JR (1979) Body weight in parous women: is there any alteration between successive pregnancies? *Acta Obstetrica et Gynecologica Scandinavica*, **58**, 45–7.

Bellisle F, Le Magnen J (1981) The structure of meals in humans: eating and drinking patterns in lean and obese subjects. *Physiology & Behavior*, **27**, 649–58.

Bellisle F, Lucas F, Le Magnen J (1984) Deprivation, palatability and the microstructure of meals in human subjects. *Appetite*, **5**, 85–94.

Bellisle F, McDevitt R, Prentice AM (1997) Meal frequency and energy balance. *British Journal of Nutrition*, **77** (Suppl 1), S57–S70.

Bellisle F, Perez C (1994) Low-energy substitutes for sugars and fats in the human diet: impact on nutritional regulation. *Neuroscience & Biobehavioral Reviews*, **18**, 197–205.

Bellisle F, Rolland-Cachera MF, Deheeger M, Guilloud-Bataille M (1988) Obesity and food intake in children: evidence for a role of metabolic and/or behavioral daily rhythms. *Appetite*, **11**, 111–18.

Bennet GA (1986) Behavior therapy for obesity: a

quantitative review of selected treatment characteristics on outcome. *Behavior Therapy,* **17**, 554–62.

Bennett N, Dodd T, Flatley J, Freeth S, Bolling K (1995) *Health Survey for England 1993.* London: HMSO.

Bennett W (1987) Dietary treatments of obesity. *Annals of the New York Academy of Sciences,* **499**, 250–63.

Berkowitz RP (1994) Relapse prevention in the treatment of obesity. In: *Obesity: Pathophysiology, Psychology and Treatment.* (eds GL Blackburn, BS Kanders). New York: Chapman and Hall.

Berman WH, Berman ER, Heymsfield S, Fauci M (1993) The effect of psychiatric disorders on weight loss in obesity clinic patients. *Behavioral Medicine,* **18** (4), 167–72.

Bhatnagar D, Anand IS, Durrington PN *et al.* (1995) Coronary risk factors in people from the Indian subcontinent living in West London and their siblings in India. *Lancet,* **345**, 405–9.

Biddle SJH (1994) What helps and hinders people being more physically active? In: *Moving on: International perspectives on promoting physical activity.* (ed. AJ Killoran, P Fentem, C Casperson), pp. 110–48. London: Health Education Authority.

Biener L, Heaton A (1995) Women dieters of normal weight: their motives, goals, and risks. *American Journal of Public Health,* **85**, 714–17.

Bingham S, Cummings J (1985) Urine nitrogen as an independent validatory measure of dietary intake: a study of nitrogen balance in individuals consuming their normal diet. *American Journal of Clinical Nutrition,* **42**, 1276–89.

Bingham S, McNeil NI, Cummings JH (1981). The diet of individuals: a study of a randomly chosen cross-section of British adults in a Cambridgeshire village. *British Journal of Nutrition,* **45**, 23–35.

Birch LL, McPhee L, Steinberg L, Sullivan S (1990) Conditioned flavor preferences in young children. *Physiology & Behavior,* **47**, 501–5.

Björkelund C, Lissner L, Anderson S, Lapidus L, Bengtsson C (1996) Reproductive history in relation to relative weight and fat distribution. *International Journal of Obesity,* **20**, 213–19.

Björntorp P (1996) The regulation of adipose tissue distribution in humans. *International Journal of Obesity,* **20**(4), 291–302.

Björntorp P, Carlgren G, Isaksson B, Krotkiewski M, Larsson B, Sjöström L (1975) Effect of an energy-reduced dietary regimen in relation to adipose tissue cellularity in obese women. *American Journal of Clinical Nutrition,* **28**, 445–52.

Björntorp P, Enzi G, Karlsson K, Krotkiewski M, Sjöström L, Smith U (1974) The effect of maternal diabetes on adipose tissue cellularity in man and rat. *Diabetologia,* **10**, 205–9.

Björvell H, Ronnberg S, Rössner S (1985) Eating patterns described by a group of treatment seeking overweight women and normal weight women. *Scandinavian Journal of Behavior Therapy,* **14**, 147–56.

Björvell H, Rössner S (1985) Long-term treatment of severe obesity: four year follow up of results of combined behavioural modification programme. *British Medical Journal,* **291**, 379–82.

Björvell H, Rössner S (1992) A ten-year follow up on weight change in severely obese subjects treated in a combined behavioural modification programme. *International Journal of Obesity,* **16**, 623–5.

Black AE, Goldberg GR, Jebb SA, Livingstone MBE, Prentice AM (1991) Critical evaluation of energy intake data using fundamental principles of energy physiology 2. Evaluating the results of dietary surveys. *European Journal of Clinical Nutrition,* **45**, 583–99.

Black AE, Prentice AM, Goldberg GR *et al.* (1993) Measurements of total energy expenditure provide insights into the validity of dietary measurements of energy intake. *Journal of the American Dietetic Association,* **93**, 572–9.

Blair SN (1993) Evidence for success of exercise in weight loss and control. *Annals of Internal Medicine,* **119**, 702–6.

Blair SN, Hardman A (1995) Special issue: physical activity, health and wellbeing – an international consensus conference. *Research Quarterly for Exercise and Sport,* **66**, 4.

Blair SN, Kampert JB, Kohl HW *et al.* (1996) Influences of cardiorespiratory fitness and other precursors on cardiovascular disease and all-cause mortality in men and women. *Journal of the American Medical Association,* **276**, 205–10.

Blair SN, Kohl HW, Paffenbarger RS Jr *et al.* (1989) Physical fitness and all-cause mortality: a prospective study of healthy men and women. *Journal of the American Medical Association,* **262**, 2392–401.

Blair SN, Kohl HW, Gorden NF (1992) Physical activity and health. A lifestyle approach. *Medicine, Exercise, Nutrition and Health,* **1**, 54–7.

Blair SN, Kohl HW, Barlow CE, Paffenbarger RS Jr, Gibbons LW, Macera CA (1995) Changes in physical fitness and all-cause mortality: a prospective study of healthy and unhealthy men. *Journal of the American Medical Association,* **273**, 1093–8.

Blitzer PH, Rimm AA, Geifer EE (1977) The effect of cessation of smoking on body weight in 57,032 women: cross-sectional and longitudinal analyses. *Journal of Chronic Disease,* **30**, 415–29.

Blundell JE, Burley VJ, Cotton JR, Lawton CL (1993) Dietary fat and the control of energy intake: evaluating the effects of fat on meal size and postmeal satiety. *American Journal of Clinical Nutrition,* **57** (Suppl 1), 772S–778S.

Blundell JE, Halford JC (1994) Regulation of nutrient supply: the brain and appetite control. *Proceedings of the Nutrition Society*, **53**, 407–18.

Blundell JE, King NA (1998) Effects of exercise on appetite control: loose coupling between energy expenditure and energy intake. *International Journal of Obesity*, **22** (Suppl 2), S22–S29.

Blundell JE, Macdiarmid JI (1997) Passive over-consumption. Fat intake and short-term energy balance. *Annals of the New York Academy of Sciences*, **827**, 392–407.

Blundell JE, Rogers PJ (1994) Sweet carbohydrate substitutes (intense sweeteners) and the control of appetite: scientific issues. In: *Appetite and Body Weight Regulation* (ed. JD Fernstrom, GD Miller), pp. 113–24. Boca Raton: CRC Press.

Boardley DJ, Sargent RG, Coker AL, Hussey JR, Sharpe PA (1995) The relationship between diet, activity and other factors and post-partum weight change by race. *Obstetrics and Gynecology*, **86**, 834–8.

Bogardus C, Lillioja S, Bennett PH (1991) Pathogenesis of NIDDM in Pima Indians. *Diabetes Care*, **14**, 689–90.

Bolton-Smith C, Smith WCS, Woodward M, Tunstall-Pedoe H (1991) Nutrient intakes of different social class groups: results from the Scottish Heart Health Study. *British Journal of Nutrition*, **65**, 321–35.

Bolton-Smith C, Woodward M (1994) Dietary composition and fat to sugar ratios in relation to obesity. *International Journal of Obesity*, **18**, 820–28.

Bolton-Smith C, Woodward M, Brown CA, Tunstall-Pedoe H (1993) Nutrient intake by duration of ex-smoking in the Scottish Heart Health Study. *British Journal of Nutrition*, **69**, 315–32.

Bonham GS, Brock DB (1985) The relationship of diabetes with race, sex, and obesity. *American Journal of Clinical Nutrition*, **41**, 776–83.

Booth DA (1985) Food-conditioned eating preferences and aversions with interoceptive elements: conditioned appetites and satieties. *Annals of the New York Academy of Sciences*, **443**, 22–41.

Booth DA (1988) Mechanisms from models – actual effects from real life: the zero-calorie drink-break option. *Appetite*, **11**(Suppl), 94–102.

Booth DA, Jarman SP (1976) Inhibition of food intake in the rat following complete absorption of glucose delivered into the stomach, intestine or liver. *Journal of Physiology*, **259**, 501–22.

Booth DA, Mather P, Fuller J (1982) Starch content of ordinary foods associatively conditions human appetite and satiation, indexed by intake and eating pleasantness of starch-paired foods. *Appetite*, **3**, 163–84.

Borecki IB, Rice T, Perusse L, Bouchard C, Rao DC (1995) Major gene influence on the propensity to store fat in trunk versus extremity depots: evidence from the Quebec family study. *Obesity Research*, **3**, 1–8.

Bortz WM (1969) A 500-pound weight loss. *American Journal of Medicine*, **47**, 325–31.

Bouchard C (1996) Can obesity be prevented? *Nutrition Reviews*, **54**, S125–S130.

Bouchard C, Perusse L (1988) Heredity and body fat. *Annual Review of Nutrition*, **8**, 258–77.

Bouchard C, Perusse L, Chagnon YC, Warden C, Ricquier D (1997) Linkage between markers in the vicinity of the uncoupling protein 2 gene and resting metabolic rate in humans. *Human Molecular Genetics*, **6**, 1887–9.

Bouchard C, Tremblay A, Despres JP *et al.* (1990) The response to long-term overfeeding in identical twins. *New England Journal of Medicine*, **322**, 1477–82.

Braddon FE, Rodgers B, Wadsworth ME, Davies J (1986) Onset of obesity in a 36 year birth cohort study. *British Medical Journal*, **293**, 299-303.

Bradley PJ (1985) Conditions recalled to have been associated with weight gain in adulthood. *Appetite*, **6**, 235–41.

Bray GA (1970) Measurement of subcutaneous fat cells from obese patients. *Annals of International Medicine*, **73**, 565–9.

Bray GA (1976) *The Obese Patient*. pp. 450. Philadelphia: Saunders.

Breeze E, Maidment A, Bennett N, Flatley J, Carey S (1994) *Health Survey for England, 1992*. London: HMSO.

British Nutrition Foundation (1992) Unsaturated fatty acids nutritional and physiological significance. The report of the British Nutrition Foundation's Task Force. London: Chapman & Hall.

Brody ML, Walsh BT, Devlin MJ (1994) Binge eating disorder: reliability and validity of a new diagnostic category. *Journal of Consulting and Clinical Psychology*, **62**, 381–6.

Broeder CE, Burrhus KA, Svanevik LS, Wilmore JH (1992) The effects of aerobic fitness on metabolic rate. *American Journal of Clinical Nutrition*, **55**, 795–801.

Brook CGD (1972) Evidence for a sensitive period in adipose-cell replication in man. *Lancet*, **2**, 624–7.

Brown JE, Kaye SA, Folsom AR (1992) Parity-related weight change in women. *International Journal of Obesity*, **16**, 627–31.

Brown JE, Potter JD, Jacobs DR, Kopher RA, Rourke MJ, Barosso GM (1996) Maternal waist-to-hip ratio as a predictor of newborn size: results of the Diana project. *Epidemiology*, **7**, 62–6.

Brownell KD, Jeffrey RW (1987) Improving long-term weight loss: pushing the limits of treatment. *Behavior Therapy*, **18**, 353–74.

Brownell KD, Kramer FM (1989) Behavioral management of obesity. *Medical Clinics of North America*, **73**, 185–201.

Brownell KD, Marlatt GA, Lichtenstein E, Wilson ET

(1986) Understanding and preventing relapse. *American Psychologist*, **41**, 765–82.

Brownell KD, Wadden TA (1992) Etiology and treatment of obesity: understanding a serious, prevalent and refractory disorder. *Journal of Clinical and Consulting Psychology*, **60**, 505–17.

Bruch H (1974) *Eating Disorders: Obesity, Anorexia Nervosa, and the Person Within*, pp. 396. London: Routledge, Kegan Paul.

Buisson D (1995) Developing new products for the consumer, In: *Food Choice and the Consumer*, (ed. D Marshall) London: Blackie.

Burr ML, Bates CJ, Fehily AM, St Leger AS (1981) Plasma cholesterol and blood pressure in vegetarians. *Journal of Human Nutrition*, **35**, 437–41.

Burr ML, Lennings CI, Milbank JE (1982b) The prognostic significance of weight and of vitamin C status in the elderly. *Age and Ageing*, **11**, 249–55.

Burr ML, Milbank JE, Gibbs D (1982a) The nutritional status of the elderly. *Age and Ageing*, **11**, 89–96.

Bush A, Webster J, Chalmers G *et al.* (1988) The Harrow slimming club: Report on 1090 enrolments in 50 courses, 1977–1986. *Journal of Human Nutrition and Dietetics*, **1**, 429–36.

Butters JW, Cash TF (1987) Cognitive-behavioral treatment of women's body-image dissatisfaction. *Journal of Consulting and Clinical Psychology*, **55**, 889–97.

Butterworth DE, Nieman DC, Butler JV, Herring JL (1994) Food intake patterns of marathon runners. *International Journal of Sport Nutrition*, **4**, 1–7.

Cade J, Barker D, Margetts B, Morris J (1988) Diet and inequalities in health in three English towns. *British Medical Journal*, **296**, 1359–62.

Campbell DM (1983) Dietary restriction in obesity and its effect on neonatal outcome. In: *Nutrition in pregnancy: proceedings of the tenth study group of the Royal College of Obstetricians and Gynaecologists*. (eds DM Campbell, MDG Gilmer) London: Royal College of Obstetricians and Gynaecologists.

Campbell RG, Hashim SA, Van Itallie TB (1971) Studies of food intake regulation in man. Responses to variations in nutritive density in lean and obese subjects. *New England Journal of Medicine*, **285**, 1402–7.

Campfield LA, Smith FJ, Guisez Y, Devos R, Burn P (1995) Recombinant mouse OB protein: evidence for a peripheral signal linking adiposity and central neural networks. *Science*, **269**, 546–9.

Cannon G (1992) *Food and Health: The Experts Agree.* London: Consumers' Association.

Caro JF, Kolaczynski JW, Nyce MR *et al.* (1996) Decreased cerebrospinal-fluid serum/leptin ratio in obesity: a possible mechanism for leptin resistance. *Lancet*, **348**, 159–61.

Casey VA, Dwyer JT, Coleman KA, Valachan I (1992) Body Mass Index from childhood to middle age: a 50 year follow-up. *American Journal of Clinical Nutrition*, **56**, 14–18.

Caspersen CJ, Powell KG, Christenson GM (1985) Physical activity, exercise and physical fitness: definitions and distinctions for health related research. *Public Health Reports*, **100**, 126–31.

Casperson CJ, Merritt (1994) Leisure-time physical activity trends by race and social status. The behavioral risk factor Surveillance System Survey, 1986–1990. *Medicine and Science in Sports and Exercise*, **26**, S80.

Catalona PM, Tyzbir ED, Allen SR, McBean JH, McAuliffe TL (1992) Evaluation of fetal growth by estimation of neonatal body composition. *Obstetrics and Gynecology*, **79**, 46–50.

Cawley D, Lee A, Lund P (1994) The Common Agricultural Policy and the UK diet. Paper presented at the 36th EAE Seminar, Reading.

Chagnon YC, Chen WJ, Perusse L *et al.* (1997) Linkage and association studies between the melanocortin receptors 4 and 5 genes and obesity-related phenotypes in the Quebec Family Study. *Molecular Medicine*, **3**, 663–73.

Chan W, Brown J, Church SM, Buss DH (1996) *Meat Products & Dishes. Supplement to McCance & Widdowson's The Composition of Foods.* London: Royal Society of Chemistry/ Ministry of Agriculture Fisheries and Food.

Chan W, Brown J, Lee SM, Buss DH (1995) *Meat, Poultry & Game. Supplement to McCance & Widdowson's The Composition of Foods.* London: Royal Society of Chemistry/ Ministry of Agriculture Fisheries and Food.

Charney E, Chamblee H, McBride M, Lyon B, Pratt R (1976) Childhood antecedents of adult obesity. Do chubby infants become obese adults? *New England Journal of Medicine*, **295**, 6–9.

Chaturvedi N, Jarrett J, Morrish N, Keen H, Fuller JH (1996) Differences in mortality and morbidity in African Caribbean and European people with non-insulin dependent diabetes mellitus: results of a 20-year follow-up of a London cohort of a multinational study. *British Medical Journal*, **313**, 848–52.

Chen LNA, Parham ES (1991) College students' use of high-intensity sweeteners is not consistently associated with sugar consumption. *Journal of the American Dietetic Association*, **91**, 686–90.

Chen Y, Rennie DC, Reeder BA (1995) Age-related association between body mass index and blood pressure: the Humbolt study. *International Journal of Obesity*, **19**, 825–31.

Ching PL, Willett WC, Rimm EB, Colditz GA, Gortmaker SL, Stampfer MJ (1996) Activity level and risk of overweight in male health professionals. *American Journal of Public Health*, **86**, 25–30.

Chouverakis C, Hojniki D (1974) Lipectomy in obese hyperglycemic mice (ob-ob). *Metabolism*, **23**, 133–7.

Chua SC, Chung WK, Wu-Peng S *et al.* (1996) Phenotypes of the mouse diabetes and rat fatty due to mutations in the ob (leptin) receptor. *Science,* **271**, 994–6.

Cioffi JA, Shafer AW, Zupancic TJ *et al.* (1996) Novel B219/ob receptor isoforms: possible role of leptin in hematopoiesis and reproduction. *Nature Medicine,* **2**, 585–8.

Clark JT, Kalra PS, Crowley WR, Kalra SP (1984) Neuropeptide Y and human pancreatic polypeptide stimulate feeding behavior in rats. *Endocrinology,* **115**, 427–9.

Clément K, Ruiz J, Cassard-Doulcier A-M *et al.* (1996) Additive effect of A->G (–3826) variant of the uncoupling protein gene and the Trp64Arg mutation of the B-adrenergic receptor gene on weight gain in morbid obesity. *International Journal of Obesity,* **20**, 1061–6.

Clément K, Vaisse C, Lahlou N *et al.* (1998) A mutation of the human leptin receptor gene causes obesity and pituitary dysfunction. *Nature,* **392**, 398–401.

Clément K, Vaisse C, Manning BS *et al.* (1995) Genetic variation in the β_3-adrenergic receptor and an increased capacity to gain weight in patients with morbid obesity. *New England Journal of Medicine,* **333**(6), 352–4.

Clissold TL, Hopkins W, Seddon RJ (1991) Lifestyle behaviours during pregnancy. *New Zealand Medical Journal,* **104**, 111–13.

Coates TJ, Jeffery RW, Wing RR (1978) The relationship between persons' relative body weights and the quality and quantity of food stored in their homes. *Addictive Behaviors,* **3**, 179–84.

Cochrane AL (1972) *Effectiveness and Efficiency: Random Reflections on Health Services,* pp. 99. London: Nuffield Provincial Hospitals Trust.

Colditz GA (1992) Economic costs of obesity. *American Journal of Clinical Nutrition,* **55**, 503S–507S.

Colditz G, Giovannucci E, Rimm E *et al.* (1991) Alcohol intake in relation to diet and obesity in men and women. *American Journal of Clinical Nutrition,* **54**, 49–55.

Colditz G, Willett W, Stampfer M *et al.* (1990) Patterns of weight change and their relation to diet in a cohort of healthy women. *American Journal of Clinical Nutrition,* **51**, 1100–1105.

Cole TJ (1990) The LMS method for constructing normalised growth standards. *European Journal of Clinical Nutrition,* **44**, 45–60.

Cole TJ, Freeman JV, Preece MA (1995) Body mass index reference curves for the UK, 1990. *Archives of Disease in Childhood,* **73**, 25–9.

Colhoun H, Prescott-Clarke P (1996) *Health Survey for England 1994.* London: HMSO.

Colman DR (1987) Consequences of national and European pricing policy for nutrition and the food industry. In: *Food and Health* (ed. R Cottrell). Carnforth: Parthenon.

Commission Directive 98/8/EC (1997) Foods intended for use in energy-restricted diets for weight reduction. Implementing regulations *The Foods Intended for Use in Energy Restricted Diets for Weight Reduction Regulations.* S.I. No. 2182.

Connolly HM, Crary JL, McGoon MD *et al.* (1997) Valvular heart disease associated with fenfluramine-phentermine. *New England Journal of Medicine,* **337**, 581–8.

Consensus Statement (1991) Gastrointestinal surgery for severe obesity. NIH Consensus Development Conference, 25–27 March, 1991.

Considine RV, Considine EL, Williams CJ *et al.* (1995) Evidence against either a premature stop codon or the absence of obese gene mRNA in human obesity. *Journal of Clinical Investigation,* **95**, 2986–8.

Cornell CE, Rodin J, Weingarten H (1989) Stimulus-induced eating when satiated. *Physiology & Behavior,* **45**, 695–704.

Cornish BH, Ward LC, Thomas BJ, Jebb SA, Elia M (1996) Evaluation of multiple frequency bioelectrical impedance and Cole–Cole analysis for the assessment of body water volumes in healthy humans. *European Journal of Clinical Nutrition,* **50**, 159–64.

Council on Scientific Affairs (1988) Treatment of obesity in adults. *Journal of the American Medical Association,* **177**, 2547–51.

Cox BD (1993) Changes in body measurements. In: *The Health and Lifestyle Survey; Seven Years on* (eds BD Cox, FA Huppert, MA Whitchelow), pp. 103–17. Aldershot: Dartmouth Publishing.

Cox BD, Blaxter H, Buckle ALJ *et al.* (1987) *The Health and Lifestyle Survey.* London: The Health Promotion Research Trust.

Cox DN, Perry L, Moore PB, Vallis L, Mela DJ (1998) Sensory and hedonic ratings of lean and obese subjects' dietary intakes. *Presented at 8th International Congress on Obesity. Paris; August/September.*

Cox DN, van Galen M, Hedderley D, Perry L, Moore P, Mela DJ (1997) Dietary, sensory and hedonic measures of lean and obese consumers' food choices. *Obesity Research,* **5** (Supp 1), 49S.

Cronk CE, Chumlea WL, Kent R (1982) Longitudinal trends of weight/stature^2 in childhood in relation to adulthood body fat measures. *Human Biology,* **54**, 751–4.

Cunningham DA, Montaye HJ, Metzer HL, Keller JB (1969) Physical activity at work and leisure as related to occupation. *Medical Science in Sport,* **1**, 165–70.

Curb JD, Marcus EB (1991) Body fat and obesity in Japanese Americans. *American Journal of Clinical Nutrition,* **53**, 1552S–1555S.

Dallosso HM, Murgatroyd PR, James WPT (1982)

Feeding frequency and energy balance in adult males. *Human Nutrition: Clinical Nutrition,* **36C**, 25–39.

Dattilo AM, Kris-Etherton PM (1992) Effects of weight reduction on blood lipids and lipoproteins: a meta-analysis. *American Journal of Clinical Nutrition,* **56**, 320–28.

Davies K, Wardle J (1994) Body image and dieting in pregnancy. *Journal of Psychosomatic Research,* **38**, 787–99.

Davies PSW, Gregory J, White A (1995) Physical activity and body fatness in pre-school children. *International Journal of Obesity* **19**, 6–10.

Davis MA, Neuhaus JM, Ettingrer WH, Mueller WH (1990) Body fat distribution and osteoarthritis. *American Journal of Epidemiology,* **132**, 701–7.

Dawson J (1995) Food retailing and the food consumer, In: *Food Choice and the Consumer,* (ed. D Marshall). London: Blackie.

de Castro JM (1997) How can energy balance be achieved by free living human subjects? *Proceedings of the Nutrition Society,* **56**, 1–14.

de Castro JM (1995) The relationship of cognitive restraint to the spontaneous food and fluid intake of free-living humans. *Physiology & Behavior,* **57**, 287–5.

de Castro JM (1990) Social facilitation of duration and size but not rate of the spontaneous meal intake of humans. *Physiology & Behavior,* **47**, 1129–35.

de Castro JM, de Castro ES (1989) Spontaneous meal patterns of humans: influence of the presence of other people. *American Journal of Clinical Nutrition,* **50**, 237–47.

de Graaf C, Drijvers JJM, Zimmermanns NJH, van het Hof KH, Weststrate JA, van den Berg H (1997) Energy and fat compensation during long term consumption of reduced fat products. *Appetite,* **29**, 305–23.

De Peuter R, Winters RT, Brinkman M, Tomas FM, Clark DG (1992) No differences in rates of energy expenditure between post obese women and their matched, lean controls. *International Journal of Obesity,* **16**, 801–8.

Department of Health (1989) *The Diets of British Schoolchildren.* Report on Health and Social Subjects: 36. London: HMSO.

Department of Health (1991) *Dietary Reference Values for Food Energy and Nutrients for the United Kingdom.* Report on Health and Social Subjects: 41. London: HMSO.

Department of Health (1992) *The Health of the Nation: A Strategy for Health in England.* London: HMSO.

Department of Health (1994) *Nutritional Aspects of Cardiovascular Disease.* Report on Health and Social Subjects: 46. London: HMSO.

Department of Health (1998) *Nutritional Aspects of the Development of Cancer.* Report on Health and Social Subjects 48. London: The Stationery Office.

Department of Health & Social Security (1972) *A Nutrition Survey of the Elderly.* Report on Health and Social Subjects: 43. London: HMSO.

Department of Health & Social Security (1975) *A Nutrition Survey of Pre-school Children, 1967–68.* Report on Health and Social Subjects: 10. London: HMSO.

Department of Health & Social Security (1979) *Nutrition and Health in Old Age.* Report on Health and Social Subjects: 16. London: HMSO.

Department of Health & Social Security (1984) *Diet and Cardiovascular Disease: Report of the Panel on Diet in Relation to Cardiovascular Disease.* Report on Health and Social Subjects: 28. London: HMSO.

Department of Health and Social Security (1987) *The Use of Very Low Calorie Diets in Obesity.* Report on Health and Social Subjects: 31. London: HMSO.

Dewey KG, Loveday CA, Nommsen-Rivers LA, McCrory MA, Lönnerdal B (1994) A randomised study of the effects of aerobic exercise by lactating women on breast-milk volume and composition. *New England Journal of Medicine,* **330**, 449–53.

Diaz EO, Prentice AM, Goldberg GR, Murgatroyd PR, Coward WA (1992) Metabolic response to experimental overfeeding in lean and overweight healthy volunteers. *American Journal of Clinical Nutrition,* **56**, 641–55.

Dibb S, Castell A (1995) *Easy to Swallow, Hard to Stomach: The Results of a Survey of Food Advertising on Television.* London: National Food Alliance.

Dibb S (1993) *Children: Advertisers' Dream, Nutrition Nightmare? The Case for more Responsibility in Food Advertising.* London: National Food Alliance.

Dietz WH (1996a) Early influences on body weight regulation. In: *Regulation of Body Weight: Biological and Behavioural Mechanisms* (eds C Bouchard, GA Bray). Chapter 9. Chichester: John Wiley and Sons Ltd.

Dietz WH (1996b) The role of lifestyle in health: the epidemiology and consequences of inactivity. *Proceedings of the Nutrition Society,* **55**, 829–40.

Dietz WH (1994) Critical periods in childhood for the development of obesity. *American Journal of Clinical Nutrition,* **59**, 955–9.

Dietz WH (1992) Childhood obesity. In: *Obesity* (eds P Björntörp, BN Brodoff), pp. 606–9. Philadelphia: Lippincott.

Dietz WH, Hartung R (1985) Changes in height velocity of obese preadolescents during weight reduction. *American Journal of Diseases of Childhood,* **139**, 705–7.

Dietz WH, Strasburger VC (1991) Children, adolescents and television. *Current Problems in Pediatrics,* **21**, 8–31.

Digby MP (1989) Marketing margins in the meat sector, England and Wales, 1978–1987. *Journal of Agricultural Economics,* **40** (2), 129–41.

DiPietro L (1995) Physical activity, body weight and

adiposity: an epidemiological perspective. *Exercise and Sport Sciences Reviews*, **23**, 275–304.

DiPietro L, Kohl HW, Barlow CE, Blair SN (1998) Improvements in cardiorespiratory fitness attenuate age-related weight gain in healthy men and women: The Aerobics Center longitudinal study. *International Journal of Obesity*, **22**, 55–62.

DiPietro L, Williamson DF, Caspersen CJ, Eaker E (1993) The descriptive epidemiology of selected physical activity and body weight among adults trying to lose weight: the behavioral risk factor surveillance system survey, 1989. *International Journal of Obesity*, **17**, 69–76.

Dishman RK (1994) *Advances in Exercise Adherence*. Champaign: Human Kinetics.

Dornhorst A, Nicholls JS, Ali K *et al.* (1994) Fetal proinsulin and birth weight. *Diabetic Medicine*, **11**, 177–81.

Dowler E, Calvert C (1995) Diet and lone parents in London. *Appetite*, **24** (3), 295.

Dreon DM, Frey-Hewitt B, Ellsworth N, Williams PT, Terry RB, Wood PD (1988) Dietary fat: carbohydrate ratio and obesity in middle-aged men. *American Journal of Clinical Nutrition*, **47**, 995–1000.

Drewnowski A (1985) Food perceptions and preferences of obese adults: a multidimensional approach. *International Journal of Obesity*, **9**, 201–12.

Drewnowski A, Brunzell JD, Sande K, Iverius PH, Greenwood MRC (1985) Sweet tooth reconsidered: taste responsiveness in human obesity. *Physiology & Behavior*, **35**, 617–22.

Drewnowski A, Holden-Wiltse J (1992) Taste responses and food preferences in obese women: effects of weight cycling. *International Journal of Obesity*, **16**, 639–48.

Drewnowski A, Kurth C, Holden-Wiltse J, Saari J (1992) Food preferences in human obesity: carbohydrate versus fats. *Appetite*, **18**, 207–21.

Drewnowski A, Kurth CL, Rahaim JO (1991) Taste preferences in human obesity: environmental and familial factors. *American Journal of Clinical Nutrition*, **54**, 635–41.

Drewnowski A, Popkin B (1997) The nutrition transition: new trends in global diet. *Nutrition Reviews*, **55**, 31–43.

Duncan KH, Bacon JA, Weinsier RL (1987) The effects of high and low energy density diets on satiety, energy intake and eating time of obese and non obese subjects. *American Journal of Clinical Nutrition*, **46**, 886–92.

Durrant ML, Royston PJ, Wlock RT (1982) Effect of exercise on energy intake and eating patterns in lean and obese humans. *Physiology & Behavior*, **29**, 449–54.

Dusdieker LB, Hemmingway DL, Stumbo PJ (1994) Is milk production impaired by dieting during lactation? *American Journal of Clinical Nutrition*, **59**, 833–40.

Edelstein SL, Barrett-Connor EL, Wingard DL, Cohn BA (1992) Increased meal frequency associated with decreased cholesterol concentrations; Rancho Bernardo, CA, 1984–1987. *American Journal of Clinical Nutrition*, **55**, 664–9.

Egger G, Swinburn B (1997) An 'ecological' approach to the obesity pandemic. *British Medical Journal*, **315**, 477–80.

Eklund RC, Crawford S (1994) Active women, social physique anxiety and exercise. *Journal of Sport and Exercise Psychology*, **16**, 431–48.

Elbers JM, Asscheman H, Seidell JC, Gooren LJ (1995) Increased accumulation of visceral fat after long-term androgen administration in women. *International Journal of Obesity*, **19** (Suppl 2), 25.

Elwood P, Bird G, Hughes S, Fehily A (1990) The nutrient intakes of women: dietary surveys in 1966 and 1983 compared. *Journal of Human Nutrition and Dietetics*, **3**, 33–7.

Emorine LJ, Marullo S, Briend-Sutren M-M *et al.* (1989) Molecular characterisation of the human β_3-adrenergic receptor. *Science*, **245**, 1118–21.

Ennew C, McDonald S, Morgan W, Strak J (1995) Overview of the UK food and drink industry. In: *The UK Food and Drink Industry – A Sector by Sector Analysis* (eds J Strak, W Morgan). Northborough: Euro PA & Associates.

Epstein LH (1996) Family-based behavioural intervention for obese children. *International Journal of Obesity*, **20** (Suppl 1), S14–S21.

Epstein LH, Valoski A, McCurley J (1993) Effect of weight loss by obese children on long-term growth. *American Journal of Diseases in Childhood*, **147**, 1076–80.

Epstein LH, Valoski AM, Vara LS *et al.* (1995) Effects of decreasing sedentary behaviour and increasing activity on weight changes in obese children. *Health Psychology*, **14**, 1–7.

Epstein LH, Valosky A, Wing RR, McCurley J (1994) Ten year outcomes of behavioural family-based treatment for childhood obesity. *Health Psychology*, **13**, 373–83.

Erickson JC, Clegg KE, Palmiter RD (1996) Sensitivity to leptin and susceptibility to seizures of mice lacking neuropeptide Y. *Nature*, **381**, 415–21.

Ernst E, Matrai A (1987) Normalisation of hemorheological abnormalities during weight reduction in obese patients. *Nutrition*, **3**, 337–9.

Evans DJ, Hoffman RG, Kalkhoff R, Kissebah AH (1983) Relationship of androgenic activity of body fat topography, fat cell morphology and metabolic aberrations in premenopausal women. *Journal of Clinical Endocrinology and Metabolism*, **57**, 307–10.

Even P, Nicolaidis S (1986) Short-term control of feeding, limitation of the glucostatic theory. *Brain Research Bulletin*, **17**, 621–6.

Eyton A (1987) Self-help lay groups. In: *Body Weight*

Control (eds AE Bender, LJ Brookes), pp. 140–46. Edinburgh: Churchill Livingstone.

Fábry P, Hejda S, Cerny K, Osankova K, Pechar J (1966) Effect of meal frequency in school children. Changes in the weight–height proportion and skin-fold thickness. *American Journal of Clinical Nutrition*, **18**, 358–61.

Fábry P, Teppermann J (1970) Meal frequency – a possible factor in human pathology. *American Journal of Clinical Nutrition*, **23**, 1059–68.

Fahlberg LL, Fahlberg LA (1990) From treatment to health enhancement: psychosocial considerations in the exercise components of health promotion programs. *The Sport Psychologist*, **4**, 168–79.

Fairburn CG (1993) Cognitive-behavioral therapy for binge eating and bulimia nervosa: a comprehensive treatment manual. In: *Binge Eating: Nature, Assessment and Treatment* (eds CG Fairburn, GT Wilson), pp. 361–404. New York: Guilford Press.

Fairburn CG, Cooper Z (1996) New perspectives on dietary and behavioural treatments for obesity. *International Journal of Obesity*, **20** (1), S9–S13.

Fairburn CG, Cooper Z (1993) The eating disorder examination. In: *Binge Eating: Nature, Assessment and Treatment* (eds CG Fairburn, GT Wilson). New York: Guilford Press.

Fairburn CG, Marcus MD, Wilson GT (1993) Cognitive behavioural therapy for binge eating and bulimia nervosa: a comprehensive treatment manual. In: *Binge Eating: Nature, Assessment and Treatment* (eds CG Fairburn, GT Wilson). New York: Guilford Press.

Fairburn CG, Wilson GT (1993) Binge eating: definition and classification. In: *Binge Eating: Nature, Assessment and Treatment* (eds CG Fairburn, GT Wilson). New York: Guilford Press.

Fan W, Boston BA, Kesterson RA, Hruby VJ, Cone RD (1997) Role of melanocortinergic neurones in feeding and the agouti obesity syndrome. *Nature*, **385**, 165–8.

Fehily AM, Barker ME, Thomson M, Yarnell JWG, Holliday RM, Thompson KA, (1990) The diets of men in four areas of the UK: The Caerphilly, Northern Ireland, Edinburgh and Speedwell Studies. *European Journal of Clinical Nutrition*, **44**, 813–17.

Fehily AM, Bird G (1986) The dietary intakes of women in Caerphilly, South Wales: a weighed and a photographic method compared. *Human Nutrition: Applied Nutrition*, **40A**, 300–307.

Fehily AM, Coles RJ, Evans WD, Elwood PC (1992) Factors affecting bone density in young adults. *American Journal of Clinical Nutrition*, **56**, 579–86.

Fehily AM, Phillips KM, Yarnell JW (1984) Diet, smoking, social class and body mass index in the Caerphilly heart disease study. *American Journal of Clinical Nutrition*, **40**, 827–33.

Feingold E, Brown PO, Siegmund D (1993) Gaussian models for genetic linkage analysis using complete high-resolution maps of identity-by-descent. *American Journal of Human Genetics*, **53**, 234–51.

Feldman M, Richardson CT (1986) Role of thought, sight, smell, and taste of food in the cephalic phase of gastric acid secretion in humans. *Gastroenterology*, **90**, 428–33.

Fentem P, Walker A (1995) Setting targets for England: Challenging, measurable and achievable. In: *Moving On: International Perspectives on Promoting Physical Activity* (eds AJ Killoran, P Fentem, C Casperson), pp. 110–48. London: Health Education Authority.

Fernstrom JD, Wurtman RJ, Hammerstrom-Wiklund B et al. (1979) Diurnal variations in plasma concentrations of tryptophan, tyrosine and other neutral amino acids: effect of dietary protein intake. *American Journal of Clinical Nutrition*, **32**, 1912–22.

Ferron F, Considine RV, Peino R, Lado IG, Dieguez C, Casanueva FF (1997) Serum leptin concentrations in patients with anorexia nervosa, bulimia nervosa and non-specific eating disorders correlate with body mass index but are independent of the respective disease. *Clinical Endocrinology*, **46**, 289–93.

Ferster CB, Nurnberger JI, Levitt EB (1962) The control of eating. *Journal of Mathematics*, **1**, 87–109.

Fichter MM, Quadflieg N, Brandl B (1993) Recurrent overeating: an empirical comparison of binge eating disorder, bulimia nervosa, and obesity. *International Journal of Eating Disorders*, **14**, 1–16.

Fine B, Heasman M, Wright J (1996) *Consumption in the Age of Affluence – the World of Food*. London: Routledge.

Finer N, Zarb P (1984) Clinical audit of an obesity clinic. *International Journal of Obesity*, **8**, 474.

Fisher JO, Birch LL (1995) Fat preferences and fat consumption of 3- to 5-year-old children are related to parental adiposity. *Journal of the American Dietetic Association*, **95**, 759–64.

Flatt JP (1987a) The difference in the storage capacities for carbohydrate and for fat and its implications for the regulation of body weight. *Annals of the New York Academy of Sciences*, **499**, 104–23.

Flatt JP (1987b) Dietary fat, carbohydrate balance and weight maintenance: effects of exercise. *American Journal of Clinical Nutrition*, **45**, 296–306.

Flatt JP, Ravussin E, Acheson KJ et al. (1985) Effects of dietary fat on postprandial substrate oxidation and on carbohydrate and fat balances. *Journal of Clinical Investigation*, **76**, 1019–24.

Flodmark CE, Pohlsson T, Ryden O, Sveger T (1993) Prevention of the progression to severe obesity in a group of obese schoolchildren treated with family therapy. *Pediatrics*, **91**, 880–84.

Forbes GB, Reina JC (1970) Adult lean body mass declines with age: some longitudinal observations. *Metabolism*, **19**, 653–63.

Forbes GB, Welle SL (1983) Lean body mass in obesity. *International Journal of Obesity*, **7**, 99–107.

Ford ES, Williamson DF, Liu S (1997) Weight change and diabetes incidence: findings from a cohort of US adults. *American Journal of Epidemiology*, **146**, 214–22.

Foreyt J, Goodrick K (1995) The ultimate triumph of obesity. *Lancet*, **346**, 134–5.

Forrester T, Wilks R, Bennett F *et al.* (1996) Obesity in the Caribbean in the origins and consequences of obesity (eds DJ Chadwick, G Cardew), pp. 17–31. Ciba Foundation Symposium 201: Chichester: John Wiley.

Forsum E, Sadurskis A, Wager J (1989) Estimation of body fat in healthy Swedish women during pregnancy and lactation. *American Journal of Clinical Nutrition*, **50**, 465–73.

Forsum E, Sadurskis A, Wager J (1988) Resting metabolic rate and body composition of healthy Swedish women during pregnancy. *American Journal of Clinical Nutrition*, **47**, 942–7.

Foster GD, Wadden TA, Feurer ID *et al.* (1990) Controlled trial of the metabolic effects of a very low calorie diet: short and long term effects. *American Journal of Clinical Nutrition*, **51**, 167–72.

Fox KR (1997) The physical self and processes in self-esteem development. In: *The Physical Self: from Motivation to Well-being* (ed. KR Fox), pp. 111–40. Champaign, IL: Human Kinetics.

Fox KR (1992) A clinical approach to exercise in the morbidly obese. In: *Treatment of the Seriously Obese Patient* (eds T Wadden, T Van Itallie), pp. 354–82. New York: Guilford Press.

Fox KR, Biddle SJH, Edmunds L, Bowler I, Kilbran A (1997) Physical activity promotion through primary health care in England. *British Journal of General Practice*, **47** (419), 367–9.

Fox PT, Elston MD, Waterlow JC (1981) Pre-school child survey. In: *Department of Health and Social Security Report on Health and Social Subjects No. 21*. Subcommittee on Nutritional Surveillance: Second Report pp. 64–84. London: HMSO.

Franks S (1995) Polycystic ovary syndrome. *New England Journal of Medicine*, **333**, 853–61.

Frederich RC, Hamman A, Anderson S, Lollman B, Lowell BB, Flier JS (1995) Leptin levels reflect body lipid content in mice: evidence for diet induced resistance to leptin action. *Nature Medicine*, **1**, 1311–14.

Freeman-Akabas S, Colt E, Kissilef HR, Pi-Sunyer FX (1995) Lack of sustained increase in metabolic rate following exercise in fit and unfit subjects. *American Journal of Clinical Nutrition*, **41**, 545–9.

Freinkel N, Metzger BE, Phelps RL *et al.* (1985) Gestational diabetes mellitus: heterogeneity of maternal age, weight, insulin secretion, HLA antigens and islet cell antibodies and the impact of maternal metabolism on pancreatic β-cell and somatic development in the offspring. *Diabetes*, **34** (Suppl 2), 1–7.

French SA, Folsom AR, Jeffery RW, Zheng W, Mink PJ, Baxter JE (1997) Weight variability and incident disease in older women: the Iowa women's health study. *International Journal of Obesity*, **21**, 217–23

French SA, Jeffery RW, Folsom AR, Williamson DF, Byers T (1995) Weight variability in a population-based sample of older women: reliability and inter-correlation of measures. *International Journal of Obesity*, **19**, 22–9.

French SA, Jeffery RW, Forster JL, McGovern PG, Kelder SH, Baxter JE (1994) Predictors of weight change over two years among a population of working adults: the healthy worker project. *International Journal of Obesity*, **18**, 145–54.

Fricker J, Giroux S, Fumeron F, Apfelbaum M (1990) Circadian rhythm of energy intake and corpulence status in adults. *International Journal of Obesity*, **14**, 387–93.

Friedlander Y, Kark JD, Kaufmann NA, Barry EM, Stein Y (1988) Familial aggregation of body mass index in ethnically diverse families in Jerusalem: the Jerusalem lipid research. *Clinical and International Journal of Obesity*, **12**, 237–47.

Friedman JM, Leibel RL, Siegel DS, Walsh J, Bahary N (1991) Molecular mapping of the mouse *ob* mutation. *Genomics*, **11**, 1054–62.

Friedman MA, Brownell KD (1995) Psychological correlates of obesity: moving to the next research generation. *Psychological Bulletin*, **117**, 3–20.

Friedman MI (1997) An energy sensor for control of energy intake. *Proceedings of the Nutrition Society*, **56**, 41–50.

Friedman MI, Ramirez I, Bowden CR, Tordoff MG (1990) Fuel partitioning and food intake: role for mitochondrial fatty acid transport. *American Journal of Physiology*, **258**, R216–R221.

Friedman MI, Stricker ME (1976) The physiological psychology of hunger, a physiological perspective. *Psychological Reviews*, **83**, 409–31.

Friedman MI, Tordoff MG (1986) Fatty acid oxidation and glucose utilization interact to control food intake in rats. *American Journal of Physiology*, **251**, R840–R845.

Frijters JER, Rasmussen-Conrad EL (1982) Sensory discrimination, intensity perception, and affective judgment of sucrose-sweetness in the overweight. *Journal of General Psychology*, **107**, 233–47.

Frost G (1989) Comparison of two different methods of energy prescription for obese non-insulin dependent diabetics. *Practical Diabetes*, **6**, 273–75.

Frost G, Masters K, King C *et al.* (1991) A new method of energy prescription to improve weight loss. *Journal of Human Nutrition and Dietetics*, **4**, 369–73.

Frühbeck G, Jebb SA, Prentice AM (1998) Leptin:

physiology and pathophysiology. *Clinical Physiology*, **18**, 399–419.

Frye CA, Crystal S, Ward KD, Kanarek RB (1994) Menstrual cycle and dietary restraint influence taste preferences in young women. *Physiology & Behavior*, **55**, 561–7.

Fulton M, Thomson M, Elton RA, Brown S, Wood DA, Oliver MF (1988) Cigarette smoking, social class and nutrient intake: relevance to coronary heart disease. *European Journal of Clinical Nutrition*, **42**, 797–803.

Fumeron F, Durack-Bown I, Betoulle D *et al.* (1996) Polymorphisms of uncoupling protein (UCP) and B-adrenoceptor genes in obese people submitted to a low calorie diet. *International Journal of Obesity*, **20**, 1051–4.

Gagnon J, Mauriege P, Roys S *et al.* (1996) The Trp64Arg mutation of the β_3 adrenergic receptor has no effect on obesity phenotypes in the Quebec family study and Swedish obese subjects cohorts. *Journal of Clinical Investigation*, **98**, 2086–93.

Galtier-Dereure F, Montpeyroux F, Boulot P, Bringer J, Jaffiol C (1995) Weight excess before pregnancy: complications and cost. *International Journal of Obesity*, **19**, 443–8.

Garbaciak JA, Richter M, Miller S, Barton JJ (1985) Maternal weight and pregnancy complications. *American Journal of Obstetrics and Gynecology*, **152**, 238–45.

Gardner Merchant (1998) What are today's children eating? *The Gardner Merchant School Meals Survey 1998*. Surrey: Gardner Merchant.

Garfinkel L (1985) Overweight and cancer. *Annals of Internal Medicine*, **103**, 1034–6.

Garn SM, Clark DC (1976) Trends in fatness and the origins of obesity. *Pediatrics*, **57**, 443–56

Garn SM, Cole PE (1980) Editorial: Do the obese remain obese and the lean remain lean? *American Journal of Public Health*, **70**, 351–53.

Garn SM, Lavelle M, Rosenburg KR, Hawthorne VM (1986) Maturational timing as a factor in female fatness and obesity. *American Journal of Clinical Nutrition*, **43**, 879–83.

Garner DM, Wooley SC (1991) Confronting the failure of behavioral and dietary treatments for obesity. *Clinical Psychology Review*, **11**, 729–80.

Garrow JS (1974) Dental splinting in the treatment of hyperphagic obesity. *Proceedings of the Nutrition Society*, **33**, 29A.

Garrow JS (1975) A survey of three slimming and weight control organisations in the U.K. In: *Recent Advances in Obesity Research* (ed. A Howard), pp. 301–4. London: Newman Publishing.

Garrow JS (1981) *Treat Obesity Seriously*, pp. 246. London: Churchill-Livingstone.

Garrow JS (1986) Effect of exercise on obesity. *Acta Medica Scandinavia Suppl*, **711**, 67–73.

Garrow JS (1987) Energy expenditure in man – an overview. *American Journal of Clinical Nutrition*, **45**, 1114–19.

Garrow JS (1988) *Obesity and Related Diseases*, London: Churchill-Livingstone.

Garrow JS (1991a) Importance of obesity. *British Medical Journal*, **303**, 704–6.

Garrow JS (1991b) The safety of dieting. *Proceedings of the Nutrition Society*, **5**, 439–93.

Garrow JS (1991c) Treating obesity. *British Medical Journal*, **302**, 803–4.

Garrow JS (1992) Treatment of obesity. *Lancet*, **340**, 409–13.

Garrow JS (1995) Obesity. In: *Oxford Textbook of Medicine*, 3 ed. (eds DJ Weatherall, JGG Ledinghaus, DA Warrell).

Garrow JS, Gardiner GT (1981) Maintenance of weight loss in obese patients after jaw wiring. *British Medical Journal*, **282**, 858–60.

Garrow JS, James WPT (eds) (1993) *Human Nutrition and Dietetics*. Ninth Edition. Edinburgh: Churchill Livingstone.

Garrow JS, Stalley SF (1975) Is there a set point for human body weight? *Proceedings of the Nutrition Society*, **34**, 84A.

Garrow JS, Stalley SF (1977) Cognitive thresholds and human body weight. *Proceedings of the Nutrition Society*, **36**, 18A.

Garrow JS, Summerbell CD (1995) Meta-analysis: effect of exercise, with or without dieting, on body composition of overweight subjects. *European Journal of Clinical Nutrition*, **49**, 1–10.

Garrow JS, Webster JD (1985) Are pre-obese people energy thrifty? *Lancet*, i, 670–71.

Garrow JS, Webster JD (1986) Long-term results of treatment of severe obesity with jaw wiring and waist cord. *Proceedings of the Nutrition Society*, **45**, 119A.

Garrow JS, Webster JD (1989) Effects on weight and metabolic rate of obese women of a 3.4 MJ (800 kcal) diet. *Lancet* **1**, 1429–31.

Garrow JS, Webster JD, Pearson M, Pacy PJ, Harpin G (1989) Inpatient-outpatient randomized comparison of Cambridge diet versus milk diet in 17 obese women over 24 weeks. *International Journal of Obesity*, **13**, 521–9.

Garry RC, Passmore R, Warnock GM, Durnin JVG (1955) *Studies on Expenditure of Energy and Consumption of Food by Miners and Clerks, Fife, Scotland, 1952*. MRC Special Report 289. London: HMSO.

Gatenby SJ, Aaron JI, Jack VM, Mela DJ (1997) Extended use of foods modified in fat and sugar content: nutritional implications in a free-living female population. *American Journal of Clinical Nutrition*, **65**, 1867–73.

Gatenby SJ, Aaron JI, Morton G, Mela DJ (1995)

Nutritional implications of reduced-fat food use by free-living consumers. *Appetite*, **25**, 241–52.

General Medical Council, (1995) *Duties of a Doctor: Good Medical Practice.* London: General Medical Council.

Georgakopoulos TA (1990) The impact of accession on food prices, inflation and food consumption in Greece. *European Review of Agricultural Economics*, **17**, 4.

Gibney M, Sigman-Grant M, Stanton J, Keast D (1995) Consumption of sugars. *American Journal of Clinical Nutrition*, **62** (Suppl), 178S–194S.

Gillett PA (1988) Self-reported factors influencing exercise adherence in overweight women. *Nursing Research*, **37**, 25–9.

Glenny AM, O'Meara S, Melville A, Sheldon TA, Wilson C (1997) The treatment and prevention of obesity: a systematic review of the literature. *International Journal of Obesity*, **21**, 715–37.

Goldberg G, Black A, Jebb S et al. (1991a) Critical evaluation of energy intake data using fundamental principles of energy physiology. *European Journal of Clinical Nutrition*, **45**, 569–81.

Goldberg GR, Prentice AM (1994) Maternal and fetal determinants of adult diseases. *Nutrition Reviews*, **52**, 191–200.

Goldberg GR, Davies HL, Murgatroyd PR, Prentice AM (1987) Overnight metabolic rate in men and women. *Proceedings of the Nutrition Society*, **46**, 118A.

Goldberg GR, Prentice AM, Coward WA et al. (1983) Beneficial health effects of modest weight loss. *International Journal of Obesity*, **16**, 397–415.

Goldberg GR, Prentice AM, Coward WA et al. (1991b) Longitudinal assessment of the components of energy balance in well-nourished lactating women. *American Journal of Clinical Nutrition*, **54**, 788–98.

Goldberg GR, Prentice AM, Coward WA et al. (1993) Longitudinal assessment of energy expenditure in pregnancy by the doubly-labelled water method. *American Journal of Clinical Nutrition*, **57**, 494–505.

Goldberg GR, Prentice AM, Davies HL, Murgatroyd PR (1990) Residual effects of graded exercise on metabolic rate. *European Journal of Clinical Nutrition*, **44**, 99–105.

Goldstein DJ (1992) Beneficial health effects of modest weight loss. *International Journal of Obesity*, **16**, 397–415.

Goodrick GK, Foreyt JP (1991) Why treatments for obesity don't last. *Journal of American Dietetic Association*, **91**(10), 1243–7.

Gordon T, Kannel WB (1973) The effects of overweight on cardiovascular disease. *Geriatrics*, **28**, 80–88.

Gordon T, Kannel WB, Dawber TR, McGee D (1975) Changes associated with quitting cigarette smoking: the Framingham study. *American Heart Journal*, **90**, 322–8.

Gortmaker SL, Must A, Perrin JM, Sobol AM, Dietz WH

(1993) Social and economic consequences of overweight in adolescence and young adulthood. *New England Journal of Medicine*, **329**, 1008–12.

Gortmaker SL, Must A, Sobol AM, Peterson K, Colditz GA, Dietz WH (1996) Television viewing as a cause of increasing obesity among children in the United States, 1986–1990. *Archives of Pediatric Adolescent Medicine*, **150**, 356–62.

Greene GW, Smiciklas-Wright H, Scholl TO, Karp RJ (1988) Post-partum weight change: how much of the weight gained in pregnancy will be lost after delivery? *Obstetrics and Gynecology*, **71**, 701–7.

Greeno CG, Wing RR (1994) Stress-induced eating. *Psychological Bulletin*, **115**, 444–64.

Greeno CG, Wing RR, Marcus MD (1995) Nocturnal eating in binge eating disorder and matched-weight controls. *International Journal of Eating Disorder*, **18**(4), 343–9.

Gregory J, Foster K, Tyler H, Wiseman M (1990) *The Dietary and Nutritional Survey of British Adults.* London: HMSO.

Gregory JR, Collins DL, Davies PSW, Hughes JM, Clarke PC (1995) *National Diet and Nutrition Survey: Children aged $1\frac{1}{2}$ to $4\frac{1}{2}$ Years.* London: HMSO.

Grilo CM, Shiffman S, Wing RR (1989) Relapse crisis and coping among dieters. *Journal of Clinical and Consulting Psychology*, **57**, 488–95.

Grinker J, Gropman-Rubin J, Bose K (1986) Sweet preference and body fatness: neonatal data. *Nutrition and Behavior*, **3**, 197–209.

Grinker J (1978) Obesity and sweet taste. *American Journal of Clinical Nutrition*, **31**, 1078–87.

Grunstein RR, Stenlöf K, Hedner J, Sjöström L (1995) Impact of obstructive apnoea and sleepiness on metabolic and cardiovascular risk factors in the Swedish Obese Subjects (SOS) study. *International Journal of Obesity*, **19**, 410–18.

Guo SS, Roche AF, Chumlea WC, Gardner JD, Siervogel RM (1994) The predictive value of childhood body mass index values for overweight at age 35 years. *American Journal of Clinical Nutrition*, **59**, 810–19.

Gurney M, Gorstein J (1988) The global prevalence of obesity – an initial overview of available data. *World Health Stat Q*, **41**, 251–4.

Gurr MI, Jung RT, Robinson MP, James WPT (1982) Adipose tissue cellularity in man: the relationship between fat cell size and number, the mass and distribution of body fat and the history of weight gain and loss. *International Journal of Obesity*, **6**, 419–36.

Gussow JD (1987) The fragmentation of need: women, food and marketing. *Heresies*, **21**, 6 (1), 39–43.

Guy-Grand B, Apfelbaum M, Crepaldi G, Gries A, Lefebvre P, Turner P (1989) International trial of long-term dexfenfluramine in obesity. *Lancet*, **2**, 1142–5.

Gwinup G (1975) Effect of exercise alone on the weight

of obese women. *Archives of Internal Medicine*, **135**, 676–80.

Haapanen N, Miilunpalo S, Pasanen M, Oja P, Vuori I (1997) Association between leisure time physical activity and 10-year body mass change among working-aged men and women. *International Journal of Obesity* **21**, 288–96.

Haarbo J, Marslew U, Gottfredsen A, Christiansen C (1995) Postmenopausal hormone replacement therapy prevents central distribution of body fat after menopause. *Metabolism*, **40**, 323–6.

Hachey DL, Silber GH, Wong WW *et al.* (1989) Human lactation II Endogenous fatty acid synthesis by the mammary gland. *Pediatric Research*, **25**, 63–8.

Hakala P (1994a) Weight reduction programmes at a rehabilitation centre and a health centre based on group counselling and individual support: short and long-term follow up study. *International Journal of Obesity*, **18**, 483–9.

Hakala P (1994b) *Conventional Treatment of Adult Obesity*. Social Insurance Institution, Finland. Publication ML 132, Turku.

Hakala P, Karvetti R, Rönnemaa T (1993) Group vs individual weight reduction programmes in the treatment of severe obesity – a five year follow up study. *International Journal of Obesity* **17**, 97–102.

Hall BD, Smith DW (1972) Prader–Willi syndrome: a resume of 32 cases including an instance of affected first cousins, one of whom is of normal stature and intelligence. *Journal of Pediatrics*, **81**, 286–93.

Han TS, Richmond P, Avenell A, Lean MEJ (1997b) Waist circumference reduction and cardiovascular benefits during weight loss in women. *International Journal of Obesity*, **21**, 127–34.

Han TS, Seidell JC, Currall JEP, Morrison CE, Deurenberg P, Lean MEJ (1997a) The influences of height and age on waist circumference as an index of adiposity in adults. *International Journal of Obesity*, **21**, 83–9.

Han TS, van Leer EM, Seidell JC, Lean MEJ (1995). Waist circumference action levels in the identification of cardiovascular risk factors: prevalence study in a random sample. *British Medical Journal*, **311**, 1401–5.

Hansen BC, Bodkin NL (1986) Heterogeneity of insulin responses: phases in the continuum leading to non-insulin-dependent diabetes mellitus. *Diabetologia*, **29**, 713–19.

Harman EM, Block AJ (1986) Why does weight loss improve the respiratory insufficiency of obesity? *Chest*, **90**, 153–4.

Harris HE, Ellison GTH (1997) Do the changes in energy balance that occur during pregnancy predispose parous women to obesity? *Nutrition Research Reviews*, **10**, 57–81.

Hartz AJ, Fischer ME, Bril G *et al.* (1986) The association of obesity with joint pain and osteoarthritis in the HANES data. *Journal of Chronic Diseases*, **39**, 311–19.

Hartz AV, Barboriak PN, Wong A *et al.* (1979) The association of obesity with infertility and related menstrual abnormalities in women. *International Journal of Obesity*, **3**, 57–73.

Harvey J, Wing RR, Mullen M (1993) Effects on food cravings of a very low calorie diet or a balanced, low calorie diet. *Appetite*, **21**(2), 105–15.

Haskell WL (1994) Health consequences of physical activity: understanding and challenges regarding dose-response. *Medicine and Science in Sports and Exercise*, **26**, 649–60.

Hausenblas HA, Carron AV, Mack DE (1997) Application of the theories of reasoned action and planned behavior to exercise behavior: a meta-analysis. *Journal of Sport and Exercise Psychology*, **19**, 36–51.

Hayaki J, Brownell KD (1996) Behaviour change in practice: group approaches. *International Journal of Obesity*, **20** (1), S27–S30.

Health Education Authority (1991) *Tomorrow's Young Adults: 9- to 15-year olds look at Alcohol, Drugs, Exercise and Smoking*. London: HEA.

Health Education Authority (1995) *Health Update: Physical Activity*. London: HEA.

Health Education Authority (1997a) *Changing what You Eat: a Guide for Professionals and Helpers*. London: HEA.

Health Education Authority (1997b) *Young and Active: Draft Policy Framework for Young People and Health-enhancing Physical Activity*. London: HEA.

Health Education Authority and Sports Council (1992) *Allied Dunbar National Fitness Survey: Main Findings*. London: Sports Council and HEA.

Heatherton TF, Polivy J, Herman CP, Baumeister RF (1993) Self-awareness, task failure, and disinhibition: how attentional focus affects eating. *Journal of Personality*, **61**, 49–61.

Heini AF, Weinsier RL (1997) Divergent trends in obesity and fat intake patterns: the American paradox. *American Journal of Medicine*, **102**, 259–64.

Heitmann BL, Lissner L, Sorensen TI, Bengtsson C (1995) Dietary fat intake and weight gain in women genetically predisposed for obesity. *American Journal of Clinical Nutrition*, **61**, 1213–17.

Heitmann BL (1994) Impedance: a valid method in assessment of body composition? *European Journal of Clinical Nutrition*, **48**, 228–40.

Heitmann BR, Lissner L (1995) Dietary under reporting by obese individuals – is it specific or non-specific. *British Medical Journal*, **311**, 986–9.

Helderstedt W, Jeffery R, Murray D (1990) The association between alcohol intake and adiposity in the general population. *American Journal of Epidemiology*, **132**, 594–611.

Heller SR, Clarke P, Daly H *et al.* (1988) Group education for obese patients with Type II diabetes: Greater success at less cost. *Diabetic Medicine*, **5**, 552–6.

Hellerstein MK, Christiansen M, Kaempfer S *et al.* (1991) Measurement of de novo hepatic lipogenesis in humans using stable isotopes. *Journal of Clinical Investment*, **87**, 1841–52.

Helmrick SP, Ragland DR, Leung RW, Paffenbarger RS (1991) Physical activity and reduced occurrence of non-insulin-dependent diabetes mellitus. *New England Journal of Medicine*, **325**, 147–52.

Henson S (1992) The CAP and healthy eating. *Nutrition and Food Science*, **4**, 2.

Herman CP (1978) Restrained eating. *Psychiatric Clinics of North America*, **1**, 593–607.

Herman CP (1996) Human eating: diagnosis and prognosis. *Neuroscience & Biobehavioral Reviews*, **20**, 107–11.

Herman CP, Mack D (1975) Restrained and unrestrained eating. *Journal of Personality*, **43**, 647 60.

Herman CP, Polivy J (1984) A boundary model for the regulation of eating. In: *Eating and its Disorders* (eds AJ Stunkard, E Stellar), pp. 141–56. New York: Raven Press.

Herman CP, Polivy J (1975) Anxiety, restraint, and eating behavior. *Journal of Abnormal Psychology*, **84**(6), 666–72.

Herman CP, Polivy J, Pliner P, Threlkeld J, Munic D (1978) Distractibility in dieters and nondieters: an alternative view of 'externality'. *Journal of Personality & Social Psychology*, **36**, 536–48.

Hetherington MM, Macdiarmid JI (1993) 'Chocolate addiction': a preliminary study of its description and its relationship to problem eating. *Appetite*, **21**, 233–46.

Hibscher JA, Herman CP (1977) Obesity, dieting and the expression of 'obese' characteristics. *Journal of Comparative and Physiological Psychology*, **91**(2), 374–80.

Hill AJ, Draper E, Stack J (1994) A weight on children's minds: body shape dissatisfaction at 9-years-old. *International Journal of Obesity*, **18**, 383–9.

Hill AJ, Magson LD, Blundell JE (1984) Hunger and palatability: tracking ratings of subjective experience before, during and after consumption of preferred and less preferred food. *Appetite*, **6**, 361–71.

Hill J, Prentice AM (1995) Sugar and body weight regulation. *American Journal of Clinical Nutrition*, **62** (Suppl), 249S–274S.

Hill JO, Schlundt DG, Sbroccot T *et al.* (1989) Evaluation of an alternating-calorie diet with and without exercise in the treatment of obesity. *American Journal of Clinical Nutrition*, **50**, 248–54.

Hill SW, McCutcheon NB (1984) Contributions of obesity, gender, hunger, food preference, and body size to bite size, bite speed, and rate of eating. *Appetite*, **5**, 73–83.

Hill SW, McCutcheon NB (1975) Eating responses of obese and non-obese humans during dinner meals. *Psychosomatic Medicine*, **37**, 395–401.

Hillman M (1993) One false move ... an overview of the findings and issues they raise. In: *Children, Transport and the Quality of Life* (ed. M Hillman). London: Policy Studies Institute.

Himms-Hagen J (1984) Thermogenesis in brown adipose tissue as an energy buffer: implications for obesity. *New England Journal of Medicine*, **311**, 1549–58.

Hirsch J (1975) Cell number and size as a determinant of subsequent obesity. In: *Childhood Obesity* (ed. M Winick), pp. 15–21. New York: John Wiley.

Hirsch J, Gallian E (1968) Methods for the determination of adipose cell size in man and animals. *Journal of Lipid Research*, **9**, 110–19.

Hodge AM, Zimmet PZ (1994) The epidemiology of obesity. *Bailliere's Clinical Endocrinology of Metabolism*, **8**, 577–99.

Hoffman RP, Armstrong PT (1996) Glucose effectiveness, peripheral and hepatic insulin sensitivity in obese and lean prepubertal children. *International Journal of Obesity*, **20**, 521–5.

Hoffmeister H, Mensink GBM, Stolzenberg H (1994) National trends in risk factors for cardiovascular disease in Germany. *Preventive Medicine*, **23**, 197–205.

Holland WW, Rona RJ, Chinn S *et al.* (1981) The national study of health and growth surveillance of primary schoolchildren (1972–1976). In: *Department of Health and Social Security Report on Health and Social Subjects No. 21*. Subcommittee on Nutritional Surveillance: Second Report pp. 85–101. London: HMSO.

Hollingsworth DR (1992) *Gestational Carbohydrate Intolerance (GCI); Gestational Diabetes Mellitus*. Baltimore: Williams & Wilkins.

Holt SHA, Brand Miller JC, Petocz P (1996) Interrelationships among post-prandial satiety, glucose and insulin responses and changes in subsequent food intake. *European Journal of Clinical Nutrition*, **50**, 788–97.

Hoogwerf BJ, Nuttall FQ (1984) Long term weight regulation in treated hyperthyroid and hypothyroid patients. *American Journal of Medicine*, **30,** 681–6.

Hortobagyi T, Israel RG, Houmard JA, McCammon MR, O'Brien KF (1992) Comparison of body composition assessment by hydrodensitometry, skinfolds, and multiple-site near-infrared spectrophotometry. *European Journal of Clinical Nutrition*, **46**, 205–12.

Hotamisligil GS, Spiegelman BM (1994) Tumor necrosis factor α: a key component of the obesity-diabetes link. *Diabetes*, **43**, 1271–8.

Howlett TA, Rees LH, Besser GM (1985) Cushing's syndrome. *Clinical Endocrinology & Metabolism*, **14**, 911–45.

Hubert HB (1986) The importance of obesity in the

development of coronary risk factors and disease: the epidemiological evidence. *Annual Reviews of Public Health,* **7**, 493–502.

Hubert HB, Feinleib M, McNamara PM, Castelli WP (1983) Obesity as an independent risk factor for cardiovascular disease: a 26-year follow-up of participants in the Framingham heart study. *Circulation,* **67**, 968–77.

Hughes JM, Li L, Chinn S, Rona RJ (1997) Trends in growth in England and Scotland, 1972 to 1994. *Archives of Diseases in Childhood,* **76**, 182–9.

Huszar D, Lynch CA, Fairchild-Huntress V *et al.* (1997) Targeted disruption of the melanocortin-4 receptor results in obesity in mice. *Cell,* **88**, 131–41.

Hytten FE (1991) Weight gain in pregnancy. In: *Clinical Physiology in Obstetrics* (eds FE Hytten, G Chamberlain), pp. 173–203. Oxford: Blackwell Scientific Publications.

IDECG (1990) *International Dietary Energy Consultancy Group. The Doubly-Labelled Water Method for Measuring Energy Expenditure: Technical recommendations for use in humans.* Vienna: IDECG/IAEA.

Institute of Medicine (1990) *Nutrition During Pregnancy.* Washington DC: National Academy Press.

Institute of Medicine (1995) Committee to develop criteria for evaluating the outcomes of approaches to prevent and treat obesity. In: *Weighing the Options – Criteria for Evaluating Weight – Management Programmes.* Washington, D.C.: National Academy Press.

Jackson RS, Creemers JW, Ohagi S *et al.* (1997) Obesity and impaired pro-hormone processing associated with mutations in the human pro-hormone convertase 1 gene. *Nature Genetics,* **16**, 218–20.

Jacobs DR, Hahn LP, Folsom AR, Hannan PJ, Sprafka JM, Burke GI (1991) Time trends in leisure-time physical activity in the upper mid-west 1957–1987. *Epidemiology,* **2**, 8–15.

Jacobsen BK, Thelle DS (1987) The Tromso heart-study – the relationship between food-habits and the body-mass index. *Journal of Chronic Diseases,* **40**, 795–800.

James WPT (1976) *Research on Obesity.* London, HMSO.

James WPT (1995) A public health approach to the problem of obesity. *International Journal of Obesity,* **19** (Suppl 3), S37–S45.

James WPT, Avenell A, Broom J, Whitehead J (1997) A one year trial to assess the value of orlistat in the management of obesity. *International Journal of Obesity,* **21** (Suppl 3), S24–S30.

Janney CA, Zhang D, Sowers M (1997) Lactation and weight control. *American Journal of Clinical Nutrition,* **66**, 1116–24.

Jebb SA, Prentice AM, Goldberg GR, Murgatroyd PR, Black AE, Coward WA (1996) Changes in macronutrient balance during over-feeding and under-feeding assessed by 12 day continuous whole-body calorimetry. *American Journal of Clinical Nutrition,* **64**, 259–66.

Jeffery RW, Gerber WM, Rosenthal BS, Lindquist RA (1983) Monetary contacts in weight control: effectiveness of group and individual contracts of varying size. *Journal of Consulting and Clinical Psychology,* **51** (2), 242–8.

Jeffery RW, Gray CW, French SA *et al.* (1995) Evaluation of weight reduction in a community intervention for cardiovascular disease risk: changes in body mass index in the Minnesota Heart Health Program. *International Journal of Obesity,* **19**, 30–39.

Jeffery RW, Hellerstedt WL, French SA, Baxter JE (1995) A randomised trial of counselling for fat restriction versus calorie restriction in the treatment of obesity. *International Journal of Obesity,* **19**, 132–7.

Jequier E (1989) Energy metabolism in human obesity. *Soz Praventivmed.* **34**, 58–62.

Johnson FE (1985) Health implications of childhood obesity. *Annals of Internal Medicine,* **103**, 1068–72.

Johnson SL, McPhee L, Birch LL (1991) Conditioned preferences: children prefer flavors associated with high dietary fat. *Physiology & Behavior,* **50**, 1245–51.

Johnstone AM, Stubbs RJ, Harbron CG (1996) Effect of overfeeding macronutrients on day-to-day food intake in man. *European Journal of Clinical Nutrition,* **50**, 418–30.

Kalvie H, White TT (1972) Pancreatic islet β-cell tumors and hyperplasia. *Annals of Surgery,* **175**, 326–35.

Kanalay JA, Andresen-Reid ML, Oenning L, Kottke BA, Jensen MD (1993) Differential health benefits of weight loss in upper body and lower body obese women. *American Journal of Clinical Nutrition,* **57**, 20–26.

Kanarek RB, Ryu M, Przypek J (1995) Preferences for foods with varying levels of salt and fat differ as a function of dietary restraint and exercise but not menstrual cycle. *Physiology & Behavior,* **57**, 821–6.

Kanders BS (1995) Pediatric obesity. In: *Weighing the options* (ed. PR Thomas), pp. 210–33. Washington DC: National Academy Press.

Kannel WB, D'Agostino RB, Cobb JL (1996) Effect of weight on cardiovascular disease. *American Journal of Clinical Nutrition,* **63** (Suppl), 419S–422S.

Kant AK, Ballard-Barbash R, Schatzkin A (1995b) Evening eating and its relation to self-reported body weight and nutrient intake in women, CSFII 1985–86. *Journal of the American College of Nutrition,* **14**, 358–63.

Kant AK, Schatzkin A, Graubard BI, Ballard-Barbash R (1995a) Frequency of eating occasions and weight change in the NHANES I Epidemiologic Follow-up Study. *International Journal of Obesity,* **19**, 468–74.

Kaplan HI, Kaplan HS (1957) The psychosomatic concept of obesity. *Journal of Nervous and Mental Diseases,* **125**, 181–201.

Karam JH, Grodsky GM, Forsham PH (1963) Excessive insulin response to glucose in obese subjects as measured by immunochemical assay. *Diabetes*, **12**, 197–204.

Karhunen L, Lappalainen R, Sipiläinen R *et al.* (1997) Serum leptin in obese women: association with eating behavior, food intake and preference for sugar and fat. *Presented at Sixth Food Choice Conference*; Uppsala, Sweden, 25–27 June.

Karlsson J, Sjöström L, Sullivan M (1998) Swedish obese subjects (SOS) – an intervention study of obesity. Two year follow-up of health-related quality of life (HRQL) and eating behaviour after gastric surgery for severe obesity. *International Journal of Obesity*, **22**, 113–26.

Kaufman NA, Poznanski R, Guggenheim K (1975) Eating habits and opinions of teenagers on nutrition and obesity. *Journal of the American Dietetic Association*, **66**, 264–8.

Kayman S, Bruvold W, Stern JS (1990) Maintenance and relapse after weight loss in women: behavioral aspects *American Journal of Clinical Nutrition*, **52**, 800–807.

Keesey RE (1986) A set-point theory of obesity. In: *Handbook of Eating Disorders* (ed. KD Brownell, JP Foreynt) New York: Basic Books.

Kennedy GC (1953) The role of depot fat in the hypothalamic control of food intake in the rat. *Proceedings of the Royal Society* (B), **140**, 578–92.

Keppel KG, Taffel SM (1993) Pregnancy-related weight gain and retention: implications of the 1990 Institute of Medicine Guidelines. *American Journal of Public Health*, **83**, 1100–1103.

Kern DL, McPhee L, Fisher J, Johnson S, Birch LL (1993) The postingestive consequences of fat condition preferences for flavors associated with high dietary fat. *Physiology & Behavior*, **54**, 71–6.

Keys A (1970) Coronary heart disease in seven countries. *Circulation*, **4** (Suppl 1), 1–91.

Keys A, Fidanza F, Karvonen MJ, Kimura N, Taylor HL (1972) Indices of relative weight and obesity. *Journal of Chronic Diseases*, **25**, 329–43.

Keys A, Menotti A, Aravanis C *et al.* (1984) The seven countries study: 2289 deaths in 15 years. *Preventive Medicine*, **13**, 141–54.

Khosla T, Lowe CR (1971) Obesity and smoking habits. *British Medical Journal*, **4**, 10–13.

Khosla T, Lowe CR (1972) Obesity and smoking habits by social class. *British Journal of Preventive and Social Medicine*, **26**, 249–56.

Killoran A, Fentem P, Casperson C (eds) (1995) *Moving on: International Perspectives on Promoting Physical Activity*. London: Health Education Authority.

King A, Coles B (1992) *The health of Canada's youth: views and behaviours of 11, 13, and 15 year olds from 11 countries*. Canada: Ministry of National Health and Welfare.

King AC (1994) Clinical and community interventions to promote and support physical activity participation. In: *Advances in Exercise Adherence* (ed. RK Dishman), pp. 183–212. Champaign, IL: Human Kinetics.

King AC, Tribble DL (1991) The role of exercise in weight regulation in nonathletes. *Sports Medicine*, **11**, 331–49.

King NA, Blundell JE, Tremblay A (1997) Effects of exercise on appetite control: implications for energy balance. *Medicine and Science in Sports and Exercise*, **29**(8), 1076–89.

King NA, Burley VJ, Blundell JE (1994) Exercise-induced suppression of appetite: effects on food intake and implications for energy balance. *European Journal of Clinical Nutrition*, **48**, 715–24.

Kirschner MA, Schneider G, Ertel NH, Worton E (1982) Obesity, androgens, oestrogens and cancer risk. *Cancer Research*, **42**, 3281–5.

Klesges R, Klesges L, Haddock C, Eck L (1992) A longitudinal analysis of the impact of dietary intake and physical activity on weight change in adults. *American Journal of Clinical Nutrition*, **55**, 818–22.

Klesges RC (1995) Cigarette smoking and body weight In: *Eating Disorders and Obesity* (eds KD Brownell, CG Fairburn), pp. 61–4. New York: Guilford Press.

Klopper A (1991) Placental metabolism. In: *Clinical Physiology in Obstetrics* (eds FE Hytten, G Chamberlain). Oxford: Blackwell Scientific Publications.

Knight I (1984) *The Heights and Weights of Adults in Great Britain*. London: HMSO.

Knight TM, Smith Z, Whittles A *et al.* (1992) Insulin resistance, diabetes and risk markers for ischaemic heart disease in Asian men and non-Asian men in Bradford. *British Heart Journal*, **67**, 343–50.

Knowler WC, Pettit DJ, Savage P, Bennett PH (1981) Diabetes incidence in Pima Indians: contributions of obesity and parental diabetes. *American Journal of Epidemiology*, **113**, 144–56.

Kopelman PG (1994) Investigation of obesity. *Clinical Endocrinology*, **41**, 703–8.

Kopelman PG (1997) The effects of weight loss treatments on upper and lower body fat. *International Journal of Obesity*, **21**, 619–25.

Kopelman PG, Pilkington TRE, White N, Jeffcoate SL (1980) Abnormal sex steroid secretion and binding in massively obese women. *Clinical Endocrinology*, **12**, 363–9.

Kopelman PG, White N, Pilkington TRE, Jeffcoate SL (1981) The effect of weight loss on sex steroid secretion and binding in massively obese women. *Clinical Endocrinology*, **14**, 113–16.

Kral JG (1995) Surgical interventions for obesity. In: *Eating Disorders and Obesity* (eds KD Brownell, CG Fairburn), pp. 510–15. New York: Guilford Press.

Krief S, Lonnqvist F, Raimbault S *et al.* (1993) Tissue

distribution of β_3-adrenergic receptor mRNA in man. *Journal of Clinical Investigation*, **91**, 344–9.

Kristal AR, White E, Shattuck AL *et al.* (1992) Long-term maintenance of a low-fat diet: durability of fat-related dietary habits in the Women's Health Trial. *Journal of the American Dietetic Association*, **92**, 553–9.

Krotkiewski M, Mandroukas L, Sjöström L *et al.* (1979) Effects of long-term physical training on body fat, metabolism, and blood pressure in obesity. *Metabolism*, **28**, 650–58.

Krotkiewski M, Sjöström L, Björntorp PB, Carlgren G, Garellick G, Smith U (1977) Adipose tissue cellularity in relation to prognosis for weight reduction. *International Journal of Obesity*, **1**, 395–416.

Kuczmarski RJ, Flegal KM, Campbell SM, Johnson CL (1994) Increasing prevalence of overweight among US adults: the national health and nutrition examination surveys 1960–1991. *Journal of the American Medical Association*, **272**, 205–11.

Kulesza W (1982) Dietary intake in obese women. *Appetite*, **3**, 61–8.

Kuskowska-Wolka A, Bergstrom R (1993a) Trends in body mass index and prevalence of obesity in Swedish men 1980–89. *Journal of the Epidemiology in Community Health*, **47**, 103–8.

Kuskowska-Wolka A, Bergstrom R (1993b) Trends in body mass index and prevalence of obesity in Swedish women 1980–89. *Journal of the Epidemiology in Community Health*, **47**, 195–99.

Kwitek-Black AE, Carmi R, Duyk GM *et al.* (1993) Linkage of Bardet–Biedl syndrome to chromosome 16q and evidence for non-allelic genetic heterogeneity. *Nature Genetics*, **5**, 392–6.

Laessle RG, Tuschl RJ, Kotthaus BC, Pirke KM (1989) Behavioral and biological correlates of dietary restraint in normal life. *Appetite*, **12**, 83–94.

Laitinen JH, Tuorila HM, Uusitupa MIJ (1991) Changes in hedonic responses to sweet and fat in recently diagnosed non-insulin-dependent diabetic patients during diet therapy. *European Journal of Clinical Nutrition*, **45**, 393–400.

Lang, T (1995) Food retailing and food poverty: of deserts and firefighting. In: *Food and Low Income: A Conference Report*. London National Food Alliance.

Lang T, Dibb S, Cole-Hamilton I, Lobstein T (1989) This food business. *New Statesman and Society*, August 11, (Suppl 2), 1–13.

Langer O (1991) Prevention of macrosomia. In: *Bailliere's Clinical Obstetrics and Gynecology. Diabetes in pregnancy* (ed. JN Oats), pp. 333–94. London: Bailliere Tindall.

Langhans W, Scharrer E (1992) Metabolic control of eating. In: *Metabolic Control of Eating, Energy Expenditure and the Bioenergentics of Obesity*. World Rev Nutrition and Diet, **70**, pp. 1–67. Basel: Karger.

Langhoff-Roos J, Lindmark G, Gebre-Medhin M (1987) Maternal fat stores and fat accretion during pregnancy in relation to infant birth weight. *British Journal of Obstetrics and Gynaecology*, **94**, 1170–77.

Langhoff-Roos J, Wibell L, Gebre-Medhin M, Lindmark G (1988) Maternal glucose metabolism and infant birth weight: a study in healthy pregnant women. *Diabetes Research*, **8**, 165–70.

Lannon J (1986) How people choose food: the role of advertising and packaging. In: *The Food Consumer* (eds C Ritson, L Gofton, J McKenzie). Chichester: John Wiley and Sons Ltd.

Lapidus L, Bengtsson C, Larsson B, Pennert K, Rybo E, Sjöström L (1984) Distribution of adipose tissue and risk of cardiovascular disease and death: a 12 year follow-up of participants in the population study of women in Gothenburg, Sweden. *British Medical Journal*, **289**, 1257–61.

LaPorte DJ (1990) A fatiguing effect in obese patients during partial fasting: increase in vulnerability to emotion-related events and anxiety. *International Journal of Eating Disorders*, **9**(3), 345–55.

Larsen F, Torgersen S (1989) Personality changes after gastric banding surgery for morbid obesity: a prospective study. *Journal of Psychosomatic Research*, **33**(3), 323–34.

Larsen PR, Inggbar SH (1992) The thyroid gland. In: *Williams Textbook of Endocrinology* (eds JD Wilson, DW Foster), pp. 357–487. Philadelphia: WB Saunders.

Larsson B (1987) Regional obesity as a health hazard in men: prospective studies. *Acta Medica Scandinavia*, **723** (Suppl), 45–51.

Larsson B, Svardsudd K, Welin L, Wilhelmsen L, Björntorp BP, Tibblin G (1984) Abdominal adipose tissue distribution, obesity, and risk of cardiovascular disease and death: 13 year follow up of participants in the study of men born in 1913. *British Medical Journal*, **288**, 1401–4.

Laurier D, Guiguet M, Chau NP, Wells JA, Valleron AJ (1992) Prevalence of obesity: a comparative study in France, the United Kingdom and the United States. *International Journal of Obesity*, **16**, 565–72.

Law CM, Barker DJ, Osmond C, Fall CH, Simmonds SJ (1992) Early growth and abdominal fatness in adult life. *Journal of the Epidemiology in Community Health*, **46**, 184–6.

Lawrence M, McKillop FM, Durnin JVGA (1991) Women who gain more fat during pregnancy may not have bigger babies: implications for recommended weight gain during pregnancy. *British Journal of Obstetrics and Gynaecology*, **98**, 254–9.

Lawson OJ, Williamson DA, Champagne CM *et al.* (1995) The association of body weight, dietary intake, and energy expenditure with dietary restraint and disinhibition. *Obesity Research*, **3**, 153–61.

Lawton CL, Blundell JE (1998) The role of reduced fat diets and fat substitutes in the regulation of energy and fat intake and body weight. *Current Opinion in Lipidology*, **9**, 41–5.

Lawton CL, Burley VJ, Ales JK, Blundell JE (1993) Dietary fat and appetite control in obese subjects: weak effects on satiation and satiety. *International Journal of Obesity*, **17**, 409–16.

Lazarus R, Baur L, Webb K, Blyth F (1996) Adiposity and body mass indices in children: Benn's index and other weight for height indices as measures of adiposity. *International Journal of Obesity*, **20**, 406–12.

Le Blanc J, Brondel L (1985) Role of palatability on meal-induced thermogenesis in human subjects. *American Journal of Physiology*, **248**, E333–E336.

Lean M, Anderson A (1988) Clinical strategies for obesity management. *Diabetic Medicine*, **5**, 515–18.

Lean MEJ, Han TS, Morrison CE (1995) Waist circumference as a measure for indicating need for weight management. *British Medical Journal*, **311**, 158–61.

Lean MEJ, Han TS, Seidall JC (1998) Impairment of health and quality of life in people with large waist circumference. *Lancet*, **351**, 853–6.

Lean MEJ, James WPT (1986) Prescription of diabetic diets in the 1980s. *Lancet*, **1**, 723–5.

Lean MEJ, Powrioge JK, Anderson AS, Garthwaite PH (1990) Obesity, weight loss and prognosis in type 2 diabetes. *Diabetic Medicine*, **7**, 228–33.

Lean M (1997) Sibutramine a review of clinical efficacy. *International Journal of Obesity*, **21**(Suppl 1), S30–S36.

Leatherhead Food Research Association (1996) *Increasing the Consumption of Vegetables amongst Target Groups*. A report of research carried out by Leatherhead Food Research Association on Behalf of the Ministry of Agriculture, Fisheries and Food.

Ledbetter DH, Riccardi VM, Airhardt SD (1981) Deletions of chromosome 15 as a cause of the Prader–Willi syndrome. *New England Journal of Medicine*, **304**, 325.

Lederman SA (1993) The effect of pregnancy weight gain on later obesity. *Obstetrics and Gynecology*, **82**, 148–55.

Lee CD, Jackson AS, Blair SN (1998). US weight guidelines: is it also important to consider cardiorespiratory fitness? *International Journal of Obesity*, **22** (Suppl 20), S2–S7.

Leibel RL, Rosenbaum M, Hirsch J (1995) Changes in energy expenditure resulting from altered body weight. *New England Journal of Medicine*, **332** (10), 621–8.

Leifer M (1977) Psychological changes accompanying pregnancy and motherhood. *Genetic Psychology Monographs*, **95**, 55–96.

Leikin EL, Jenkins JH, Pomerantz GA, Klein L (1987) Abnormal glucose screening tests in pregnancy. A risk factor for fetal macrosomia. *Obstetric Gynecology*, **69**, 570–73.

Leitch CA, Jones PJH (1993) Measurement of human lipogenesis using deuterium incorporation. *Journal of Lipid Research*, **34**, 157–63.

LeMagnen J (1983) Body energy balance and food intake: a neuroendocrine regulatory mechanism. *Physiological Reviews*, **63**, 314–86.

LeMagnen J (1985) *Hunger*. Cambridge: Cambridge University Press.

Leon GR, Roth L (1977) Obesity: causes, correlations, and speculations. *Psychological Bulletin* **84**, 117–39

Leppert M, Baird L, Anderson KL, Otterud B, Lupski JR, Lewis RA (1994) Bardet–Biedl syndrome is linked to DNA markers on chromosome 11q and is genetically heterogeneous. *Nature Genetics*, **7**, 108–12.

Lessan NG, Finer N (1996) Is hypothyroidism a cause of obesity? *Clinical Endocrinology*, **151**, 106 (Abstract).

Leveille G (1970) Adipose tissue metabolism. Influence of periodicity of eating and diet composition. *Federation Proceedings*, **29**, 1294–1301.

Lévy E, Lévy P, Le Pen C, Badsdevant A (1995) The economic cost of obesity: the French situation. *International Journal of Obesity*, **19**, 788–92.

Lew EA (1985) Mortality and weight: insured lives and the American Cancer Society study. *Annals of Internal Medicine*, **103**, 1024–9.

Lichtman S, Pisarka K, Berman F et al. (1992) Discrepancy between self-reported and actual caloric intake and exercise in obese subjects. *New England Journal of Medicine*, **327**, 1893–8.

Liebowitz SF, Hoebel BG (1998) Behavioural neuroscience of obesity. In: *Handbook of Obesity*. (eds GA Bray, C Bouchard, WPT James). New York: Marcel Dekker.

Lightman SW, Pisarska K, Berman ER et al. (1992) Discrepancy between self-reported and actual caloric intake and exercise in obese subjects. *New England Journal of Medicine*, **327**, 1893–8.

Lindroos A-K, Lissner L, Sjöström L (1996) Weight change in relation to intake of sugar and sweet foods before and after weight reducing gastric surgery. *International Journal of Obesity*, **20**, 634–43.

Lissau I, Sorensen TIA (1994) Parental neglect during childhood and increased risk of obesity in young adulthood. *Lancet*, **343**, 324–7.

Lissner L, Brownell KD (1992) Weight cycling, mortality and cardiovascular disease: a review of epidemiologic findings In: *Obesity* (eds PB Björntorp, BN Brostoff), pp. 653–61. Philadelphia: Lippincott.

Lissner L, Heitmann BL (1995) Dietary fat and obesity: evidence from epidemiology. *European Journal of Clinical Nutrition*, **49**, 79–90.

Lissner L, Bengtsson C, Lapidus L, Larsson B, Bengtsson B, Brownell K (1989) Body weight variability and mortality in the Gothenburg prospective studies of men and women. In: *Obesity in Europe 88* (eds PB Björntorp, S Rossner), pp. 55–60. London: Libbey.

Lissner L, Levitsky DA, Strupp BJ, Kalkwarf HJ, Roe DA (1987) Dietary fat and the regulation of energy intake in human subjects. *American Journal of Clinical Nutrition,* **46**, 886–92.

Lissner L, Odell PM, D'Agostino RB *et al.* (1991) Variability of body weight and health outcomes in the Framingham population. *New England Journal of Medicine,* **324**, 1839–44.

Livingstone MBE, Strain JJ, Prentice AM, Coward WA, Nevin GB, Barker ME, Hickey RJ, McKenna PG, Whitehead RG (1991) Potential contribution of leisure activity to the energy expenditure patterns of sedentary populations. *British Journal of Nutrition,* **65**, 145–55.

Lluch A, Stricker-Krongrad A, Michel F, Méjean L (1995) Food preferences and food intake in French obese consultants. *Appetite,* **24**, 193 (Abstract).

Lonnqvist F, Arner P, Nordfors L, Schalling M (1995) Overexpression of the obese (*ob*) gene in adipose tissue of human obese subjects. *Nature Medicine,* **1**, 950–53.

Louis-Sylvestre J, LeMagnen J (1980) A fall in blood glucose level precedes meal onset in free feeding rats. *Neuroscience and Behavioural Research,* **4**, 13–15.

Löffler G, Herberg L, Bachmeier M, Maier M, Laub R (1994) Regulation of adipose tissue growth. In: *Obesity in Europe 1993* (ed. H Ditschuneit), pp. 41–9. London: Libbey.

Lucas A (1991) Programming by early nutrition in man. In: *The Childhood Environment and Adult Disease* (eds GR Bock, J Whelan), pp. 38–55. Chichester: John Wiley.

Luciano A, Bressan F, Zoppi G (1997) Body mass index reference curves for children aged 3–19 years from Verona, Italy. *European Journal of Clinical Nutrition,* **51**, 6–10.

Lusky A, Barell V, Lubin F *et al.* (1996) Relationship between morbidity and extreme values of body mass index in adolescents. *International Journal of Epidemiology,* **25**, 829–34.

Lustig A (1991) Weight loss programmes: failing to meet ethical standards. *Journal of the American Dietetic Association,* **91** (10), 1252–4.

Lyle BJ, McMahon KE, Kreutler PA (1991) Assessing the potential dietary impact of replacing dietary fat with other macronutrients. *Journal of Nutrition,* **122**, 211–16.

Lyon XH, DiVetta V, Milon H, Jéquier E, Schutry Y (1995) Compliance to dietary advice directed towards increasing the carbohydrate to fat ratio of the everyday diet. *International Journal of Obesity,* **19**, 260–69.

Macdiarmid JI, Hetherington MM (1995) Mood modulation by food: an exploration of affect and cravings in 'chocolate addicts'. *British Journal of Clinical Psychology,* **34**, 129–38.

MacFie HJH, Thomson DMH (1994) *Measurement of Food Preferences.* London: Blackie.

Maddox GL, Back K, Liederman V (1968) Overweight as social deviance and disability. *Journal of Health and Social Behaviour,* **9**, 287–98.

Maehlum S, Grandmontagne M, Newsholme EA, Sejersted OM (1986) Magnitude and duration of excess postexercise oxygen consumption in healthy young subjects. *Metabolism,* **35**, 425–9.

Maffei M, Halaas J, Ravussin E, Pratley RE, Lee GH (1995) Leptin levels in human and rodent: measurement of plasma leptin and *ob* RNA in obese and weight-reduced subjects. *Nature Medicine,* **1**, 1155–61.

Mahoney MJ, Mahoney K (1976) Cognitive ecology: cleaning up what you say to yourself. In: *Permanent Weight Control,* pp. 46–68. New York, Norton.

Malcolm R, O'Neill PM, Hirsch AA, Currey HS, Moskowitz G (1980) Taste hedonics and thresholds in obesity. *International Journal of Obesity,* **4**, 203–12.

Manson JE, Colditz GA, Stampfer MJ (1994) Parity, ponderosity and the paradox of a weight-preoccupied society (Editorial). *Journal of the American Medical Association,* **271**, 1788–90.

Manson JE, Colditz GA, Stamfer MJ *et al.* (1990) A prospective study of obesity and risk of coronary heart disease in women. *New England Journal of Medicine,* **322**, 822–9.

Manson JE, Willett WC, Stamfer MJ *et al.* (1995) Body weight and mortality among women. *New England Journal of Medicine,* **333**, 677–85.

Marcus CL, Curtis S, Koerner CB, Joffe A, Serwint JR, Loughlin GM (1996) Evaluation of pulmonary function and polysomnography in obese children and adolescents. *Pediatric Pulmonology,* **21**, 176–83.

Marcus MD, Wing RR (1987) Binge eating among the obese. *Annals of Behavioral Medicine,* **9**, 23–7.

Marcus MD (1993) Binge eating in obesity. In: *Binge Eating: Nature, Assessment and Treatment* (eds CG Fairburn, GT Wilson,), pp. 77–96. New York: Guilford Press.

Marcus MD, Wing RR, Lamparski DM (1985) Binge eating and dietary restraint in obese patients. *Addictive Behaviours,* **10**, 163–8.

Maresh M, Beard RW, Bray CS, Elkeles RS, Wadsworth J (1989) Factors predisposing to and outcome of gestational diabetes. *Obstetric Gynecology,* **74**, 342–6.

Marmot MG, Davey Smith G, Stanfeld S *et al.* (1991) Health inequalities among British civil servants: the Whitehall II study. *Lancet,* **337**, 1387–93.

Martin WH III (1996) Effects of acute and chronic exercise on fat metabolism. *Exercise and Sports Science Reviews,* **24**, 203–31.

Martinson EW, Morgan WP (1997) Antidepressant effects of physical activity. In: *Physical Activity and Mental Health* (ed. WP Morgan), pp. 93–106. Washington, DC: Taylor and Francis.

Mason EE (1982) Vertical banded gastroplasty for morbid obesity. *Archives of Surgery*, **117**, 701–6.

Mattes RD (1993) Fat preference and adherence to a reduced-fat diet. *American Journal of Clinical Nutrition*, **57**, 373–81.

Maxfield E, Konishi F (1966) Patterns of food intake and physical activity in obesity. *Journal of the American Dietetic Association*, **49**, 406–8.

Mayer J (1953) Glucostatic mechanism of regulation of food intake. *New England Journal of Medicine*, **249**, 13–16.

Mayer J, Marshall ND *et al.* (1954) Exercise, food intake, and body weight in normal and genetically obese adult mice. *American Journal of Physiology*, **77**, S44.

McAuley E, Courneya K (1993) Adherence to exercise and physical activity as health promoting behaviors: attitudinal and self-efficacy influences. *Applied and Preventive Psychology*, **2**, 65–77.

McCance RA, Widdowson EM (1974) The determinants of growth and form. *Proceedings of the Royal Academy of London B*, **185**, 1–17.

McCann BS, Warnick GR, Knopp RH (1990) Changes in plasma lipids and dietary intake accompanying shifts in perceived workload and stress. *Psychosomatic Medicine*, **52**, 97–108.

McGandy RB, Barrows CH, Spanias A, Meredith A, Stone JL, Norris JH (1966) Nutrient intakes and energy expenditure in men of different ages. *Journal of Gerontology*, **21**, 581–7.

McKeigue PM, Shah B, Marmot MG (1991) Relation of central obesity and insulin resistance with high diabetes prevalence and cardiovascular risk in South Asians. *Lancet*, **337**, 382–6.

McMurray RG, Harrell JS, Levine AA, Gansky SA (1995) Childhood obesity elevates blood pressure and total cholesterol independent of physical activity. *International Journal of Obesity*, **19**, 881–6.

McNeill G, Morrison DC, Davidson L, Smith JS (1992) The effect of changes in dietary carbohydrate v fat intake on 24 hour energy expenditure and nutrient oxidation in post-menopausal women. *Proceedings of the Nutrition Society*, **51**, 91A.

Meade TW, Ruddock V, Stirling Y, Chakrabati R, Miller GJ (1993) Fibrinolytic activity, clotting factors and long-term incidence of ischaemic heart disease in the Northwick Park study. *Lancet*, **342**, 1076–9.

Meichenbaum D (1977) *Cognitive-behavior Modification.* New York: Plenum Press.

Meiselman HL, Wyant KW (1981) Food preferences and flavor experiences. In: *Criteria of Food Acceptance* (eds J Solms, RL Hall), pp. 144–52. Zurich: Forster Verlag.

Meiselman HL (1977) The role of sweetness in the food preference of young adults. In: *Taste and development. The genesis of sweet taste preference* (ed. JM Weiffen-

bach), pp. 269–79. Washington DC: US Government Printing Office.

Meisler JG, St Jeor S (1996) Summary and recommendations from the American Health Foundation's expert panel on healthy weight. *American Journal of Clinical Nutrition*, **63** (Suppl 3), 474S–477S.

Mela DJ (1992) Sensory evaluation methods in nutrition and dietetics research. In: *Research: Successful Approaches* (ed. ER Monsen), pp. 220–47. Chicago: American Dietetic Association.

Mela DJ (1995) Understanding fat preference and consumption: applications of behavioural sciences to a nutritional problem. *Proceedings of the Nutrition Society*, **54**, 453–64.

Mela DJ (1996a) Assessing the dietary implications of macronutrient substitutes. In: *Progress in Obesity Research 7* (ed. A Angel), Chapter 59, pp. 423–30. London: John Libbey.

Mela DJ (1996b) Eating behaviour, food preferences and dietary intake in relation to obesity and body weight status. *Proceedings of the Nutrition Society*, **55**, 803–16.

Mela DJ (1996c) Implications of fat replacement for nutrition and food intake. *Fett/Lipid*, **98**, 50–55.

Mela DJ (1997a) Impact of macronutrient-substituted foods on food choice and dietary intake. *Annals of the New York Academy of Sciences*, **819**, 96–107.

Mela DJ (1997b) Fat and sugar substitutes: implications for dietary intakes and energy balance. *Proceedings of the Nutrition Society*, **56**, 827–40.

Mela DJ, Aaron JI (1997) 'Honest but invalid': What the subjects say about recording their food intake. *Journal of the American Dietetic Association*, **97**, 791–3.

Mela DJ, Catt SL (1996) Ontogeny of human taste and smell preferences and their implications for food selection. In: *Long Term Consequences of Early Environments* (eds CJK Henry, SJ Ulijaszek), pp. 137–52. Cambridge: Cambridge University Press.

Mela DJ, Langley K, Martin A (1994) Sensory assessment of fat content: effect of emulsion and subject characteristics. *Appetite*, **22**, 67–81.

Mela DJ, Rogers PJ (1998) *Food & Obesity: The Psychobiological Basis of Appetite and Weight Control.* London: Chapman & Hall.

Mela DJ, Sacchetti DS (1991) Sensory preferences for fats in foods: relationships to diet and body composition. *American Journal of Clinical Nutrition*, **53**, 908–15.

Mela DJ, Trunck F, Aaron JI (1993) No effect of extended home use on liking for sensory characteristics of reduced-fat foods. *Appetite*, **21**, 117–29.

Mellinkoff S, Frankland S, Boyle D *et al.* (1956) Relationship between serum amino acid concentration and fluctuations in appetite. *Journal of Applied Physiology*, **8**, 535–8.

Metzger BE, Silverman BL, Freinkel N, Dooley SL,

Ogata ES, Green OC (1990) Amniotic fluid concentration as a predictor of obesity. *Archives of Disease in Childhood*, **65**, 1050–52.

Metzner HL, Lamphiear DE, Wheeler NC, Larkin FA (1977) The relationship between frequency of eating and adiposity in adult men and women in the Tecumseh Community Health Study. *American Journal of Clinical Nutrition*, **30**, 712–15.

Michener W, Rozin P (1994) Pharmacological versus sensory factors in the satiation of chocolate craving. *Physiology & Behavior*, **56**(3), 419–22.

Miller DS, Mumford P (1967) Gluttony 1: An experimental study of overeating on high protein diets. *American Journal of Clinical Nutrition*, **20**, 1212–22.

Miller DS, Mumford P, Stock MJ (1967) Gluttony 2: Thermogenesis in overeating man. *American Journal of Clinical Nutrition*, **20**, 1223–9.

Miller GJ, Kotecha S, Wilkinson WH *et al.* (1988) Dietary and other characteristics relevant for coronary heart disease in men of Indian, West Indian and European descent in London. *Atherosclerosis*, **70**, 63–72.

Miller WR (1996) Motivational interviewing: Research, practice and puzzles. *Addictive Behaviors*, **21**, 835–42.

Mills JK (1994) The obese personality: defense, compromise, symbiotic arrest, and the characterologically depressed self. *Issues in Psychoanalytic Psychology*, **16**(1), 67–80.

Ministry of Agriculture, Fisheries and Food (1993) *National Food Survey 1992*. Annual Report on Household Food Consumption and Expenditure. London: HMSO.

Ministry of Agriculture, Fisheries and Food (1995) *National Food Survey 1994*. Annual Report on Household Food Consumption and Expenditure. London: HMSO.

Ministry of Agriculture, Fisheries and Food (1996) *National Food Survey 1995*. Annual Report on Household Food Consumption and Expenditure. London: HMSO.

Ministry of Agriculture, Fisheries and Food (1997) *National Food Survey 1996*. Annual Report on Household Food Consumption and Expenditure. London: HMSO.

Ministry of Agriculture, Fisheries and Food (1998) *National Food Survey 1997*. Annual Report on Household Food Consumption and Expenditure. London: HMSO.

Monroe KB, Petroshius SM (1981) Buyers' perceptions of price: an update of the evidence. In: *Perspectives in Consumer Behaviour*, 3rd ed. (eds HH Kassarjan, TS Pobertsin), pp. 43–4. London: Scott, Foresman and Company.

Montague CT, Farooqi IS, Whitehead JP *et al.* (1997a) Congenital leptin deficiency is associated with severe early-onset obesity in humans. *Nature,* **387**, 903–8.

Montague CT, Prins JB, Sanders L, Digby JE, O'Rahilly S (1997b) Depot- and sex-specific differences in human leptin mRNA expression: implications for the control of regional fat distribution. *Diabetes*, **46**(3), 342–7.

Moore L (1994) *Health-related behaviours in Wales, 1985–93: findings from the Health in Wales Surveys.* Cardiff: Health Promotion Wales.

Morgan KJ, Johnson SR, Stampley GL (1983) Children's frequency of eating, total sugar intake and weight/height stature. *Nutrition Research,* **3**, 635–52.

MRC Epidemiology Unit (1991) *Epidemiological Studies of Cardiovascular Diseases. Progress Report VII*. Cardiff: MRC Epidemiology Unit.

Muls E, Kempen K, Vansant G, Saris W (1995) Is weight cycling detrimental to health? A review of the literature in humans. *International Journal of Obesity,* **19** (Suppl 3), S46–S50.

Murgatroyd PR, Shetty PS, Prentice AM (1993a) Techniques for measurement of human energy expenditure: a practical guide. *International Journal of Obesity,* **17**, 549–68.

Murgatroyd PR, Souko BJ, Wittekind A, Goldberg GR, Ceesay SM, Prentice AM (1993b) Non-invasive techniques for assessing carbohydrate flux: 1. Measurement of depletion by indirect calorimeter. *Acta Physiologica Scandinavica,* **147**, 91–8.

Mussell MP (1995) Onset of binge eating, dieting, obesity and mood disorders among subjects seeking treatment for binge eating disorder. *International Journal of Eating Disorders,* **17**(4), 395–401.

Must A, Jacques PF, Dallal GE, Bajema CJ, Dietz WH (1992) Long-term morbidity and mortality of overweight adolescents. A follow-up of the Harvard Growth study of 1922 to 1935. *New England Journal of Medicine,* **327**, 1350–55.

Naeye RL (1979) Weight gain and the outcome of pregnancy. *American Journal of Obstetrics and Gynecology,* **135**, 3–9.

Naeye RL (1990) Maternal body weight and pregnancy outcome. *American Journal of Clinical Nutrition,* **52**, 273–9.

National Advisory Committee on Nutrition Education (1983) *Proposals for Nutritional Guidelines for Health Education in Britain*. London: Health Education Council.

National Task Force on the Prevention and Treatment of Obesity (1993a) Weight Cycling. *Journal of the American Medical Association,* **272**(15), 1196–1202.

National Task Force on the Prevention and Treatment of Obesity (1993b) Very low-calorie diets. *Journal of the American Medical Association,* **270**(8), 967–74.

Neggers Y, Goldenburg RL, Cliver SP, Hoffman HJ, Cutter GR (1995) The relationship between maternal and neonatal anthropometric measurements in term newborns. *Obstetric Gynecology,* **85**, 192–6.

New SA, Grubb DA (1996) Relationship of biscuit, cake and confectionery consumption to body mass index and energy intake in Scottish women. *Proceedings of the Nutrition Society,* **55**, 122A.

Newcombe RG (1982) Development of obesity in parous women. *Journal of Epidemiology and Community Health,* **36**, 306–9.

Newmark SR, Williamson B (1983) Survey of very-low-calorie weight reduction diets, novelty diets. *Archives of Internal Medicine,* **143**, 1195–8.

Newsholme EA, Leech AR (1983) *Biochemistry for the Medical Sciences.* Chichester: John Wiley.

Ni Mhurchu C, Margetts BM, Speller VM (1997) Applying the stages of change model to dietary change. *Nutrition Reviews,* **55** (1), 10–16.

Nicholls RD, Knoll J, Butler MG, Karam S, Lalande M (1989) Genetic imprinting suggested by maternal heterodisomy in non-deletion Prader–Willi syndrome. *Nature,* **342**, 281–5.

Nicolaidis S, Rowland N (1976) Metering of intravenous versus oral nutrients and regulation of energy balance. *American Journal of Physiology,* **231**, 661–8.

NIH Technology Assessment Conference Panel (1992) Methods for voluntary weight loss and control. *Annals of Internal Medicine,* **116** (11), 941–9.

NIH Technology Assessment Conference Panel (1993) Methods for voluntary weight loss and control. *Annals of Internal Medicine,* **119**, 764–70.

Nisbett RE (1968) Taste, deprivation, and weight determinants of eating behavior. *Journal of Personality and Social Psychology,* **10**, 107–16.

Novin D, Robinson K, Culbreth LA *et al.* (1985) Is there a role for the liver in control of food intake? *American Journal of Clinical Nutrition,* **42**, 1050–62.

O'Leary KD, Wilson GT (1975) *Behavior Therapy: Application and Outcome.* Englewood Cliff: Prentice Hall.

O'Neill O, Fehily A (1991) Nutrient intakes of men in South Wales: a comparison of surveys taken in 1980–1983 and 1990. *Journal of Human Nutrition and Dietetics,* **4**, 413–19.

Ockene J, Kristellar J, Ockene I (1992) Smoking cessation in cardiac patients: the coronary artery smoking intervention study. *Health Psychology,* **11** (2), 119–26.

Office of Health Economics (1994) *Obesity.* London: Office of Health Economics.

Office of Population Censuses and Surveys (1990) *The General Household Survey.* London: HMSO.

Office of Population, Censuses and Surveys (1994) *The General Household Survey.* London: HMSO.

Ohlin A, Rossner S (1996) Factors related to body weight changes during and after pregnancy: the Stockholm pregnancy and weight development study. *Obesity Research,* **4**, 271–6.

Ohlin A, Rossner S (1994) Trends in eating patterns, physical activity and sociodemographic factors in relation to post-partum body weight development. *British Journal of Nutrition,* **71**, 457–70.

Ohlin A, Rossner S (1990) Maternal body weight development after pregnancy. *International Journal of Obesity,* **14,** 159–73.

Oppert J-M, Vohl M-C, Chagnon M, Dionne FT *et al.* (1994) DNA polymorphism in the uncoupling protein (UCP) gene and human body fat. *International Journal of Obesity,* **18**, 526–31.

Orbach S (1978) *Fat is a Feminist Issue,* pp. 192. London: Hamlyn.

Orford J (1984) *Excessive Appetites,* Chichester: Wiley.

Ortega RM, Requejo AM, Andrés P *et al.* (1995) Relationship between diet composition and body mass index in a group of Spanish adolescents. *British Journal of Nutrition,* **74**, 765–73.

Ortega RM, Requejo AM, Quintas E *et al.* (1996) Estimated energy balance in female university students: differences with respect to body mass index and concern about body weight. *International Journal of Obesity,* **20**, 1127–9.

Ortmeyer HK, Bodkin NL, Varghese SS, Hansen BC (1996) Glycogen phosphorylase activity and glycogen concentration in muscle of normal to overtly diabetic rhesus monkeys. *International Journal of Obesity,* **20**, 98–105.

Pacy PJ, Barton N, Webster JD, Garrow JS (1985) The energy cost of aerobic exercise in fed and fasted normal subjects. *American Journal of Clinical Nutrition,* **42**, 764–8.

Pangborn RM, Bos KEO, Stern JS (1985) Dietary fat intake and taste responses to fat in milk by under, normal, and overweight women. *Appetite,* **6**, 25–40.

Parham ES, Astrom MF, King SH (1990) The association of pregnancy weight gain with the mothers post-partum weight. *Journal of the American Dietetic Association,* **90**, 550–54.

Parker DR, Gonzalez S, Derby CA, Gans KM, Lasater TM, Carleton RA (1997) Dietary factors in relation to weight change among men and women from two southeastern New England communities. *International Journal of Obesity,* **21**, 103–9.

Parker JD, Abrams B (1993) Differences in post-partum weight retention between black and white mothers. *Obstetrics and Gynecology,* **81**, 768–74.

Pascale RW, Wing RR, Butler BA, Mullen MM, Bononi P (1995) Effects of a behavioural weight loss program stressing calorie restriction versus calorie plus fat restriction in obese individuals with NIDDM or a family history of diabetes. *Diabetes Care,* **18**, 1241–8.

Passmore R (1973) Energy balance and control of body weight. In: *Human Nutrition and Dietetics,* 4th ed. (eds S Davidson, R Passmore, JF Brock), pp. 27–33. Edinburgh: Churchill-Livingstone.

Pate RR, Pratt M, Blain SN *et al.* (1995) Physical activity and public health: A recommendation from the Centers for Disease Control and Prevention and the American College of Sports Medicine. *Journal of the American Medical Association,* **273**, 402–8.

Pate RR, Long BJ, Heath G (1994) Descriptive epidemiology of physical activity in adolescents. *Pediatric Exercise Science,* **6**, 434–47.

Patrick JM, Bassey EJ, Irving JM, Blecher A, Fentem PA (1986) Objective measurements of customary physical activity in elderly men and women before and after retirement. *Quarterly Journal of Experimental Physiology,* **71**, 47–58.

Paul AA, Southgate DAT (1978) *McCance & Widdowson's 'The Composition of Foods',* 4th ed. London: HMSO.

Pavlou KN, Krey S, Steffee WP (1989) Exercise as an adjunct to weight loss and maintenance in moderately obese subjects. *American Journal of Clinical Nutrition,* **49**, 1115–23.

Payne JH, De Wind LT (1969) Surgical treatment of obesity. *American Journal of Surgery,* **118**, 141–7.

Pears J, Jung RT, Gunn A (1990) Long term weight changes in treated hypothyroid and hyperthyroid patients. *Scottish Medical Journal,* **35**, 180–82.

Pelleymounter MA, Cullen MJ, Baker MB *et al.* (1995) Effects of the obese gene product on body weight regulation in *ob/ob* mice. *Science,* **269**, 540–42.

Perri MG (1992) Improving maintenance of weight loss following treatment by diet and lifestyle modification. In: *Treatment of the Seriously Obese Patient* (eds TA Wadden, TB Van Italie), pp. 456–77. London: Guilford Press.

Perri MG, McAdoo WG, McAllister DA, Laver JB, Yancey DZ (1986) Enhancing the efficacy of behavior therapy for obesity: effects of aerobic exercise and a multicomponent treatment maintenance program. *Journal of Consulting and Clinical Psychology,* **54,** 670–75.

Perri MG, McAllister PA, Gange JJ, Jordan RC, McAdoo WG, Neyu AM (1988) Effects of four maintenance programs on long term maintenance of obesity. *Journal of Consulting and Clinical Psychology,* **56** (4), 529–34.

Perri MG, Neyu AM, Patti ET, McCann LL (1989) Effect of length of treatment on weight loss. *Journal of Consulting and Clinical Psychology,* **57** (3), 450–52.

Perri MG, Shapiro RM, Warren WL, McAdoo WG (1984) Maintenance strategies for the treatment of obesity: an evaluation of relapse prevention training and post treatment contact by mail and telephone. *Journal of Consulting and Clinical Psychology,* **52** (3), 404–13.

Peters ETHJ, Seidell JC, Menotti A *et al.* (1995) Changes in body weight in relation to mortality in 6441 European middle-aged men: The Seven Countries Study. *International Journal of Obesity,* **19**, 862–8.

Peters JC, Harper AE (1981) Protein and energy consumption, plasma amino acids ratios and brain neurotransmitter concentrations. *Physiology & Behavior,* **27**, 287–98.

Pettitt DJ, Baird HR, Aleck KA, Bennett PH, Knowler WC (1983) Excessive obesity in offspring of Pima Indian women with diabetes during pregnancy. *New England Journal of Medicine,* **308**, 242.

Pettitt DJ, Bennett PH, Knowler WC, Baird HR, Aleck KA (1985) Gestational diabetes mellitus and impaired glucose tolerance during pregnancy. Long-term effects on obesity and glucose tolerance in the offspring. *Diabetes,* **34** (Suppl 2), 119–22.

Pettitt DJ, Knowler WC, Bennett PH, Aleck KA, Baird HR (1987) Obesity in offspring of diabetic Pima Indian women despite normal birth weight. *Diabetes Care,* **10**, 76–80.

Pettitt DJ, Nelson RG, Saad MF, Bennett PH, Knowler WC (1993) Diabetes and obesity in the offspring of Pima Indian women with diabetes during pregnancy. *Diabetes Care,* **16** (Suppl 1), 310–17.

Pfohl M, Luft D, Blomberg I, Schmollimg RM (1994) Long-term changes of body weight and cardiovascular risk factors after weight reduction with group therapy and dexfenfluramine. *International Journal of Obesity,* **18**, 391–5.

Phinney SD, LaGrange BM, O'Connell M, Danforth R Jr. (1988) Effects of aerobic exercise on energy balance and nitrogen balance during very low calorie dieting. *Metabolism,* **37**, 758–65.

Plante TG, Rodin J (1990) Physical fitness and enhanced psychological health. *Current Psychology: Research and Reviews,* **9,** 3–24.

Platte P, Wurmser H, Wade SE, Mecheril A, Pirke KM (1996) Resting metabolic rate and diet-induced thermogenesis in restrained and unrestrained eaters. *International Journal of Eating Disorders,* **20**, 33–41.

Plummer WA (1940) *Body Weight in Spontaneous Myxoedema,* pp. 88–98. Transactions of the American Association for the Study of Goiter.

Podar T, Solutsev A, Väli M, Vinogradova T, Podar I (1996) No deterioration of glucose tolerance in weight cycling obese. *International Journal of Obesity,* **20**, 921–4.

Polivy J (1976) Perception of calories and regulation of intake in restrained and unrestrained subjects. *Addictive Behaviors,* **1**, 237–43.

Polivy J, Herman CP, Younger JC, Erskine B (1979) Effects of a model on eating behavior: the induction of a restrained eating style. *Journal of Personality,* **47**, 100–114.

Pollack CP, Green J, Smith GP (1989) Blood glucose prior to meal request in humans isolated from all temporal cues. *Physiology & Behavior,* **46**, 529–34.

Poppitt SD, Prentice AM (1996) Energy density and its role in the control of food intake: evidence from metabolic and community studies. *Appetite*, **26**, 153–74.

Poppitt SD, Prentice AM, Goldberg GR, Whitehead RG (1994) Energy-sparing strategies to protect human fetal growth. *American Journal of Obstetrics and Gynecology*, **171**, 118–25.

Poppitt SD, Swann D, Black AE, Prentice AM (1998) Assessment of selective under-reporting of food intake by both obese and non-obese women in a metabolic facility. *International Journal of Obesity*, **221** C4, 303–11.

Porzelius LK, Houston C, Smith M, Arfken C, Fisher E Jr. (1995) Comparison of a standard behavioral weight loss treatment and a binge eating weight loss treatment. *Behavior Therapy*, **26**, 119–34.

Poskitt EM, Cole TJ (1977) Do fat babies stay fat? *British Medical Journal*, **1**, 7–9.

Poskitt EME, Cole TJ (1984) Do fat babies stay fat? *British Medical Journal*, **1**, 7–9.

Post GB, Kemper HCG (1993) Nutrient intake and biological maturation during adolescence. The Amsterdam Growth and Health Study. *European Journal of Clinical Nutrition*, **47**, 400–408.

Post GB, Welton DC (1995) The development of nutritional intake during 15 years of follow-up. In: *The Amsterdam Growth and Health Study. A Longitudinal Analysis of Health, Fitness and Lifestyle* (ed. HGC Kemper) Vol. 6, pp. 108–34. Champaign IL: Human Kinetics.

Powell KE, Blair S (1994) The public health burdens of sedentary living habits: theoretical but realistic estimates. *Medicine and Science in Sports and Exercise*, **26**, 851–6.

Powell KE, Thompson PD, Coopersen CJ, Kendrick JS (1987) Physical activity and the incidence of coronary heart disease. *Annual Review of Public Health*, **8**, 253–87.

Power C, Moynihan C (1988) Social class and changes in weight-for-height between childhood and early adulthood. *International Journal of Obesity*, **12**, 445–53.

Power C, Lake JK, Cole TJ (1998) Measurements and long-term health risks of child and adolescent fatness. *International Journal of Obesity*, **22**, 507–26.

Prader A, Labhart A, Willi H (1956) Ein syndrome von adipositas, kleinwuchs, kryptorchismus, und oligophrnie nach myoonieartigem zustand im neugeborenenalter. *Schweiz Med. Wochenschr.*, **86**, 1260.

Prentice AM (1992) Energy expenditure in the elderly. *European Journal of Clinical Nutrition*, **46** (Suppl 3), S21–S28.

Prentice AM (1995a) Alcohol and obesity. *International Journal of Obesity*, **19**, (Suppl 5), S44–S51.

Prentice AM (1995b) Are all calories equal? In *Weight Control* (ed. R Cottrell), pp. 8–33. London: Chapman & Hall.

Prentice AM, Black AE, Goldberg GR *et al.* (1986) High levels of energy expenditure are in obese women. *British Medical Journal*, **292**, 983–7.

Prentice AM, Black AE, Murgatroyd PR, Goldberg GR, Coward WA (1989) Metabolism or appetite: questions of energy balance with particular reference to obesity. *Journal of Human Nutrition and Dietetics*, **2**, 95–104.

Prentice AM, Goldberg GR (1996) Maternal obesity increases congenital malformations. *Nutrition Reviews*, **54**, 146–52.

Prentice AM, Jebb SA (1995a) Obesity in Britain: gluttony or sloth? *British Medical Journal*, **311**, 437–9.

Prentice AM, Jebb SA (1995b) *British Medical Journal*, **311**, 1568–9.

Prentice AM, Poppitt SD (1996) Importance of energy density and macronutrients in the regulation of energy intake. *International Journal of Obesity* (Suppl 2), S18–23.

Prentice AM, Diaz EO, Murgatroyd PR, Goldberg GR, Sonko BJ, Black AE, Coward WA (1991a) Doubly-labelled water measurements and calorimetry in practice. In: *New Techniques in Nutritional Research* (eds RG Whitehead, A Prentice), pp. 177–206 (Bristol-Myers Squibb/Mead Johnson Nutrition Symposia), Academic Press Inc.

Prentice AM, Goldberg GR, Jebb SA, Black AE, Murgatroyd PR, Diaz EO (1991b) Physiological responses to slimming. *Proceedings of the Nutrition Society*, **50**, 441–58.

Prentice AM, Jebb SA, Cole TJ (1996) Paradoxical associations between alcohol consumption and obesity in men and women. *International Journal of Obesity*, **19** (Suppl 4), 138.

Prentice AM, Jebb SA, Goldberg GR *et al.* (1992) Effects of weight cycling on body composition. *American Journal of Clinical Nutrition*, **56**, 209S–216S.

Prescott-Clarke P, Primatesta P (1998) *Health Survey for England 1996*. London: HMSO.

Prins JB, O'Rahilly S (1997) Regulation of adipose cell number in man. *Clinical Science*, **92**, 3–11.

Prochaska JO (1991) Assessing how people change. *Cancer*, **67**, 805–7.

Prochaska JO, DiClemente CC (1986) Towards a comprehensive model of change. In: *Treating Addictive Behaviours: Processes of Change* (eds WR Miller, N Heather). New York: Plenum.

Prochaska JO, Marcus BH (1994) The transtheoretical model: applications to exercise. In: *Advances in Exercise Adherence* (ed. RK Dishman), pp. 161–80. Champaign, IL: Human Kinetics.

Prochaska JO, Velicer WF, Rossi JS *et al.* (1994) Stages of change and decisional balance for 12 problem behaviors. *Health Psychology*, **13**, 39–46.

Pudel V, Westenhoefer J (1992) Dietary and behavioural principles in the treatment of obesity. In: *International*

Monitor on Eating Patterns and Weight Control. Medicom/Servier.

Raglin JS (1997) Anxiolytic effects of physical activity. In: *Physical Activity and Mental Health* (ed. WP Morgan), pp. 107–27. Washington, DC: Taylor and Francis.

Ramirez I, Friedman M (1982) Glycerol is not a physiologic signal in the control of food intake in rats. *Physiology & Behaviour*, **29**, 921–5.

Rand DSW, MacGregor AMC (1991) Successful weight loss following obesity surgery and the perceived liability of morbid obesity. *International Journal of Obesity*, **15**, 577–79.

Ravelli J-P, Stein ZA, Susser MW (1976) Obesity in young men after famine exposure in utero and early infancy. *New England Journal of Medicine*, **295**, 349–53.

Ravussin E (1993) Energy metabolism in obesity. Studies in the Pima Indians. *Diabetes Care*, **16**, 232–8.

Ravussin E, Bogardus C (1987) Relationship of genetics, age, and physical fitness to daily energy expenditure and fuel utilization. *American Journal of Clinical Nutrition*, **49**, 968–75.

Ravussin E, Burnand B, Schutz Y, Jequier E (1982) Twenty-four hour energy expenditure and resting metabolic rate in obese, moderately obese, and control subjects. *American Journal of Clinical Nutrition*, **35**, 566–73.

Ravussin E, Fontvieille AM, Swinburn BA, Bogardus C (1993) Risk factors for the development of obesity. *Annals NY Academy of Sciences*, 141–50.

Ravussin E, Lilioja S, Knowler W.C. *et al.* (1988) Reduced rate of energy expenditure as a risk factor for body-weight gain. *New England Journal of Medicine*, **318**, 467–72.

Raymond NC, Mussell MP, Mitchell JE, de Zwaan M, Crosby RD (1995) An age-matched comparison of subjects with binge eating disorder and bulimia nervosa. *International Journal of Eating Disorders*, **18**(2), 135–43.

Reaven GM (1995) Are insulin resistance and/or compensatory hyperinsulinaemia involved in the aetiology and clinical course of patients with hypertension? *International Journal of Obesity*, **19** (Suppl 1), S2–S5.

Rebuffé-Scrive M (1987) Regional adipose tissue metabolism in women during and after reproductive life and in men. In: *Recent Advances in Obesity V* (eds EM Berry, *et al.*), pp. 82–91. London: Libbey.

Rebuffé-Scrive M, Enk L, Crona N *et al.* (1985) Fat cell metabolism in different regions in women. Effects of menstrual cycle, pregnancy and lactation. *Journal of Clinical Investigations*, **75**, 1973–6.

Rebuffé-Scrive M, Lonnroth P, Marin P, Wesslau C, Björntorp P, Smith U (1987) Regional adipose tissue metabolism in men and postmenopausal women. *International Journal of Obesity*, **11**, 347–55.

Rebuffé-Scrive M, Walsh UA, McEwen B, Rodin J (1992) Effect of chronic stress and exogenous glucocoticoids on regional fat distribution and metabolism. *Physiology Behaviour*, **52** (3), 583–90.

Reed DR, Ding Y, Xu W, Cather C, Price RA (1995) Human obesity does not segregate with the chromosomal regions of Prader–Willi, Bardet–Biedl, Cohen, Borjeson or Wilson–Turner syndromes. *International Journal of Obesity*, **19**, 599–603.

Reinus JF, Heymsfield SB, Wiskind R, Casper K, Galambos JT (1989) Ethanol: relative fuel value and metabolic effects *in vivo*. *Metabolism*, **38**, 125–35.

Rice T, Borecki IB, Bouchard C, Rao DC (1992) Commingling analysis of regional fat distribution measures: the Quebec Family Study. *International Journal of Obesity*, **16**, 831–44.

Richardson JS (1952) The treatment of maternal obesity. *Lancet*, **1**, 525–8.

Riddoch C, Mahoney C, Murphy N, Boreham C, Cran G (1991) The physical activity patterns of Northern Irish schoolchildren ages 11–16 years. *Pediatric Exercise Science*, **3**, 300–309.

Ries W (1973) Feeding behaviour in obesity. *Proceedings of the Nutrition Society*, **32**, 187–93.

Rink TJ (1994) In search of a satiety factor. *Nature*, **372**, 406–7.

Risch N (1990) Linkage strategies for genetically complex traits II. The power of affected relative pairs. *American Journal of Human Genetics*, **46**, 229–41.

Rising R, Harper IT, Fontvieille AM, Ferraro RT, Spraul M, Ravussin E (1994) Determinants of total daily energy expenditure: variability in physical activity. *American Journal of Clinical Nutrition*, **59**, 800–804.

Rissanen AM, Heliovaara M, Knekt P, Reunanen A, Aromaa A (1991) Determinants of weight gain and overweight in adult Finns. *European Journal of Clinical Nutrition*, **45**, 419–30.

Rissanen AM, Heliovaara M, Knekt P, Reunanen A, Aromaa A, Maatela J (1990) Risk of disability and mortality due to overweight in a Finnish population. *British Medical Journal* **301**, 835–6

Ritson C (1983) A coherent food and nutrition policy: the ultimate goal. In: *The Food Industry, Economics and Politics* (eds J Burns, J McInerney, A Swinbank). London: Heinemann.

Ritson C (1992) Non-price effects of the CAP on food markets. In: *Proceedings of the CAP and Healthy Eating* workshop (ed S Henson). Reading: University of Reading.

Ritson C (1997a) The CAP and the consumer. In: *The Common Agricultural Policy* (eds C Ritson, D Harvey). Wallingford: CAB International.

Ritson C (1997b) Introduction. In: *The Common Agricultural Policy* (eds C Ritson, D Harvey), Chapter 1, pp. 1–8. Wallingford: CAB International.

Ritson C, Hutchins R (1991) The consumption revolution. In: *Fifty Years of the National Food Survey* (ed. JM Slater). London: HMSO.

Ritson C, Hutchins R (1995) Food choice and the demand for food. In: *Food Choice and the Consumer* (ed. D Marshall). London: Blackie.

Ritson C, Swinbank A (1997) Europe's green money. In: *The Common Agricultural Policy* (eds C Ritson, D Harvey), Chapter 6, pp. 115–37. Wallingford: CAB International.

Rizek RL, Welsch SO, Marston RM, Jackson EM (1983) Levels and sources of fat in the US food supply and diets of individuals. In: *Dietary Fats and Health* (eds EG Perkins, WJ Visek) pp. 13–43. Champaign II: American Chemists Society.

Robbins TW, Fray PJ (1980) Stress-induced eating: fact, fiction or misunderstanding. *Appetite*, **1**, 103–33.

Roberts SB, Savage J, Coward WA, Chew B, Lucas A (1988) Energy expenditure and energy intake in infants born to lean and overweight mothers. *New England Journal of Medicine*, **318**, 461–6.

Robison JI, Hoerr SL, Petersmarck KA, Anderson JV (1995) Redefining success in obesity intervention: the new paradigm. *Journal of the American Dietetic Association*, **95**(4), 422–3.

Rodgers S, Burnet R, Goss A *et al.* (1977) Jaw wiring in the treatment of obesity. *Lancet*, **1**, 1221–3.

Rodin J (1981) Current status of the internal–external hypothesis for obesity: what went wrong? *American Psychologist*, **36**, 361–72.

Rodin J (1980) The externality theory today. In: *Obesity* (ed. AJ Stunkard). Philadelphia: Saunders.

Rodin J, Bray GA, Atkinson RL *et al.* (1977) Predictors of successful weight loss in an outpatient obesity clinic. *International Journal of Obesity*, **1**, 79–87.

Rodin J, Schank D, Striegel-Moore R (1989) Psychological features of obesity. *Medical Clinics of North America*, **73**, 47–66.

Rodin J, Slochower J (1976) Externality in the nonobese: the effects of environmental responsiveness on weight. *Journal of Personal. and Social Psychology*, **29**, 557–65.

Rogers PJ, Hill AJ (1989) Breakdown of dietary restraint following mere exposure to food stimuli: interrelationships between restraint, hunger, salivation, and food intake. *Addictive Behaviors*, **14**, 387–97.

Rolland-Cachera M (1995) Prediction of adult body composition from infant and child measurements. In: *Body Composition Techniques in Health and Disease* (eds P Davies, T Cole). Cambridge: Cambridge University Press.

Rolland-Cachera M, Bellisle F, Pequignot F, Deheeger M, Sempe M (1990) Influence of body fat distribution during childhood on body fat distribution during adulthood: a two-decade follow-up study. *International Journal of Obesity*, **14**, 473–81.

Rolland-Cachera MF, Deheeger M, Guilloud-Bataille M, Avons P, Patois E, Sempe M (1987) Tracking the development of adiposity rebound from one year of age to adulthood. *Annals of Human Biology*, **14**, 219–29.

Rolland-Cachera MF, Deheeger M, Bellisle F, Sempe M, Guilloud-Bataille M, Patois E (1984) Adiposity rebound in children: a simple indicator for predicting obesity. *American Journal of Clinical Nutrition*, **39**, 129–35.

Rollnick S (1996) Behavioural change in practice: targeting individuals. *International Journal of Obesity*, **20** (Suppl. 1), S22–S26.

Rollnick S, Kinnersley P, Stott N (1993) Methods of helping people with behaviour change. *British Medical Journal*, **307**, 188–90.

Rollnick S, Heather N, Bell A (1992) Negotiating behaviour change in medical settings: the development of brief motivational interviewing. *Journal of Mental Health*, **1**, 25–37.

Rolls B (1994) Changing the preference for fat in foods. *Nutrition Reviews*, **52**, 21–3.

Rolls BJ (1991a) Effects of intense sweeteners on hunger, food intake and body weight: a review. *American Journal of Clinical Nutrition*, **53**, 872–8.

Rolls BJ (1991b) The impact of low-fat foods on energy and nutrient intakes. *Trends in Food Science & Technology*, **2**, 325–8.

Rolls BJ, Kim-Harris S, Fischman MW, Foltin RW, Moran TH, Stoner SA (1994) Satiety after preloads with different amounts of fat and carbohydrate: implications for obesity. *American Journal of Clinical Nutrition*, **60**, 476–87.

Rolls BJ, Rolls ET, Rowe EA *et al.* (1981) Sensory specific satiety in man. *Physiology & Behavior*, **27**, 137–42.

Roncari DA, Kindler S, Hollenberg CH (1986) Excessive proliferation of cultured adipocytes from massively obese persons. *Metabolism*, **35**, 1–4.

Rookus MA, Burema J, Deurenberg P, van der Wiel-Wetzels WAM (1985) The impact of adjustment of a weight-height index (W/H^2) for frame size on the prediction of body fatness. *British Journal of Nutrition*, **54**, 335–42.

Rookus MA, Rokerbrand P, Burema J, Duerenberg P (1987) The effect of pregnancy on the body mass index 9 months post-partum in 49 women. *International Journal of Obesity*, **11**, 609–18.

Rose G, Marmot MG (1981) Social class and coronary heart disease. *British Heart Journal*, **45**, 13–19.

Rosen JC, Srebnik D, Saltzberg E, Wendt S (1991) Development of a body image avoidance questionnaire. *Psychological Assessment*, **3**, 1–6.

Rosenbaum S, Skinner RK, Knight IB, Garrow JS (1985) A survey of heights and weights of adults in Great Britain. *Annals of Human Biology*, **12**, 115–27.

Ross R, Pedwell H, Rissanen J (1995) Response of total and regional lean tissue and skeletal muscle to a program of energy restriction and resistance exercise. *International Journal of Obesity,* **19**, 781–7.

Rossner S (1995) Long-term intervention strategies in obesity treatment. *International Journal of Obesity,* **19**, S29–S33.

Rossner S, Lagerstrand L, Persson HE, Sachs C (1991) The sleep apnoea syndrome in obesity: risk of sudden death. *Journal of International Medicine,* **230**, 135–41.

Rothschild M, Peterson HR, Pfeifer MA (1989) Depression in obese men, *International Journal of Obesity,* **13**, 479–85.

Rothwell NJ, Stock MJ (1979) A role for brown adipose tissue in diet-induced thermogenesis. *Nature,* **281**, 31–5.

Rothwell NJ, Stock MJ (1986) Brown adipose tissue and diet-induced thermogenesis. In: *Brown Adipose Tissue* (eds P Trayhurn, DC Nicholls). pp. 269–98. London: Arnold.

Royal College of Physicians (1983) *Obesity: A Report of the Royal College of Physicians.* Reprinted from the Journal of the Royal College of Physicians of London **17** (1).

Rozen R, Brigant L, Apfelbaum M (1994) Effects of cycles of food restriction followed by *ad libitum* refeeding on body composition and energy expenditure in obese rats. *American Journal of Clinical Nutrition,* **59**, 560–65.

Rozin, P, Levine E, Stoess C (1991) Chocolate craving and liking. *Appetite,* **17**, 199–212.

Rozin PN, Schulkin J (1990) Food selection. In: *Handbook of Behavioral Neurobiology* (ed. EM Stricker). pp. 297–328. New York: Plenum.

Ruderman AJ, Belzer LJ, Halperin A (1985) Restraint, anticipated consumption, and overeating. *Journal of Abnormal Psychology,* **94**, 547–55.

Russek M (1963) A hypothesis on the participation of hepatic glucoreceptors in the control of food intake. *Nature,* **197**, 79–80.

Ruxton CHS, Kirk TR, Belton NR (1996) The contribution of specific dietary patterns to energy and nutrient intakes in 7- to 8-year-old Scottish schoolchildren. III. Snacking habits. *Journal of Human Nutrition and Dietetics,* **9**, 23–31.

Sakurai Y, Kono S, Honjo S *et al.* (1995) Relation of waist–hip ratio to glucose tolerance, blood pressure, and serum lipids in middle-aged Japanese males. *International Journal of Obesity,* **19**, 632–7.

Sallis J, Patrick K (1994) Physical activity guidelines for adolescents: consensus statement. *Pediatric Exercise Science,* **6**, 299–301.

Samra JS, Tang LCH, Obhrai MS (1988) Changes in body weight between consecutive pregnancies. *Lancet,* **2**, 1420–21.

Schachter S (1971) Some extraordinary facts about obese humans and rats. *American Psychologist,* **26**, 129–44.

Schachter S, Goldman R, Gordon A (1968) Effects of fear, food deprivation, and obesity on eating. *Journal of Personality and Social Psychology,* **10**(2), 91–7.

Schachter S, Rodin J (1974) *Obese Humans and Rats.* Washington DC: Erlbaum/Halsted.

Schauberger CW, Rooney BL, Brimer LM (1992) Factors that influence weight loss in the puerperium. *Obstetrics and Gynecology,* **79**, 424–9.

Scheen AJ, Paquot N, Letiexhe MR, Paolisso G, Castillo MJ, Lefebvre PJ (1995) Glucose metabolism in obese subjects: lessons from OGTT, IVGTT and clamp studies. *International Journal of Obesity,* **19** (Suppl. 3), S14–S20.

Schenck CH, Mahowald MW (1994) Review of nocturnal sleep-related eating disorders. *International Journal of Eating Disorders,* **15**, 343–56.

Schoeller DA (1990) How accurate is self-reported dietary energy intake? *Nutrition Reviews,* **48**, 373–9.

Schoeller DA, Fjeld CR (1991) Human energy metabolism: what have we learned from the doubly labeled water method? *Annual Review of Nutrition,* **11**, 355–73.

Schofield WN (1985) Predicting basal metabolic rate, new standards and review of previous work. *Human Nutrition: Clinical Nutrition,* **39C** (1), 5–41.

Schofield WN, Schofield C, James WPT (1985) Basal metabolic rate, *Human Nutrition: Clinical Nutrition,* **39C** (Suppl. 1), 1–96.

Scholl TO, Hediger ML, Schall JI, Ances IG, Smith WK (1995) Gestational weight gain, pregnancy outcome and post-partum weight retention. *Obstetrics and Gynecology,* **86**, 423–7.

Schulz LO, Schoeller DA (1994) A compilation of total daily energy expenditure and body weights in healthy adults. *American Journal of Clinical Nutrition,* **60**, 676–81.

Schutz HG, Diaz-Knauf KV (1989) The role of the mass media in influencing eating. In: *Handbook of the Psychophysiology of Human Eating* (ed. R Shepherd). Chichester: Wiley.

Schutz Y, Bessard T, Jequier E (1987) Exercise and postprandial thermogenesis in obese women before and after weight loss. *American Journal of Clinical Nutrition,* **45**, 1424–32.

Schutz Y, Ravussin E, Diethelm R, Jequier E (1982) Spontaneous physical activity measured by radar in obese and control subjects studied in a respiration chamber. *International Journal of Obesity,* **6**, 23–8.

Schwartz MB, Brownell KO (1995) Matching individuals to weight loss treatments: a summary of obesity experts. *Journal of Consulting and Clinical Psychology,* **63** (1), 149–53.

Sclafani A (1995) How food preferences are learned: laboratory and animal models. *Proceedings of the Nutrition Society,* **54**, 419–27.

Scottish Office Home and Health Department (1993) *The*

Scottish Diet. Report of a Working Party to the Chief Medical Officer for Scotland. Edinburgh: Scottish Office Home and Health Department.

Scottish Intercollegiate Guidelines Network (SIGN) (1996) Obesity in Scotland: integrating prevention with weight management. Edinburgh: Royal College of Physicians.

Serignan CB (1980) Mandatory weight control program for 550 police officers choosing either behaviour modification or 'willpower'. *Obesity and Bariatric Medicine*, **9**, 88–92.

Segal KR, Pi-Sunyer FX (1989) Exercise and obesity. *Medical Clinics of North America*, **73**, 217–36.

Segal KR, Chun A, Coronel P, Valdez V (1992) Effects of exercise mode and intensity on postprandial thermogenesis in lean and obese men. *Journal of Applied Physiology*, **72**, 1754–63.

Seidell JC (1998) Epidemiology – definition and classification of obesity. In: *Clinical Obesity* (eds P Kopelman, M Stock). Oxford: Blackwell Science.

Seidell JC (1997) What is the cost of obesity? *International Journal of Obesity*, **21** (Suppl. 2), S1.

Seidell JC (1995) The impact of obesity on health status: some implications for health care costs. *International Journal of Obesity*, **19** (Suppl. 6, S13–S16.

Seidell JC, Bakx KC, Deureonberg P, van den Hoogen HJM, Hautvast JGAJ, Stijnen T (1986) Overweight and chronic illness – a retrospective cohort study, with a follow-up of 6–17 years, in men and women initially 20–50 years of age. *Journal of Chronic Diseases*, **39**, 585–93.

Seidell JC, Björntorp P, Sjöström L, Sannerstedt R, Krotkiewski M, Kvist H (1989) Regional distribution of muscle and fat mass in men – new insight into the risk of abdominal obesity using computed tomography. *International Journal of Obesity*, **13**, 289–303.

Seidman DS, Laor A, Gale R, Stevenson DK, Danon YL (1991) A longitudinal study of birth weight and being overweight in late adolescence. *American Journal of Disease in Children*, **145**, 782–5.

Shah M, McGovern P, French S, Baxter J (1994) Comparison of a low fat, *ad libitum* complex carbohydrate diet with a low-energy diet in moderately obese women. *American Journal of Clinical Nutrition*, **59**, 980–84.

Shaper A, Wannamethee SG, Walker M (1997) Body weight: implications for the prevention of coronary heart disease, stroke, and diabetes mellitus in a cohort study of middle aged men. *British Medical Journal*, **314**, 1311–17.

Shaper AG, Pocock SJ, Walker M, Cohen NM, Wale CJ, Thomson AG (1981) British Regional Heart Study: cardiovascular risk factors in middle-aged men in 24 towns. *British Medical Journal*, **283**, 179–86.

Shaw GM, Velie EM, Schaffer D (1996) Risk of neural tube defect-affected pregnancies among obese women. *Journal of the American Medical Association*, **275**, 1093–6.

Sheldon JH (1949) Maternal obesity. *Lancet*, **2**, 869–73.

Shelmet JJ, Reichard GA, Skutches CL, Hoeldtke RD, Owen OE, Boden G (1988) Ethanol causes acute inhibition of carbohydrate, fat and protein oxidation and insulin resistance. *Journal of Clinical Investment*, **81**, 1137–45.

Shepherd R (1990) Overview of factors influencing food choice. In: *Why We Eat What We Eat* (ed. M Ashwell), Proceedings of the Twelfth British Nutrition Foundation Annual Conference,

Shepherd R (1989) Factors influencing food preferences and choice. In: *Handbook of the Psychophysiology of Human Eating* (ed. R Shepherd). Chichester: Wiley.

Shetty POS, Prentice AM, Goldberg GR *et al.* (1994) Alterations in fuel selection and voluntary food intake in response to isoenergetic manipulation of glycogen stores in humans. *American Journal of Clinical Nutrition*, **60**, 534–43.

Shock NW (1972) Energy metabolism, caloric intake and physical activity of the aging. In: *Nutrition In Old Age* (ed. LA Carlson). Symposium of the Swedish Nutrition Foundation X. Uppsala: Almquist & Wiksell.

Shwartz M, Brownell KD (1995) Matching individuals to weight loss treatments: a survey of obesity experts. *Journal of Consulting and Clinical Psychology*, **63**(1), 149–53.

Siggaard R, Raben A, Astrup A (1996) Weight loss during 12 weeks of *ad libitum* carbohydrate-rich diet in overweight and normal-weight subjects at a Danish work site. *Obesity Research*, **4**, 347–56.

Silliman K, Kretchmer N (1995) Maternal obesity and body composition of the neonate. *Biology of the Neonate*, **68**, 384–93.

Silverman BL, Rizzo T, Green OC *et al.* (1991) Long-term prospective evaluation of offspring of diabetic mothers. *Diabetes*, **40** (Suppl. 2), 121–5.

Silverstone JT, Goodall E (1987) Recent studies in the clinical pharmacology of anorectic drugs. In: *Recent Advances in Obesity Research:V* (eds EM Berry, SH Blondheim, HE Eliahou, E Shafrir), pp. 285–9. London: Libbey.

Silverstone T (1992) Appetite suppressants: a review. *Drugs*, **43**, 820–36.

Simon C, Schlienger JL, Sapin R, Imler M (1986) Cephalic phase insulin secretion in relation to food presentation in normal and overweight subjects. *Physiology & Behavior*, **36**, 465–9.

Sims EAH, Danforth E Jr, Horton ES, Bray GA, Glennon JA, Salans LB (1973) Endocrine and metabolic effects of experimental obesity in man. *Recent Progress in Hormone Research*, **29**, 457–96.

Simson PC, Booth DA (1973) Subcutaneous release of

amino acids loads on food and water intakes in the rat. *Physiology & Behavior,* **11**, 329–36.

Sjöström L (1976) Comments on adipocyte sizing. *Clinica Chimica Acta,* **74**, 89–91.

Sjöström L, Narbro K & Sjöström D (1995) Costs and benefits when treating obesity. *International Journal of Obesity,* **19** (Suppl 6), S9–S12.

Smith DE, Lewis CE, Caveny JL, Perkins LL, Burke GL, Bild DE (1994) Longitudinal changes in adiposity associated with pregnancy: The CARDIA Study. *Journal of the American Medical Association,* **271**, 1747–51.

Smith DE, Marcus MD, Kaye W (1992) Cognitive behavioral treatment of obese binge eaters. *International Journal of Eating Disorders,* **12** (3), 257–62.

Smith Z, Knight T, Sahota P, Kernohan E, Baker M (1993) Dietary patterns in Asian and Caucasian men in Bradford: differences and implications for nutrition education. *Journal of Human Nutrition and Dietetics,* **6**, 323–33.

Snehalatha C, Ramachandran A, Vijay V, Viswanathan M (1994) Differences in plasma insulin responses in urban and rural Indians: a study in Southern Indians. *Diabetes Medicine,* **11**, 445–8.

Sniderman AD, Cianflone K (1994) The adipsin-ASP pathway and regulation of adipocyte function. *Annals of Medicine,* **26**, 389–93.

Sobal J (1991) Obesity and nutritional sociology: a model for coping with the stigma of obesity. *Clinical Sociology Review,* **9**, 125–41.

Sobal J, Stunkard AJ (1989) Socioeconomic status and obesity: a review of the literature. *Psychological Bulletin,* **105**(2), 260–75.

Society of Actuaries (1959) *Build and Blood Pressure Study 1959.* Chicago: Society of Actuaries.

Sohlstrom A, Forsum E (1995) Changes in adipose tissue volume and distribution during reproduction in Swedish women as assessed by magnetic resonance imaging. *American Journal of Clinical Nutrition,* **61**, 287–95.

Sonko BJ, Prentice AM, Murgatroyd PR, Goldberg GR, van de Ven M, Coward WA (1994) The influence of alcohol on postmeal fat storage. *American Journal of Clinical Nutrition,* **59**, 619–25.

Sonne-Holm S, Sorensen TI (1986) Prospective study of attainment of social class of severely obese subjects in relation to parents social class, intelligence and education. *British Medical Journal,* **29**, 2586–9.

Sonstroem RJ (1997a) Physical activity and self-esteem. In: *Physical Activity and Mental Health* (ed. WP Morgan), pp. 127–44. Washington DC: Taylor & Francis.

Sonstroem RJ (1997b) The physical self-system: a mediator of exercise and self-esteem. In: *The Physical Self: From Motivation to Well Being* (ed. KR Fox), pp. 3–26. Champaign, IL: Human Kinetics.

Sonstroem RJ, Potts SA (1996) Life adjustment correlates of physical self-concepts. *Medicine and Science in Sports and Exercise,* **28**, 619–25.

Sonstroem RK, Potts SA (1997) Life adjustment correlates of physical self-concepts. *Medicine and Science in Sports and Exercise,* **2**, 329–37.

Sorensen TIA (1995) The genetics of obesity. *Metabolism,* **44**, 4–6.

Sorensen TIA, Price RA (1990) Secular trends in body mass index among Danish young men. *International Journal of Obesity,* **14**, 411–19.

Sorensen TIA, Price RA, Stunkard AJ, Schulsinger F (1989) Genetics of obesity in adult adoptees and their biological siblings. *British Medical Journal,* **298**, 87–90.

Southgate DAT (1986) Obese deceivers? *British Medical Journal,* **292**, 1692–3.

Southgate DAT, Durnin JVGA (1970) Calorie conversion factors: an experimental reassessment of the factors used in the calculations of the energy value of human diets. *British Journal of Nutrition,* **24**, 517–35.

Specker S, de Zwaan M, Raymond N, Mitchell J (1994) Psychopathology in subgroups of obese women with and without binge eating disorder. *Comprehensive Psychiatry,* **35** (3), 185–90.

Spirt BA, Graves LW, Weinstock R, Bartlett SJ, Wadden TA (1995) Gallstone formation in obese women treated by a low-calorie diet. *International Journal of Obesity,* **19**, 593–5.

Spitzer RL, Devlin M, Walsh BT *et al.* (1992) Binge eating disorder: a multisite field trial of the diagnostic criteria. *International Journal of Eating Disorders,* **11**, 191–203.

Spitzer RL, Rodin J (1981) Human eating behavior: a critical review of studies in normal weight and overweight individuals. *Appetite,* **2**, 293–329.

Spitzer RL, Yanovski S, Wadden T *et. al.* (1993) Binge eating disorder: its further validation in a multisite study. *International Journal of Eating Disorders,* **13**, 137–53.

Spring B, Maller O, Wurtman J *et al.* (1982) Effects of protein and carbohydrate meals on mood and performance: interactions with sex and age. *Journal of Psychiatric Research,* **17**, 155–67.

Stacey TE (1991) Placental transfer. In: *Clinical Physiology in Obstetrics* (eds F Hytten, G Chamberlain), Chapter 18, 2nd ed. Oxford: Blackwell Scientific Publications.

Stamler J, Farinaro E, Mojonnier LM, Hall Y, Moss D, Stamler R (1980) Prevention and control of hypertension by nutritional-hygienic means. Long-term experience of the Chicago Coronary Prevention Evaluation Program. *Journal of the American Medical Association,* **243**, 1819–23.

Stefanick ML (1993) Exercise and weight control. *Exercise and Sport Sciences Reviews,* **21**, 363–96.

Stephens TW, Basinski M, Bristow PK *et al.* (1995) The role of neuropeptide Y in the antiobesity action of the obese gene product. *Nature,* **377**, 530–32.

Stock MJ (1999) Physiology of oxygen balance from cachexia to obesity. In: *Appetite, Obesity and Disorders of Over and Under Eating* (ed. P. Kopelman). London: Royal College of Physicians. In press.

Stock M, Rothwell N (1982) *Obesity and Leanness: Basic Aspects*, pp. 98. London: Libbey.

Storlien LH, James DE, Burleigh KM, Chisholm DJ, Kraegen EW (1986) Fat feeding causes widespread in vivo insulin resistance, decreased energy expenditure and obesity in rats. *American Journal of Physiology,* **251**, E576–83.

Storlien LH, Jenkins AB, Chisholm DJ, Pascoe WS, Khouri S, Kraegen EW (1991) Influence of dietary fat composition on development of insulin resistance in rats. *Diabetes,* **40**, 280–89.

Strobel A, Issad T, Camoin L, Ozata M, Strosberg AD (1998) A leptin missense mutation associated with hypogonadism and morbid obesity. *Nature Genetics,* **18**, 213 15.

Stuart RB (1967) Behavioural control over eating. *Behaviour Research and Therapy,* **5,** 357–65.

Stubbs RJ (1995) Macronutrient effects on appetite. *International Journal of Obesity,* **19** (Suppl. 5), S11–S19.

Stubbs RJ, Harbron CG, Murgatroyd PR, Prentice AM (1995a) The effect of covert manipulation of the dietary fat and energy density on food intake and substrate flux in ad libitum. *American Journal of Clinical Nutrition,* **62**, 316 29.

Stubbs RJ, Harbron CG, Prentice AM (1996) Covert manipulation of the dietary fat to carbohydrate ratio of isoenergetically dense diets: effect on food intake of men feeding *ad libitum. International Journal of Obesity,* **20**, 651–60.

Stubbs RJ, Ritz P, Coward WA, Prentice AM (1995b) The effect of covert manipulation of the dietary fat to carbohydrate ratio and energy density on food intake and energy balance in 'free living' men, feeding *ad libitum. American Journal of Clinical Nutrition,* **62**, 330–37.

Stunkard AJ (1959) Eating patterns and obesity. *Psychiatric Quarterly,* **33**, 284–94.

Stunkard AJ (1995) Prevention of obesity. In: *Eating Disorders and Obesity* (eds KD Brownell, CG Fairburn), pp. 572–6. New York: Guilford Press.

Stunkard AJ, Berkowitz R, Wadden T, Tanrikut C, Reiss E, Young L (1996) Binge eating disorder and the night-eating syndrome. *International Journal of Obesity,* **20**, 1–6.

Stunkard AJ, Harris JR, Pedersen NL, McClearn GE (1990) The body mass index of twins who have been reared apart. *New England Journal of Medicine,* **322**, 1483–7.

Stunkard AJ, Messick S (1985). The three-factor eating questionnaire to measure dietary restraint, disinhibition and hunger. *Journal of Psychosomatic Research,* **29**, 71–8.

Stunkard AJ, Wadden TA (1992) Psychological aspects of severe obesity. *American Journal of Clinical Nutrition,* **55**, S524–S532.

Stunkard AJ, Sorensen TIA, Hanis C *et al.* (1986) An adoption study of human obesity. *New England Journal of Medicine,* **314**, 193–8.

Sullivan M, Karlsson J, Sjöström L *et al.* (1993) Swedish obese subjects (SOS) – an intervention study of obesity. Baseline evaluation of health and psychosocial functioning in the first 1743 subjects examined. *International Journal of Obesity,* **17**, 503–12.

Summerbell CD (1989) Feeding pattern and body weight in humans. PhD thesis, CNAA, London.

Summerbell CD, Moddy RC, Shanks J, Stock MJ, Geissler C (1996) Relationship between feeding pattern and body mass index in 220 free-living people in four age-groups. *European Journal of Clinical Nutrition,* **50**, 513–19.

Summerbell CD, Watts C, Higgins JPT, Garrow JS (1998) Randomised controlled trial of novel, simple and well-supervised weight reducing diets in outpatients. *British Medical Journal,* **317**, 1487–9.

Suter PM, Schutz Y, Jequier E (1992) The effect of ethanol on fat storage in healthy subjects. *New England Journal of Medicine,* **326**, 983–7.

Sutcliffe JF (1996) A review of *in vivo* experimental methods to determine the composition of the human body. *Physics in Medicine & Biology,* **41**, 791–833.

Svendsen OL, Hassager C, Christiansen C (1994) Six months follow-up on exercise added to a short-term diet in overweight postmenopausal women – effects on body composition, resting metabolic rate, cardiovascular risk factors and bone. *International Journal of Obesity,* **18**, 692–8.

Swinbank A (1992) The CAP and food prices. In: *Proceedings of the CAP and Healthy Eating Workshop* (ed. S Henson). Reading: University of Reading.

Tambe K, Moun T, Eaves L *et al.* (1991) Genetic and environmental contributions to the variance of the body mass index in a Norwegian sample of first and second degree relatives. *American Journal of Human Biology,* **3**, 257–67.

Tanner JM, Whitehouse RH (1975) Revised standards for triceps and subscapular skinfolds in British children. *Archives of Disease in Childhood,* **50**, 142–5.

Tanner JM (1962) *Growth at Adolescence.* Oxford: Blackwell.

Tartaglia LA, Dempski M, Weng X, Deng N, Culpepper J, Devos R (1995) Identification and expression cloning of a Leptin receptor, OB-R. *Cell,* **83**, 1263–71.

Taylor CB, Fortmann SP, Flora J *et al.* (1991) Effect of

long-term community health education on body mass index. *American Journal of Epidemiology, 134,* 235–49.

Teff KL, Engelman K (1996) Palatability and dietary restraint: effect on cephalic phase insulin release in women. *Physiology & Behavior, 60,* 567–73.

Telch CF, Agras WS (1994) Obesity, binge eating and psychopathology: are they related? *International Journal of Eating Disorders, 15,* 53–61.

Thomas CD, Peters JC, Reed GW, Abumrad NN, Sun M, Hill JO (1992) Nutrient balance and energy expenditure during *ad libitum* feeding of high-fat and high-carbohydrate diets in humans. *American Journal of Clinical Nutrition, 55,* 934–42.

Thompson DA, Moskowitz HR, Campbell RG (1977) Taste and olfaction in human obesity. *Physiology & Behavior, 19,* 335–7.

Thorogood M (1995) The epidemiology of vegetarianism and health. *Nutrition Research and Reviews, 8,* 179–92.

Thorogood M, Carter R, Benfield L, McPherson K, Mann JI (1987) Plasma lipids and lipoprotein cholesterol concentrations in people with different diets in Britain. *British Medical Journal, 295,* 351–3.

Tokunaga K, Matzuzawa Y, Kotani Y *et al.* (1991) Ideal body weight estimated from the body mass index with the lowest morbidity. *International Journal of Obesity, 15,* 1–5.

Tordoff MG, Friedman MI (1986) Hepatic portal glucose infusions decrease food intake and increase food preference. *American Journal of Physiology, 251,* R192–R196.

Toubro S, Astrup A (1997) Randomised comparison of diets for maintaining obese subjects weight after major weight loss: ad lib, low fat, high carbohydrate diet vs fixed energy intake. *British Medical Journal, 314,* 29–34.

Trayhurn P (1986) Brown adipose tissue and energy balance. In: *Brown Adipose Tissue* (eds P Trayhurn, DG Nicholls). London: Arnold, pp. 299–338.

Trayhurn P (1996) Socratic debate: obesity is predominantly a problem of food intake – the case against. In: *Progress in Obesity Research: 7* (eds A Angel, H Anderson, C Bouchard, D Lau, L Leiter, R Mendelson). London: Libbey, pp. 475–9.

Treasure DC, Lox CL, Lawton BR (1998) Determinants of physical activity in a sedentary obese female population. *Journal of Sport and Exercise Psychology, 20,* 218–24.

Tremblay A, Buemann B (1995) Exercise training, macronutrient balance and body weight control. *International Journal of Obesity, 19,* 79–86.

Tremblay A, Leblanc C, Sevigny J, Savoie JP, Bouchard C (1983) The relationship between energy intake and expenditure: a sex difference. In: *Health Risk Estimation, Risk Reduction and Health Promotion* (ed. Landry F). Ottawa: Canadian Public Health Association.

Troisi RJ, Wolf AM, Manson JE, Klinger KM, Colditz GA (1995) Relation of body fat distribution to reproductive factors in pre- and postmenopausal women. *Obesity Research, 3,* 143–51.

Tuschl RJ, Platte P, Laessle RG, Stichler W, Pirke KM (1990) Energy expenditure and everyday eating behavior in healthy young women. *American Journal of Clinical Nutrition, 52,* 81–6.

US Department of Health and Human Services (PHS) (1996). *Physical activity and health. A report of the Surgeon General (Executive Summary).* Superintendent of Documents, Pittsburgh, PA.

Vague J (1953) *La differenciation sexuelle humaine: ses incidences en pathologie,* pp. 386. Paris: Masson.

Valdez R, Athens M, Thompson GH, Bradshaw BS, Stern MP (1994) Birthweight and adult health outcomes in a biethnic population in the USA. *Diabetologia, 37,* 624–31.

van Dale D, Saris WHM, ten Hoor F (1990) Weight maintenance and resting metabolic rate 18–40 months after a diet/exercise treatment. *International Journal of Obesity, 14,* 347–60.

Van Lethe FJ, Kempner CG, van Mechelan W *et al.* (1996a) Rapid maturation in adolescence results in greater obesity in adulthood: The Amsterdam Growth and Health Study. *American Journal of Clinical Nutrition, 64,* 18–24.

Van Lethe FJ, Kempner CG, van Mechelan W *et al.* (1996b) Biological maturation and the distribution of subcutaneous fat from adolescence into adulthood: The Amsterdam Growth and Health Study. *International Journal of Obesity, 20,* 121–9.

Van Loan MD (1996) Body fat distribution from subcutaneous to intra-abdominal: a perspective. *American Journal of Clinical Nutrition, 64,* 787–8.

Van Stratum P, Lussenburg RN, van Wezel LA, Vergroesen AJ, Cremer HD (1978) The effect of dietary carbohydrate: fat ratio on energy intake by adult women. *American Journal of Clinical Nutrition, 31,* 206–21.

Van Strien T, Frijters JE, Roosen RG, Knuiman-Hijl WJ, Defares PB (1985) Eating behavior, personality traits and body mass in women. *Addict Behavior, 10* (4), 333–43.

Van Strien T, Rookus MA, Bergers GP, Frijters JE, Defares PB (1986a) Life events, emotional eating and change in body mass index. *International Journal of Obesity, 10* (1), 29–35.

Van Strien T, Schippers GM, Cox WM (1986b) The Dutch eating behaviour questionnaire (DEBQ) for assessment of restrained, emotional, and external eating behaviour. *International Journal of Eating Disorders, 5,* 295–315.

Van Raaij JMA, Schonk CM, Vermaat-Miedema SH, Peek MEM, Hautvast JGA (1989) Body fat mass and basal metabolic rate in Dutch women before, during and after pregnancy; a reappraisal of the energy cost of pregnancy. *American Journal of Clinical Nutrition,* **49,** 765–72.

Verboeket-van de Venne WPHG, Westerterp KR, Kester ADM (1993) Effect of the pattern of food intake on human energy metabolism. *British Journal of Nutrition,* **70,** 103–15.

Verger P, Lanteaume MT, Louis-Sylvestre JL (1994) Free food choice after exercise in men. *Appetite,* **22,** 159–64.

Verschuur R, Kemper HCG (1985) The pattern of daily physical activity. *Medicine and Sport Science,* **20,** 169–86.

Vohr BR, McGarvey ST, Coll CG (1995) Effects of maternal gestational diabetes and adiposity on neonatal adiposity and blood pressure. *Diabetes Care,* **18,** 467–75.

Wadden TA, Bartlett S, Letizia K, Foster GD, Stunkard AJ, Conill A (1992a) Relationship of dietary history to resting metabolic rate, body composition, eating behaviour, and subsequent weight loss. *American Journal of Clinical Nutrition,* **56,** 2035–85.

Wadden TA, Foster GD, Wang J *et al.* (1992b) Clinical correlates of short and long-term weight loss. *American Journal of Clinical Nutrition,* **56,** 271S–274S.

Wadden TA, Foster GD, Stunkard AJ, Linowitz JR (1989) Dissatisfaction with weight and figure in obese girls; discontent but not depression. *International Journal of Obesity,* **13,** 89–97.

Wadden TA, Steen SN (1996) Improving the maintenance of weight loss: the ten per cent solution. In: *Progress in Obesity Research 7* (eds A Angel, H Anderson, C Bouchard, D Lau, L Leiter, R Mendelson). London: Libbey.

Wadden TA, Steen SN, Wingate BJ, Foster GG (1996) Psychosocial consequences of weight reduction: how much weight loss is enough? *American Journal of Clinical Nutrition,* **63** (Suppl. 3), 461S–465S.

Wadden TA, Sternberg JA, Letizia KA, Stunkard AJ, Foster GD (1989) Treatment of obesity by very low calorie diet, behaviour therapy, and their combination: a five year perspective. *International Journal of Obesity,* **13** (2), 39–46.

Wadden TA, Stunkard AJ (1985) Social and psychological consequences of obesity. *Annals of Internal Medicine,* **103,** 1062–7.

Wadden TA, Stunkard AJ (1987) Psychopathology and obesity. *Annals of the New York Academy of Sciences,* **55,** 55–65.

Wadden TA, Stunkard AJ (1993) Psychosocial consequences of obesity and dieting: research and clinical findings. In: *Obesity: Theory and Therapy* (Eds TA Wadden, AJ Stunkard), pp 163–77. New York: Raven Press.

Wadden TA, Stunkard AJ, Liebschutz J (1992b) Etiology and treatment of obesity: understanding a serious, prevalent and refractory disorder. *Journal of Clinical and Consulting Psychology,* **60,** 505–17.

Walberg JL (1989) Aerobic exercise and resistance weight-training during weight reduction. Implications for obese persons and athletes. *Sports Medicine,* **47,** 343–56.

Walston J, Silver K, Bogardus C *et al.* (1995) Time of onset of non-insulin-dependent diabetes mellitus and genetic variation in the β_3-adrenergic-receptor gene. *New England Journal of Medicine,* **333,** 343–7.

Wankel LM, Mummery WK, Stephens T, Craig CL (1994) Prediction physical activity intention from social psychological variables: results from the Campbell's Survey of Wellbeing. *Journal of Sport and Exercise Psychology,* **16,** 56–69.

Wannamethee G, Shaper AG (1990) Weight change in middle-aged British men: implications for health. *European Journal of Clinical Nutrition,* **44,** 133–42.

Wardle J (1980) Dietary restraint and binge eating. *Behaviour Analysis and Modification,* **4** (3), 201–9.

Wardle J (1987) Compulsive eating and dietary restraint. *British Journal of Clinical Psychology,* **26,** 47–55.

Wardle J, Beinart H (1981) Binge eating: a theoretical review. *British Journal of Clinical Psychology,* **20,** 97–109.

Wardle J, Marsland L, Sheikh Y, Quinn M, Fedoroff I, Ogden J (1992) Eating style and eating behaviour in adolescents. *Appetite,* **18,** 167–83.

Warwick ZS, Hall WG, Pappas TN, Schiffman SS (1993) Taste and smell sensations enhance the satiating effect of both a high carbohydrate and a high-fat meal in humans. *Physiology & Behavior,* **53,** 553–6.

Waterlow JC (1976) *Research on obesity: a report of a DHSS/MRC Group,* pp. 94. London: HMSO.

Webster JD, Hesp R, Garrow JS (1984) The composition of excess weight in obese women estimated by body density, total body water and total body potassium. *Human Nutrition: Clinical Nutrition,* **38C,** 299–306.

Weingarten HP, Elston D (1991) Food cravings in a college population. *Appetite,* **17,** 167–75.

Weissenburger J, Rush AJ, Giles DE, Stunkard AJ (1986) Weight change in depression. *Psychiatry Research,* **17,** 275–83.

Werler MM, Louik C, Shapiro S, Mitchell AA (1996) Prepregnant weight in relation to risk of neural tube defects. *Journals of the American Medical Association,* **275,** 1089–92.

West DB, Prinz WA, Greenwood MRC (1989) Regional changes in adipose tissue blood flow and metabolism in rats after a meal. *American Journal of Physiology,* **257,** R711–R716.

West DL, Brans YW (1986) Maternal diabetes and neonatal macrosomia. Dynamic skinfold thickness measurements. *American Journal of Perinatology*, **3**, 9–13.

Westerterp KR, Meijer GAL, Janssen GME, Saris WHM, ten Hoor F (1992) Long-term physical activity on energy balance and body composition. *British Journal of Nutrition*, **68**, 21–30.

Westerterp KR, Verboeket-van de Venne WPHG, Westerterp-Plantenga MS, Velthuis-te Wierik EJM, de Graaf C, Weststrate JA (1996) Dietary fat and body fat: an intervention study. *International Journal of Obesity*, **20**, 1022–6.

Westerterp-Plantenga MS, van den Heuvel E, Wouters L, ten Hoor F (1992) Diet-induced thermogenesis and cumulative food intake curves as a function of familiarity with food and dietary restraint in humans. *Physiology & Behavior*, **51**, 457–65.

Westerterp-Plantenga MS, Wijckmans-Duysens NA, ten Hoor F (1994) Food intake in the daily environment after energy-reduced lunch, related to habitual meal frequency. *Appetite*, **22**, 173–82.

Weststrate JA (1992) Effect of nutrients on the regulation of food intake: can a reduced fat diet reduce energy intake? Unpublished Unilever Research Report, Unilever Laboratories, The Netherlands.

Weststrate JA, Dopheide T, Robroch L, Deurenberg P, Hautvast JGA (1990a) Does variation in palatability affect the postprandial response in energy expenditure? *Appetite*, **15**, 209–19.

Weststrate JA, Weys P, Poortvliet E, Deurenberg P, Hautvast JGAJ (1990b) Lack of a systematic sustained effect of prolonged exercise bouts on resting metabolic rate in fasting subjects. *European Journal of Clinical Nutrition*, **44**, 91–7.

White A, Nicolaas G, Foster K, Browne F, Carey S (1993) *Health Survey for England, 1991*. London: HMSO.

White M, Raybould S, Foy C, Harrington B, Harland J (1996) Who eats a healthy diet? Spatial and socio-economic patterning of dietary behaviour in Newcastle upon Tyne. Conference paper presented by White M to the Human Nutrition Research Centre Inaugural Symposium *Cells to Populations – Improving Nutrition*, University of Newcastle upon Tyne.

Whiting MJ, Hall JC, Iannos J, Roberts HG, Watts JMCK (1984) The cholesterol saturation of bile and its reduction by chendeoxycholic acid in massively obese patients. *International Journal of Obesity*, **8**, 681–8.

Widdowson EM, McCance RA (1975) A review: new thoughts on growth. *Pediatric Research*, **9**, 154–6.

Widén E, Lehto M, Kanninen T, Walston J, Shuldiner AR, Groop LC (1995) Association of a polymorphism in the β_3-adrenergic-receptor gene with features of the insulin resistance syndrome in Finns. *New England Journal of Medicine*, **333**, 348–51.

Wilding J (1997) Science, medicine and the future: Obesity Treatment. *British Medical Journal*, **315**, 997–1000.

Wilfley DE, Brownell KD (1994) Physical activity and diet in weight loss. In: *Advances in Exercise Adherence* (ed. RK Dishman) pp. 361–93. Champaign, IL: Human Kinetics.

Wilks R, McFarlane-Anderson N, Bennett F *et al.* (1996) Obesity in peoples of the African diaspora. In: *The Origins and Consequences of Obesity*, pp. 37–53. Chichester: Wiley (Ciba Foundation Symposium 201).

Willett WC (1998) Dietary fat and obesity: an unconvincing relation. *American Journal of Clinical Nutrition*, **68**, 1149–50.

Willett WC, Manson JE, Stampfer MJ *et al.* (1995) Weight, weight change and coronary heart disease in women. *Journal of the American Medical Association*, **273**, 461–5.

Williamson DF, Madans J, Anda RF, Kleinman JC, Biovino GA, Byers T (1991) Smoking cessation and severity of weight gain in a national cohort. *New England Journal of Medicine*, **324**, 739–45.

Williamson DF, Madans J, Anda, RF, Kleinman JC, Kahn HS, Byers T (1993) Recreational physical activity and 10-year weight change in a US national cohort. *International Journal of Obesity*, **17**, 279–86.

Williamson DF, Madans J, Pamuk E, Flegal KM, Kendrick JS, Serdula MK (1994) A prospective study of childbearing and 10-year weight gain in US white women 25 to 45 years of age. *International Journal of Obesity*, **18**, 561–9.

Williamson DF, Pamuk E, Thun M, Flanders D, Byers T, Heath C (1995) Prospective study of intentional weight loss and mortality in never-smoking overweight US white women aged 40–64 years. *American Journal of Epidemiology*, **141**, 1128–41.

Wilson GT, Fairburn CG (1993) Cognitive treatments for eating disorders. *Journal of Consulting and Clinical Psychology*, **61**, 261–9.

Wilson GT (1993) Behavioural Treatment of Obesity: thirty years and counting. *Advances in Behavioural Research Therapy*, **16**, 31–75.

Wilson GT (1994) Behavioral treatment of obesity: thirty years and counting. *Advances in Behaviour Research and Therapy*, **16**, 31–75.

Wing RR, Jeffery RW, Burton LR *et al.* (1996) Food provision vs structured meal plans in the behavioural treatment of obesity. *International Journal of Obesity*, **20**, 56–62.

Wisen O, Hellstrom PM (1995) Gastrointestinal motility in obesity. Journal of Internal Medicine, **237**, 411–18.

Wolfe BL (1992) Long term maintenance following attainment of goal weight: a preliminary investigation. *Addictive Behaviours*, **17**, 469–77.

Wolfe WS, Sobal J, Olson CM, Frongilla EA (1997) Parity-associated body weight: modification by socio-demographic and behavioural factors. *Obesity Research*, **5**, 131–41.

Womersley J, Durnin JVGA (1977) A comparison of the skinfold method with extent of 'overweight' and various weight-height relationships in the assessment of obesity. *British Journal of Nutrition*, **38**, 271–84.

Woo R, Garrow JS, Pi-Sunyer FX (1982a) Voluntary food intake during prolonged exercise in obese women. *American Journal of Clinical Nutrition*, **36**, 478–84.

Woo R, Garrow JS, Pi-Sunyer FX (1982b) Effect of increased physical activity on voluntary intake in lean women. *Metabolism*, **34**, 836–41.

Wood PD, Stefanick ML, Dreon DM *et al.* (1988) Changes in plasma lipids and lipoproteins in overweight men during weight loss through dieting and compared with exercise. *New England Journal of Medicine*, **319**, 1173–79.

Wood PD, Stefanick ML, Williams PT, Haskell WL (1991) The effects on plasma lipoproteins of a prudent weight-reducing diet, with or without exercise, in overweight men and women. *New England Journal of Medicine*, **325**, 461–6.

Woods S, Decke E, Vasselli J (1974) Metabolic hormones and regulation of body weight. *Psychological Review*, **81**, 26–43.

Wooley OW, Wooley SC, Dunham RB (1972) Can calories be perceived and do they affect hunger in obese and non obese humans? *Journal of Comparative and Physiological Psychology*, **80**, 250–58.

Wooley SC, Garner DM (1991) Obesity treatment: the high cost of false hope. *Journal of the American Dietetic Association*, **91** (10), 1248–51.

Wooley SC, Garner DM (1994) Dietary treatments for obesity are ineffective. *British Medical Journal*, **309**, 655–6.

Woolfolk RL, Lehrer PM (1984) *Principles and Practices of Stress Management*. Guilford: New York.

World Health Organisation (WHO) (1995) Exercise for health. WHO/FIMS Committee on Physical Activity for Health. *Bulletin of the World Health Organisation*, **73** (2), 135–6.

World Health Organisation (WHO) (1997) *Obesity: Preventing and Managing the Global Epidemic*. Geneva: WHO.

World Health Organisation (WHO) MONICA Project (1988) Geographical variation in the major risk factors of coronary heart disease in men and women aged 35–64 years. *World Health Statistics Quarterly*, **41**, 115–40.

Wurtman JJ (1988) Carbohydrate craving, mood changes, and obesity. *Journal of Clinical Psychiatry*, **49**, 37–9.

Wurtman R, Wurtman J (1986) Carbohydrate craving, obesity and brain serotonin. In: *Serotonergic System, Feeding and Body Weight Regulation* (ed S Nicolaidis). London: Academic Press.

Yarnell JWG, Fehily AM, Milbank J, Kubicki AJ, Eastham R, Hayes TM (1983) Determinants of plasma lipoproteins and coagulation factors in men from Caerphilly, South Wales. *Journal of the Epidemiology in Community Health*, **37**, 137–40.

Yarnell JWG, Milbank J, Walker CL, Fehily AM, Hayes TM (1982) Determinants of high density lipoprotein and total cholesterol in women. *Journal of the Epidemiology in Community Health*, **36**, 167–71.

Young B, Webley P, Hetherington M, Zeedyk S (1995) *The Role of Television Advertising in Children's Food Choice*. Report prepared for the Ministry of Agriculture, Fisheries and Food.

Zeffler A, Adamson AJ (1995) Access to and cost of healthy eating in Newcastle. Student Report, Human Nutrition Research Centre, University of Newcastle.

Zeigler EE, O'Donnell AM, Nelson SE, Fomon SJ (1976) Body composition of the reference fetus. *Growth*, **40**, 329–41.

Zhang Y, Proenca R, Maffei M, Barone M, Leopold L, Friedman JM (1994) Positional cloning of the mouse obese gene and its human homologue. *Nature*, **372**, 425–32.

Zumoff B, Strain GW, Miller LK *et al.* (1988) Partial reversal of the hypogonadotrophic hypogonadism of obese men by administration of corticosuppressive doses of dexmethasone. *International Journal of Obesity*, **12**, 525–31.

Index

For definitions, *see also glossary of terms*, 213–15